The Neuroscience of Social Interaction

The Neuroscience of Social Interaction

Decoding, imitating, and influencing the actions of others

Edited by

CHRISTOPHER D. FRITH

Wellcome Department of Imaging Neuroscience,
Institute of Neurology, University College London, London

and

DANIEL M. WOLPERT

Sobell Department of Motor Neuroscience and Movement Disorders,
Institute of Neurology, University College London, London

Originating from a Theme Issue first published by Philosophical
Transactions of the Royal Society, Series B.

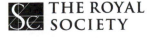 THE ROYAL SOCIETY

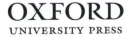
UNIVERSITY PRESS

OXFORD

UNIVERSITY PRESS

Great Clarendon Street, Oxford OX2 6DP

Oxford University Press is a department of the University of Oxford.
It furthers the University's objective of excellence in research, scholarship,
and education by publishing worldwide in

Oxford New York

Auckland Cape Town Dar es Salaam Hong Kong Karachi
Kuala Lumpur Madrid Melbourne Mexico City Nairobi
New Delhi Shanghai Taipei Toronto

With offices in

Argentina Austria Brazil Chile Czech Republic France Greece
Guatemala Hungary Italy Japan South Korea Poland Portugal
Singapore Switzerland Thailand Turkey Ukraine Vietnam

Oxford is a registered trade mark of Oxford University Press
in the UK and in certain other countries

Published in the United States
by Oxford University Press Inc., New York

© The Royal Society, 2003

The moral rights of the author have been asserted
Database right Oxford University Press (maker)

First published by the Royal Society 2003

First published by Oxford University Press 2004
Reprinted 2004, 2005

A catalogue record for this title is available
from the British Library

ISBN 0 19 852925 2 (Hbk)
0 19 852926 0 (Pbk)

10 9 8 7 6 5 4 3

Typeset by Newgen Imaging Systems (P) Ltd., Chennai, India
Printed in Great Britain
on acid-free paper by
Biddles Ltd., King's Lynn, Norfolk

Preface

A key question for science to explore in the twenty-first century concerns the mechanism that allows skilful social interaction. Although enormous advances in our understanding of the links between the mind, the brain, and behaviour have been made in the last few decades, these are based on studies in which people are considered as strictly isolated units. For example, studies might typically examine the brain activity when volunteers press a button when they are aware of seeing a visual stimulus. Outside the laboratory, in contrast, we spend most of our time thinking about and interacting with other people rather than looking at abstract shapes and pushing buttons. One of the major functions of our brains must be to facilitate such social interactions. It is the mental and neural mechanisms that underlie this social interaction which forms the main theme of this book.

We have concentrated on two-person social interactions in which one person, either implicitly or explicitly, tries to 'read' the hidden mental states of the other; their goals, beliefs or feelings. In this book we have brought together scientists from many different disciplines, but all concerned with the same problems. These problems include how goals and intentions can be read from watching another person's movements, how movements that we see can be converted into movements that we make, and how our own behaviour can be used to influence the behaviour of others. The book reviews the general principles concerning the cognitive and neural bases of social interactions that have emerged. Within this framework the authors discuss many different aspects of social interaction, demonstrating the excitement and vigour of this emerging discipline.

This book was originally published as an issue of the Philosophical Transactions of the Royal Society, Series B, *Phil. Trans. R. Soc. Lond. B* (2003) **358**, 429–602.

Christopher D. Frith   *London*
Daniel M. Wolpert   *August 2003*

Contents

List of Contributors

Harold Bekkering, Nijmegen Institute for Cognition and Information, University of Nijmegen, Montessorilaan 3, NL-6525 HR, Nijmegen, The Netherlands

Aude Billard, Computer Science and Neuroscience, University of Southern California, 3641 Watt Way, Los Angeles, CA 90089-2520, USA and School of Engineering, Swiss Federal Institute of Technology, Lausanne, CH 1015 Lausanne, Switzerland

R. J. R. Blair, Unit on Affective Cognitive Neuroscience, Mood and Anxiety Disorders Program, National Institute of Mental Health, National Institute of Health, Department of Health and Human Services, 15K North Drive, Bethesda, MD 20892-2670, USA

Andrew Blake, Microsoft Research, 7 JJ Thomson Avenue, Cambridge CB3 0FB, UK

R. W. Byrne, School of Psychology, University of St Andrews, St Andrews, Fife KY16 9JU, UK

Gergely Csibra, Centre for Brain and Cognitive Development, School of Psychology, Birkbeck College, Malet Street, London WC1E 7HX, UK

Jean Decety, Center for Mind, Brain and Learning, University of Washington, Seattle, WA 98195, USA

Kenji Doya, ATR Human Information Science Laboratories and CREST, Japan Science and Technology Corporation, 2-2-2 Hikaridai, Seika-cho, Soraku-gun, Kyoto 619-0288, Japan.

Christopher D. Frith, Wellcome Department of Imaging Neuroscience, Institute of Neurology, University College London, Queen Square, London WC1N 3AR, UK

Uta Frith, Institute of Cognitive Neuroscience, University College London, Queen Square, London WC1N 3AR, UK

Vittorio Gallese, Istituto di Fisiologia Umana, Università di Parma, Via Volturno, 39, 43100 Parma, Italy

Merideth Gattis, School of Psychology, University of Cardiff, Cardiff CF10 3XQ, UK

Dale Griffin, Graduate School of Business, Stanford University, Stanford, CA 94305, USA

Richard Gonzalez, Department of Psychology, University of Michigan, Ann Arbor, MI 48109, USA

Anthony Hoogs, GE Global Research, One Research Circle, Niskayuna NY 12309, USA

Auke Ijspeert, Computer Science and Neuroscience, University of Southern California, 3641 Watt Way, Los Angeles, CA 90089-2520, USA and School of Computer and Communication Sciences, Swiss Federal Institute of Technology, Lausanne, CH 1015 Lausanne, Switzerland

Susan C. Johnson, Department of Psychology, Jordan Hall, Building 420, Stanford University, Stanford, CA 94305, USA

Mitsuo Kawato, ATR Human Information Science Laboratories, Japan Science and Technology Corporation, 2-2-2 Hikaridai, Seika-cho, Soraku-gun, Kyoto 619-0288, Japan.

Andrew N. Meltzoff, Center for Mind, Brain and Learning, University of Washington, Seattle, WA 98195, USA

David Perrett, School of Psychology, University of St Andrews, St Andrews, Fife, KY16 9JU, UK

Aina Puce, Centre for Advanced Imaging, Department of Radiology, West Virginia University, PO Box 9236, Morgantown, WV 26506-9236, USA

Jens Rittscher, GE Global Research, One Research Circle, Niskayuna NY 12309, USA

David Sally, Cornell University, Johnson Graduate School of Management, 371 Sage Hall, Ithaca, NY 14853 6201, USA

Stefan Schaal, Computer Science and Neuroscience, University of Southern California, 3641 Watt Way, Los Angeles, CA 90089-2520, USA and ATR Human Information Sciences, 2-2 Hikaridai, Seika-cho, Soraku-gun, Kyoto 619-0218, Japan

Tania Singer, Wellcome Department of Imaging Neuroscience, Institute of Neurology, University College London, Queen Square, London WC1N 3AR, UK

Gees Stein, GE Global Research, One Research Circle, Niskayuna NY 12309, USA

Andreas Wohlschläger, Department of Cognition and Action, Max Planck Institute for Psychological Research, Amalienstrasse 33, D-80799 Munich, Germany

Daniel M. Wolpert, Sobell Department of Motor Neuroscience and Movement Disorders, Institute of Neurology, University College London, Queen Square, London WC1N 3AR, UK

Introduction: the study of social interactions

Tania Singer, Daniel Wolpert, and Chris Frith

In the last few decades there have been enormous advances in our understanding of the links between the mind, the brain, and behaviour. Sensory systems, especially the visual system, have been explored in detail leading to a much greater understanding of the mechanisms underlying visual perception (Zeki 1993). We also know much more about the mechanisms by which our motor system allows us to reach and grasp objects (Jeannerod *et al.* 1995). Progress has also been made in our understanding of the higher cognitive functions involved in the solving of novel problems (Shallice 1988). Most remarkable of all, has been the enthusiasm with which neuroscientists have embarked on the search for the neural correlates of consciousness (Crick and Koch 1998).

However, a striking feature of these approaches is that people are considered as strictly isolated units. For example, in a typical experiment a volunteer might sit at a bench or lie in a brain scanner, watching abstract shapes appear on a screen and pressing a button when a target shape appears. In contrast, outside the laboratory we spend most of our time thinking about and interacting with other people rather than looking at abstract shapes and pushing buttons. It is this social interaction which forms the main theme of this volume.

Humans, like other primates, are intensely social creatures. One of the major functions of our brains must be to enable us to be as skilful in social interactions as we are in recognizing objects and grasping them. Furthermore, any differences between human brains and those of our nearest relatives, the great apes, are likely to be linked to our unique achievements in social interaction and communication rather than our motor or perceptual skills. In particular, humans have the ability to mentalize, that is to perceive and communicate mental states, such as beliefs and desires. The acid test of this ability is the understanding that behaviour can be motivated by a false belief (Dennett 1978). Deception, for example, depends upon such understanding. This ability is absent in monkeys and exists in only rudimentary form in apes (Povinelli and Bering 2002). A key problem facing neuroscience therefore, and one that is at least as important as the problem of consciousness, is to uncover the neural mechanisms underlying our ability to read other minds and to show how these mechanisms evolved. To solve this problem experiments are needed in which people (or animals) interact with one another rather than behave in isolation.

The emergence of social cognitive neuroscience

In the past few years a new interdisciplinary field of research has emerged from a union between cognitive neuroscience and social psychology. Although, the inaugural 'Social Cognitive Neuroscience' conference was held in California in 2001, the first articles and books referring to the 'social brain' had appeared a number of years earlier. Leslie Brothers, for example, proposed a model of a neuronal circuitry subserving social cognition in 1990 (see also Brothers 1997) and nine years later Ralph Adolphs wrote an influential overview article on 'social cognition and the human brain' (Adolphs, 1999). The popularity of the new field has generated a rapidly growing number of focused conferences, special issues of journals, and books (e.g., Adolphs 2003; Allison, Puce, and McCarthy 2000; Cacioppo *et al.* 2001; Harmon-Jones and Devine, in press; Heatherton and Macrae 2003; Ochsner and Lieberman 2001). The agenda of social cognitive neuroscience has been described in terms of seeking 'to understand phenomena in terms of interactions between three levels of analysis: the social level, which is concerned with the motivational and social factors that influence behaviour and experience; the cognitive level, which is concerned with the information-processing mechanisms that give rise to social-level phenomena; and the neural level, which is concerned with the brain mechanisms that instantiate cognitive-level processes' (Ochsner and Lieberman 2001: p.717 ff).

Social psychology and social cognition

The field of *social psychology* traditionally focused on the investigation of one level: the influence of socio-cultural factors on behaviour. The level of cognitive processes was only added to the study of social behaviour in the late 1970s when the field of *social cognition* emerged as a sub-field of social psychology. This inclusion was greatly influenced by the 'cognitive revolution' that took place in the neighbouring discipline of cognitive psychology during the 1960s and 1970s (the first issue of the journal *'Social Cognition'* appeared in 1982, the first edition of the *'Handbook for social cognition'* in 1984). Theoretically, and methodologically, the intellectual movement of social cognition strongly relied on the information-processing approach and the new experimental paradigms developed in this context. Concepts such as inhibition and activation, automaticity and control, search set and task set, interference and facilitation were introduced into social psychology. Nowadays, most social psychologists have integrated these concepts into their everyday vocabulary and empirical practice.

Broadly defined, the field of social cognition attempts to understand and explain how the thoughts, feelings, and behaviour of individuals are influenced by the actual, imagined, or implied presence of others (e.g., Allport

1985). Prototypical topics in social cognition are the study of attitude formation and attitude change, person perception and person stereotyping, causal
attribution and social inferences, self-knowledge, self-concept, and self-
deception as well as the study of the influence of motivation and emotions on
cognition and behaviour. It is important to keep in mind that the field of traditional social psychology embraces a much broader scope of more complex
themes ranging from the study of gender differences, sexism, racism, through
media persuasion, propaganda, international negotiation, non-verbal communication to group dynamics, social bonding, family, and partnership relations.
Although the complex nature of the topics addressed in social psychology carries the danger of an associated lack of precision with regard to their empirical assessment, the experimental precision gained in social cognition through
the introduction of well-controlled experimental techniques borrowed from
cognitive psychology carries the risk of loosing ecological validity at the
expense of internal validity.

Social cognitive neuroscience

In contrast to social psychology, which is concerned with the study of complex real-life social phenomena, social cognitive neuroscience has investigated quite basic social abilities such as attending to, recognizing, and
remembering socio-emotionally relevant stimuli. Functional imaging studies
on *person perception*, for example, have focused on implicit or explicit judgements on the basis of socially relevant cues in the human face such as emotional expressions (Morris *et al.* 1996; Phillips *et al.* 1997; Sprengelmeyer *et
al.* 1998), facial attractiveness (O'Doherty *et al.* 2003), trustworthiness
(Winston *et al.* 2002) or racial identity (Hart *et al.* 2000; Phelps *et al.* 2000,
2001). In addition, a stream of studies has investigated our ability to decode
social signals on the basis of *biological motion*. These have included stimuli
depicting body gestures and body movements (hands, mouth, and whole body)
as well as complex movements of interacting geometrical shapes (for reviews
see Allison *et al.* 2000; Chapters 1 and 3 in this volume).

    Another important line of research in social cognitive neuroscience is
closely linked to the discovery of *'mirror neurons'* in monkeys (Gallese *et al.*
1996, Rizzolatti *et al.* 1996). These neurons respond when monkeys see someone else performing a specific action as well as when the monkey itself performs that particular action. The discovery of mirror neurons aroused great
interest owing to their obvious relevance for social interactions. In particular,
such neurons provide a neural mechanism that may be a critical component of
imitation and our ability to represent the goals and intentions of others.
Although the early functional imaging studies have mostly focused on understanding how we represent the *simple actions* of others (for a review see
Blakemore and Decety 2001; Grezes and Decety 2001), recent articles have

proposed that similar mechanisms are involved in understanding the *feelings and sensations* of others (e.g., Gallese 2001; Gallese and Goldman 1998; Preston and de Waal 2002; Chapter 7 of this volume). The growing interest in the phenomena of empathy has led to the recent emergence of imaging studies investigating sympathetic or empathetic reactions in response to others making emotional facial expressions or telling sad versus neutral stories (e.g., Carr *et al.* 2003; Decety and Chaminade 2003; Farrow *et al.* 2001).

Our ability to make attributions about the mental states (desires, beliefs, intentions) of others based on complex behavioural cues has also been studied in the context of research on *'theory of mind'* or *'mentalizing'*. This line of research was inspired by primatology (e.g., Premack and Woodruff 1978; Tomasello *et al.* 1993, 2003; Povinelli and Bering 2002; Povinelli and Vonk 2003), developmental psychology (Astington 2001; Leslie 1987; Wimmer and Perner 1983; Wellman 2001), as well as by neuropsychological research on autism (Baron-Cohen 1995; Frith 2003). In particular, it has been hypothesized that autistic children lack a theory of mind. This lack can explain their failures in communication and social interaction (Baron-Cohen *et al.* 1985). Recent imaging studies on normal healthy adults have focused on the ability to 'mentalize', that is, to automatically attribute mental states to others. These studies have used stories, cartoons, picture sequences, and animated geometric shapes (Brunet *et al.* 2000; Castelli *et al.* 2000; Gallagher *et al.* 2000, 2002; Goel *et al.* 1995; Schultz *et al.* 2003; Vogeley *et al.* 2001).

Finally, social cognitive neuroscience has started to investigate *social reasoning* in various ways. Some researchers have focused on the study of social exchange and mutual co-operation using social dilemma tasks developed in the framework of game theory and economy. In general, these tasks involve a dyad or a group of people playing games for monetary reward and losses. The pay-off matrices of these games are usually designed such that they allow for different playing strategies. Some are selfish strategies leading to the maximization of the individual's gain at the expense of the group's profit, others are co-operative strategies involving fair but less profitable choices for the single individual. These social dilemma games in their various forms allow for the investigation of social reasoning (working out what the other player will do), social emotions (emotional responses to cooperation, defection, and cheating), and their interaction. So far, functional imaging studies have focused on three different types of game, the simultaneous Prisoner Dilemma Game (Rilling *et al.* 2002), the sequential Trust and Reciprocity Game (McCabe 2001) and the Ultimatum Game (Sanfey *et al.* 2003). The significance of these studies derives not so much from the results they produced as from their innovative paradigms that introduce realistic social interactions into the scanner environment. All of the studies using social dilemma paradigms involved subjects in the scanner playing interactive games with what they believed to be real persons situated outside the scanner (for a related interactive game situation involving the children's game 'stone, paper, scissors' see also Gallagher *et al.* 2002). A related line of research focuses on the study of neuronal correlates of human morality by investigating moral emotions (Moll *et al.* 2002*a,b*, 2003) and moral reasoning (Greene *et al.* 2001, 2002). Moral reasoning is studied in moral dilemma tasks that involve situations in which all possible solutions to a given problem are associated with undesirable outcomes. Although the functional imaging studies using social and moral dilemmas pose slightly different questions, they share a common aim, namely understanding how emotional and cognitive processes relate to each other and to decision making. This topic has always been a core concern of traditional social psychology.

Despite the impressive amount of research generated, social cognitive neuroscience is still in its infancy and has so far focused on the study of very basic social abilities. For example, neuroscience has mostly ignored the study of self-concept and self-esteem and their relation to cognitive processing and behaviour—core topics of social cognition. Similarly, even more complex real-life phenomena studied by traditional social psychology such as the origin and consequences of prejudice and the development of interpersonal relationships have yet to be addressed.

The simplicity of the studies to date may reflect the early stage of development in the field and the methodological limits imposed by neuroimaging and other neurophysiological techniques. However, it could also be argued that the desire for simplicity reflects the ethos of cognitive neuroscience. Cognitive neuroscience aims to isolate universal cognitive and neural processes. The social cognitive tradition, in contrast, strives to study the interplay of ecologically valid and hence complex and context dependent, social, motivational, and cultural factors.

From an uni-directional to a bi-directional account

Most of the neuroimaging studies that investigate social phenomena do so from an uni-directional perspective. The focus has been on understanding the effects of socially relevant stimuli on the mind of a single person. In contrast, the study of social interaction involves by definition a bi-directional perspective and is concerned with the question of how two minds shape each other mutually through reciprocal interactions. To understand interactive minds we have to understand how thoughts, feelings, intentions, and beliefs can be transmitted from one mind to the other. Therefore, it is not sufficient to understand how our own thoughts, feelings, and beliefs are represented and biased as a function of our social context. We also have to study how we can communicate these thoughts and feelings to another mind to enable another person to build a representation of our thoughts and feelings in his or her own brain. The communication loop is closed when, in a second step, the other mind is able to feed back the created representation to us so that we, in turn, can try to correct it in case it does not match with our own representation. The mechanisms underlying such social interactions (Neural Hermeneutics, Frith 2003) ultimately enable social and cultural learning (e.g., Tomasello *et al.* 1993). Delineation of these mechanisms is an important and promising goal for research in social cognitive neuroscience. This will have to be accompanied, however, by the development of new methods and paradigms, such as the involvement of more than one person in experimental tasks or the simultaneous recording of dyadic brain interactions using techniques such as EEG or fMRI (Montague *et al.* 2002).

Mechanisms of social interaction

It is not our aim in this book to represent the whole field of social cognitive neuroscience. We have concentrated on two-person social interactions in which one person, either implicitly or explicitly, tries to 'read' the hidden mental states of the other; their goals, beliefs, or feelings. Although spoken dialogue is the most obvious example of such an interaction, we have only considered situations in which communication is not carried by words. We made this decision in the, no doubt naïve, belief that non-verbal interactions will be simpler to explain. For an account of exciting developments in the understanding the mechanisms underlying spoken dialogue we recommend Pickering and Garrod (2003).

The book is organized in terms of three stages in the interaction between an 'observer' and an 'actor'. First, the observer watches the movements of the actor and infers goals, beliefs, and feelings. Second, the observer generates behaviour in response to that of the actor. In the simplest case the observer imitates the actor. Successful imitation often indicates some understanding of the goals of the actor. Third, the communicative loop is closed so that the actor, in turn, interprets and responds to the behaviour of the observer. Within this framework the authors discuss many different aspects of social interactions, demonstrating the excitement and vigour of this emerging discipline. Here we will highlight some of the key ideas that emerge in the chapters that follow.

A) Biological motion and the decoding of social signals

The term 'biological motion' was coined by Johansson in 1973. He attached small points of light at the joints of human actors and filmed them moving about in the dark. Typically all that is presented in such point light displays is few moving dots, but the observer can instantly perceive the motion as a human figure, can see what the figure is doing, and can tell whether it is male or female (Kozlowski and Cutting 1977). This demonstrates that there is something special about the motion of living things. This motion, in the absence of any other cues, can convey detailed and specific information about what other organisms are doing. At the lowest level we can detect whether or not an object is animate. The movement of inanimate objects like billiard balls is determined by outside forces while animate objects are self-propelled. At the next level we can detect agency. The movements of agents are determined by their goals. At the highest level we can detect intentionality. The movements of intentional agents are determined by their beliefs and desires.

In Chapter 1, Puce and Perrett present evidence that there is a dedicated neural system in the brains of primates, both human and non-human, for detecting and interpreting biological motion. Movements of hands, faces, and eyes are of particular interest to this system, which lies in the superior temporal sulcus (STS) adjacent to V5, an area concerned with visual motion in general. This region of STS does more than simply detect biological motion, it also distinguishes between different types of biological motion such as whether eyes are looking towards or away from the observer. Furthermore, the late components of EEG potentials evoked by biological motion are altered by the context in which the motion occurs.

Csibra reports in Chapter 2 that, before they are 1 year old, human infants can follow another person's gaze direction or pointing gesture. This behaviour implies that they are already interpreting actions in terms of goals. In this case the goal is communicative ('there is something interesting over here'). These infants can also interpret non-communicative actions as goal-directed, such as when a ball jumps over a barrier 'in order to reach a target'. These attributions are not based solely on the nature of the movements observed, but also on the end state of the movement and the context in which it occurs. However, although infants under one year can attribute goals to moving objects, they do not seem to attribute mental states such as beliefs and desires.

In Chapter 3, Frith and Frith outline the developmental trajectory of the ability to mentalize. This trajectory parallels the analysis of different levels of decoding social signals, starting with biological motion, followed by agency detection, and finally attribution of intentionality or mentalizing. Mentalizing becomes explicit at the age of 4 to 6 years when children are able to explain the misleading events that give rise to a false belief. Mentalizing depends upon a more complex brain system than the detection of biological motion. However, the mentalizing system includes STS as one of its components. Another component is located in the temporal poles and may be concerned with the context in which the observed behaviour is occurring. Medial pre-frontal cortex seems to have a special role in the mentalizing system. This area is activated when mental states of the self, as well as others, are represented and may have a role in signalling that mental representations do not necessarily correspond to the actual state of the world.

Rittscher and his colleagues describe computational approaches that have been used for the machine recognition and interpretation of human actions in Chapter 4. They use, for example, motion contour tracking (examining how a smooth curve that encompasses the outline of an actor changes over time) to identify the nature of biological motion. They suggest that semantic context needs to be taken into account to provide a higher-level interpretation of the observed motion. Their approach uses a small collection of low-level models encoding set of motion primitives that are then interpreted in terms of the semantic context in which they occur. Detection of biological motion seems to be sufficient for the attribution of animacy, but, for the attribution of goals and intentions, the context in which the movement occurs must also be taken into account.

B) Mirror neurons and the imitation of behaviour

In 1996 Giacomo Rizzolatti's group at the University of Parma reported the serendipitous discovery of neurons that respond when monkeys see someone else performing a specific action as well as when they do the particular action themselves (Gallese *et al.* 1996). These mirror neurons are thought to represent the neural basis for imitation. Studies in humans have shown that observing someone else's action facilitates the neural circuits the observer would use to perform the same action (Fadiga *et al.* 1995), and it has long been known that patients with frontal lobe lesions may sometimes automatically and inappropriately imitate the actions of others (Lhermitte *et al.* 1986).

When we imitate someone we take the next step beyond the simple observation of biological motion. We observe the action and then we try to reproduce it. This leads to a fundamental problem. What we see is a series of configurations of the person in space, but what we have to do is to issue a series of motor commands. How can we translate what we see into what we need to do? The discovery of mirror neurons demonstrated that a mechanism for translation is present in the primate brain and is automatically elicited when viewing the actions of others. A frequent theme in the contributions to this special issue is that this mirroring system could underlie the development of empathy and other forms of inter-subjectivity.

In Chapter 5, Meltzoff and Decety illustrate how much can be gained by combining insights from developmental psychology and neuroscience. They argue that perception and action are not independent entities that must be 'associated' during a lengthy postnatal learning period. New-born imitation is the best evidence to date that some neurally-based mirroring ability is innately wired and ready to interact with others at birth. Meltzoff and Decety show how the basic mechanisms involved in infant imitation provide the foundation for understanding that others are 'like me'. They hypothesize that the primitive 'like me' understanding of infants is a vital building block for the later ability to adopt the perspective of others—a fundamental mechanism for empathy. The authors emphasize not only on the similarity between self and other (the focus of debates about 'mirror neurons') but also on how humans differentiate their own acts and intentions from those of others. Neuroimaging studies from their lab suggest that the right inferior parietal lobe has a critical role in distinguishing the self from others. The combination of systems that represent others as both 'like me' and as 'different from me' is fundamental for a mature intersubjectivity.

Wohlschläger and his colleagues show in Chapter 6, that children clearly make attributions about intentions when imitating the actions of others. As a result they make predictable 'mistakes' during imitation. On seeing an adult press a button with her left hand, children interpret the task to be imitated as 'pressing the button' and use whichever hand is most convenient. In this respect, they are behaving like Csibra's infants who expect goals to be achieved by the most efficient means. However, if the form of the movement is seen as the goal of the action, then the movement will be imitated exactly. Here again the context in which the movement is made has a role in determining the goal that will be attributed and hence the level at which the imitation occurs.

In Chapter 7, Gallese proposes that the mirroring system in the brain applies to emotions and intentions as well as to actions. These mirror effects are automatic and unconscious simulations. When we see an action, this automatically triggers action simulation at a covert level. This involves, not only the motor system, but also systems concerned with the sensory conse-quences of the action being simulated. Similar effects occur when we see an expression of emotion. These automatic effects ensure that we share, to some degree, the inner states of the people with whom we are interacting, a necessary starting point for attributing mental states to others.

In spite of their mirror neurons, there is no evidence that monkeys can learn new skills by imitation and it has been suggested that true imitation learning cannot occur unless the learner can attribute intentions and understand cause-effect relationships. In Chapter 8, Byrne analyses in detail the processes by which mountain gorillas might use imitation to learn how to prepare nettles for eating and proposes that this learning occurs without any attribution of intentions or causal understanding. He suggests that imitation in this case depends on the perceptual ability to parse a complex action into a sequence of more primitive actions, and detect hierarchical organization underlying the action's original production. This ability might be a necessary preliminary to attributing intention and cause.

In Chapter 9, Schaal and his colleagues discuss the computational methods that have been used to control robots that can learn by imitation. Such learn-ing seems to be best achieved if movements are decomposed into a set of movement primitives that can be observed in the robot teacher as well as gen-erated in the robot student. A common framework for observation and pro-duction can be achieved by expressing these movement primitives in task space, i.e. the series of movements made by the pole in a pole-balancing task. Such task-level imitation requires prior knowledge of how movements of the pole can be converted into movements of the arm that is doing the balancing.

Using this method, robots can successfully learn by imitation. This learning, sometimes called 'mimicking' can occur without any knowledge of goals, but cannot generalize to new contexts. Much more robust learning by imitation can be achieved if the task goal is known so that imitated movement trajectories can be improved by trial and error learning. Even better imitation can be achieved if the movement primitives are used to make predictions about the behaviour of the robot teacher (see also Chapter 14).

C) Closing the communication loop.

The most remarkable feature of social interactions is how skilled we are in correctly inferring the goals, beliefs, and feelings of others. How is it possible to read these mental states? They are fundamentally hidden and can never be checked by an outside observer. We believe that to discover the mechanisms that underlie this mentalizing, it will be necessary to study the closed the loop of social interactions. In most studies of imitation this loop remains open. The transmitter (or teacher) displays some action and then the receiver (or learner) imitates that action. To close the loop the transmitter must observe the imitation and then respond in some way to the receiver. A prototype of such a communicative loop is seen when a mother teaches her infant to pronounce a word correctly by exaggerating certain acoustic features of the word (Burnham *et al*. 2002). Through a series of iterations the transmitter and receiver can reach a consensus as to the nature of the action being imitated. Through this mutually contingent behaviour the hidden purpose of the action is passed from transmitter to receiver. The contributors to the final part of this volume are concerned with interactions in which the communicative loop is closed in this way.

Johnson shows in Chapter 10 that infants will treat a novel, amorphously-shaped object as an agent with goals if it interacts contingently with them or with another person, i.e. if it moves in response to another agent's actions. Infants can use the object's environmentally directed behaviour to determine its attentional orientation and object-oriented goals. Adults will also treat objects that behave contingently as agents in spite of knowing that the objects are artefacts. This suggests that this agent-detection mechanism is a module that is hard wired in the brain. However, while this mechanism may be necessary, it does not seem to be sufficient to support advanced mentalizing ability.

In Chapter 11, Blair shows that emotional expressions are communicative gestures with specific roles in social interactions. Confronted with an expression of anger the receiver will stop performing his current action in order to change the expression of the transmitter. Expressions of embarrassment after the commission of a social solecism are designed by the transmitter to prevent further criticism from the receiver. Thus emotional expressions and empathy permit the rapid modification of behaviour during social interactions. Disorders in the perception of emotional expressions involve a failure to recognize the intention behind these expressions and can have devastating effects leading to persistent anti-social behaviour as in psychopathy.

While social interactions may be a novel topic for study for neuroscientists, well-established techniques for such studies have been developed in the social sciences. In Chapter 12, Griffin and Gonzalez describe a series of formal approaches for the design and analysis of studies of dyadic interactions. They show how these methods permit the measurement of interdependence and social influence.

Sally considers the various interactive games that have been developed by economists, such as the prisoners' dilemma, in Chapter 13. These games require that each player predict what the other will do in order to work out an appropriate strategy. A consistent observation is that most players do not adopt the optimum strategy as defined by the Nash equilibrium. In part this seems to be due to the players attributing beliefs and intentions to each other that extend beyond the narrow confines of the game. Sally considers the various factors that cause players not to adopt the optimum economic strategy.

In Chapter 14, Wolpert and his colleagues present a computational account of interactions that can be applied to robots as well as to people. Fundamental to this account is the idea of the 'forward model' that predicts the consequences of issuing a particular command to the motor system. The current context in which the agent is acting can be discovered by running multiple forward models to see which one gives the best prediction. Each forward model (or predictor) is paired with a controller that is used to issue motor commands. Through prediction, the most appropriate controller can be identified for any point in an action sequence. These multiple predictor-controller pairs can also be used for imitation. Through prediction the receiver (or learner) can estimate which controller he must use to generate what the transmitter (or teacher) is doing at each point in the movement sequence. As long as the motor control system in the learner is sufficiently similar to that in the teacher, then the learner can reproduce the movement by using this sequence of controllers. However, the teacher can also observe the learner and, in the same way, estimate the sequence of controllers the teacher would use to generate the learner's movement. If communication has been successful, then the sequence that the teacher estimates should correspond to the sequence he originally used. In this way the communicative loop is closed and the success of the communication can be checked. We suggest that we have here the rudiments of mechanism by which intentions can be transmitted from one mind to another. Such a mechanism could be the basis for some of the most intricate and complex human social interactions.

References

Adolphs, R. (1999). Social cognition and the human brain. *Trends Cogn. Sci.* **3**, 469–79.

Allison, T., Puce, A., and McCarthy, G. (2000). Social perception from visual cues: role of the STS region. *Trends Cogn. Sci.* **4**, 267–78.

Allport, A. (1985). The historical background of social psychology. In: *Handbook of social psychology*, (ed. G. Lindzey and E. Aronson) pp. 1–46. New York: Random House.

Astington, J. W. (2001). The future of theory-of-mind research: understanding motivational states, the role of language, and real-world consequences. *Child Dev.* **72**, 685–7.

Baron-Cohen, S. (1995). Mindblindness: an essay on autism and theory of mind. Cambridge, MA: MIT Press/Bradford Books.

Baron-Cohen, S., Leslie, A. M., and Frith, U. (1985). Does the autistic child have a "theory of mind"? *Cognition* **21**, 37–46.

Blakemore, S. J. and Decety, J. (2001). From the perception of action to the understanding of intention. *Nat. Rev. Neurosci.* **2**, 561–7.

Brothers, L. (1990). The social brain: A project for integrating primate behavior and neurophysiology in a new domain. *Concepts in Neuroscience* **1**, 27–51.

Brothers, L. (1997). *Friday's footprint: How society shapes the human mind*. New York: Oxford University Press.

Brunet, E., Sarfati, Y., Hardy-Bayle, M. C., and Decety, J. (2000). A PET investigation of the attribution of intentions with a nonverbal task. *Neuroimage* **11**, 157–66.

Burnham, D., Kitamura, C., and Vollmer-Conna, U. (2002). What's New Pussycat? On talking to babies and animals. *Science* **296**, 1435.

Cacioppo, J. (2001). *Foundations in Social Neuroscience*. Cambridge, MA: MIT Press.

Carr, L., Iacoboni, M., Dubeau, M. C., Mazziotta, J. C., and Lenzi, G. L. (2003). Neural mechanisms of empathy in humans: a relay from neural systems for imitation to limbic areas. *Proc. Natl. Acad. Sci. USA* **100**, 5497–502.

Castelli, F., Happe, F., Frith, U., and Frith, C. (2000). Movement and mind: a functional imaging study of perception and interpretation of complex intentional movement patterns. *Neuroimage* **12**, 314–25.

Crick, F. and Koch, C. (1998). Consciousness and neuroscience. *Cerebral Cortex* **8**, 97–107.

Decety, J. and Chaminade, T. (2003). Neural correlates of feeling sympathy. *Neuropsychologia* **41**, 127–38.

Dennett, D. C. (1978). Beliefs About Beliefs. *Behavioral and Brain Sciences* **1**, 568–70.

Fadiga, L., Fogassi, L., Pavesi, G., and Rizzolatti, G. (1995). Motor facilitation during action observation: a magnetic stimulation study. *Journal of Neurophysiol* 73: 2608–11.

Farrow, T. F., Zheng, Y., Wilkinson, I. D., Spence, S. A., Deakin, J. F., Tarrier, N., *et al.* (2001). Investigating the functional anatomy of empathy and forgiveness. *Neuroreport* **12**, 2433–8.

Frith, C. D. (2003). Neural Hermeneutics: How Brains Interpret Minds. Keynote Lecture, *9th Annual Meeting of the Organization of Human Brain Mapping*, New York.

Frith, C. D. and Frith, U. (1999). Interacting minds—a biological basis. *Science* **286**, 1692–5.

Frith, U. (2003). Autism: Explaining the Enigma (2nd edition). Oxford: Blackwell.

Gallagher, H. L., Happé, F., Brunswick, N., Fletcher, P. C., Frith, U., and Frith, C. D. (2000). Reading the mind in cartoons and stories: an fMRI study of 'theory of mind' in verbal and nonverbal tasks. *Neuropsychologia* **38**, 11–21.

Gallagher, H. L., Jack, A. I., Roepstorff, A., and Frith, C. D. (2002). Imaging the intentional stance in a competitive game. *Neuroimage* **16**, 814–21.

Gallese, V. (2001). The "Shared Manifold" Hypothesis: from mirror neurons to empathy. *Journal of Consciousness Studies* **8**, 33–50.

Gallese, V., Fadiga, L., Fogassi, L., and Rizzolatti, G. (1996). Action recognition in the premotor cortex. *Brain* **119**, 593–609.

Gallese, V. and Goldman, A. (1998). Mirror neurons and the simulation theory of mind-reading. *Trends in Cognitive Sciences* **12**, 493–501.

Goel, V., Grafman, J., Sadato, N., and Hallett, M. (1995). Modeling other minds. *Neuroreport* **6**, 1741–6.

Greene, J. and Haidt, J. (2002). How (and where) does moral judgment work? *Trends Cogn. Sci.* **6**, 517–23.

Greene, J. D., Sommerville, R. B., Nystrom, L. E., Darley, J. M., and Cohen, J. D. (2001). An fMRI investigation of emotional engagement in moral judgment. *Science* **293**, 2105–8.

Grezes, J. and Decety, J. (2001). Functional anatomy of execution, mental simulation, observation, and verb generation of actions: a meta-analysis. *Hum. Brain Mapp.* **12**, 1–19.

Harmon-Jones, E. and Devine, T. (2003). Special issue on social neuroscience. *Journal of Personality and Social Psychology* **85**(4), 589–776.

Hart, A. J., Whalen, P. J., Shin, L. M., McInerney, S. C., Fischer, H., and Rauch, S. L. (2000). Differential response in the human amygdala to racial outgroup vs ingroup face stimuli. *Neuroreport* **11**, 2351–5.

Heatherton, R. F. and Macrae, C. N. (2003). *Social Cognitive Neuroscience: A Reader*. Cambridge, MA: Blackwell.

Jeannerod, M., Arbib, M. A., Rizzolatti, G., and Sakata, H. (1995). Grasping objects: the cortical mechanisms of visuomotor transformation. *Trends Neurosci.* **18**, 314–20.

Johansson, G. (1973). Visual perception of biological motion and a model of its analysis. *Percept. Psychophys.* **14**, 202–11.

Kozlowski, L. T. and Cutting, J. E. (1977). Recognizing the sex of a walker from a dynamic point-light display. *Perc. Psychophys.* **21**, 575–80.

Leslie, A. M. (1987). Pretence and representation. The origins of 'theory of mind'. *Psychological Review* **94**, 412–26.

Leslie, A. M. (1994). Pretending and believing: issues in the theory of ToMM. *Cognition* **50**, 211–38.

Lhermitte, F., Pillon, B., and Serdaru, M. (1986). Human autonomy and the frontal lobes. Part I: Imitation and utilization behavior: a neuropsychological study of 75 patients. *Annals of Neurology* **19**, 326–34.

McCabe, K., Houser, D., Ryan, L., Smith, V., and Trouard, T. (2001). A functional imaging study of cooperation in two-person reciprocal exchange. *Proc. Natl. Acad. Sci. USA* **98**, 11832–5.

Moll, J., Oliveira-Souza, R., Bramati, I. E., and Grafman, J. (2002a). Functional networks in emotional moral and nonmoral social judgments. *Neuroimage* **16**, 696–703.

Moll, J., Oliveira-Souza, R., Eslinger, P. J., Bramati, I. E., Mourao-Miranda, J., Andreiuolo, P. A., *et al.* (2002b). The neural correlates of moral sensitivity: a functional magnetic resonance imaging investigation of basic and moral emotions. *J. Neurosci.* **22**, 2730–6.

Moll, J., Oliveira-Souza, R., and Eslinger, P. J. (2003). Morals and the human brain: a working model. *Neuroreport* **14**, 299–305.

Morris, J. S., Frith, C. D., Perrett, D. I., Rowland, D., Young, A. W., Calder, A. J., *et al.* (1996). A differential neural response in the human amygdala to fearful and happy facial expressions. *Nature* **383**, 812–15.

O'Doherty, J., Winston, J., Critchley, H., Perrett, D., Burt, D. M., and Dolan, R. J. (2003). Beauty in a smile: the role of medial orbitofrontal cortex in facial attractiveness. *Neuropsychologia* **41**, 147–55.

Ochsner, K. N. and Lieberman, M. D. (2001). The emergence of social cognitive neuroscience. *American Psychologist* 717–34.

Phelps, E. A. (2001). Faces and races in the brain. *Nat. Neurosci.* **4**, 775–6.

Phelps, E. A., Cannistraci, C. J., and Cunningham, W. A. (2003). Intact performance on an indirect measure of race bias following amygdala damage. *Neuropsychologia* **41**, 203–8.

Phillips, M. L., Young, A. W., Senior, C., Brammer, M., Andrew, C., Calder, A. J., *et al.* (1997). A specific neural substrate for perceiving facial expressions of disgust. *Nature* **389**, 495–8.

Pickering, M. J. and Garrod, S. (2003). Toward a mechanistic psychology of dialogue. *Behav Brain Sci* **26**, in press.

Povinelli, D. J. and Bering, J. M. (2002). The mentality of apes revisited. *Current Directions in Psychological Science* **11**, 115–19.

Povinelli, D. J. and Vonk, J. (2003). Chimpanzee minds: suspiciously human? *Trends Cogn. Sci.* **7**, 157–60.

Premack, D. and Woodruff, G. (1978). Does the chimpanzee have a theory of mind? *Behavioral-and-Brain-Science* **1**, 515–26.

Preston, S. D. and de-Waal, F. B. M. (2002). Empathy: Its ultimate and proximate bases. *Behavioral-and-Brain-Science* **25**, 1–72.

Montague, P. R., Berns, G. S., Cohen, J. D., McClure, S. M., Pagnoni, G., Dhamala, M., *et al.* (2002). Hyperscanning: Simultaneous fMRI during linked social interactions. *Neuroimage* **16**, 1159–64.

Rilling, J., Gutman, D., Zeh, T., Pagnoni, G., Berns, G., and Kilts, C. (2002). A neural basis for social cooperation. *Neuron* **35**, 395–405.

Rizzolatti, G., Fadiga, L., Gallese, V., and Fogassi, L. (1996). Premotor cortex and the recognition of motor actions. *Brain Res. Cogn.* **3**, 131–41.

Sanfey, A. G., Rilling, J. K., Aronson, J. A., Nystrom, L. E., and Cohen, J. D. (2003). The neural basis of economic decision-making in the Ultimatum Game. *Science* **300**, 1755–8.

Schultz, R. T., Grelotti, D. J., Klin, A., Kleinman, J., Van der, G. C., Marois, R., *et al.* (2003). The role of the fusiform face area in social cognition: implications for the pathobiology of autism. *Philos. Trans. R. Soc. Lond. B. Biol. Sci.* **358**, 415–27.

Shallice, T. (1988). *From Neuropsychology to Mental Structure*. Cambridge: Cambridge University Press.

Tomasello, M., Kruger, A. C., and Ratner, H. H. (1993). Cultural learning. *Behavioral-and-Brain-Science* **16**, 495–552.

Tomasello, M., Call, J., and Hare, B. (2003). Chimpanzees understand psychological states – the question is which ones and to what extent. *Trends Cogn. Sci.* **7**, 153–6.

Vogeley, K., Bussfeld, P., Newen, A., Herrmann, S., Happé, F., Falkai, P., *et al.* (2001). Mind reading: neural mechanisms of theory of mind and self-perspective. *Neuroimage* **14**, 170–81.

Wellman, H. M., Cross, D., and Watson, J. (2001). Meta-analysis of theory-of-mind development: the truth about false belief. *Child Dev.* **72**, 655–84.

Wimmer, H. and Perner, J. (1983). Beliefs about beliefs: representation and constraining function of wrong beliefs in young children's understanding of deception. *Cognition* **13**, 103–28.

Winston, J. S., Strange, B. A., O'Doherty, J., and Dolan, R. J. (2002). Automatic and intentional brain responses during evaluation of trustworthiness of faces. *Nat. Neurosci.* **5**, 277–83.

Zeki, S. (1993). *A Vision of the Brain*. Oxford: Blackwell.

1

Electrophysiology and brain imaging of biological motion

Aina Puce and David Perrett

The movements of the faces and bodies of other conspecifics provide stimuli of considerable interest to the social primate. Studies of single cells, field potential recordings and functional neuroimaging data indicate that specialized visual mechanisms exist in the superior temporal sulcus (STS) of both human and non-human primates that produce selective neural responses to moving natural images of faces and bodies. STS mechanisms also process simplified displays of biological motion involving point lights marking the limb articulations of animate bodies and geometrical shapes whose motion simulates purposeful behaviour. Facial movements such as deviations in eye gaze, important for gauging an individual's social attention, and mouth movements, indicative of potential utterances, generate particularly robust neural responses that differentiate between movement types. Collectively such visual processing can enable the decoding of complex social signals and through its outputs to limbic, frontal and parietal systems the STS may play a part in enabling appropriate affective responses and social behaviour.

Keywords: biological motion; event related potentials; functional magnetic resonance imaging; humans; single-unit electrophysiology; animals

1.1 Introduction

Primates, being social animals, continually observe one another's behaviour so as to be able to integrate effectively within their social living structure. At a non-social level, successful predator evasion also necessitates being able to 'read' the actions of other species in one's vicinity. The ability to interpret the motion and action of others in human primates goes beyond basic survival and successful interactions with important conspecifics. Many of our recreational and cultural pursuits would not be possible without this ability. Excellent symphony orchestras exist not only owing to the exceptional musicians, but also their ability to interpret their conductors' non-verbal instructions. Conductors convey unambiguously not only the technical way that the orchestra should execute the piece of music, but modulate the mood and emotional tone of the music measure by measure. The motion picture industry owes much of its success today to its silent movie pioneers, who could entertain with their non-verbal antics. The world's elite athletes rely on the interpretation of other's movements to achieve their team's goals successfully and foil opponents.

1.2 Human behavioural studies of biological motion perception

The perception of moving biological forms can rely on the ability to integrate form and motion but it can also rely on the ability to define form from motion (Oram and Perrett 1994, 1996). The latter is evident in the ingenious work of Johansson who filmed actors dressed in black with white dots attached to their joints on a completely black set (Johansson 1973). With these moving dots human observers could reliably identify the walking or running motions, for example, of another human or an animal (Fig. 1.1). This type of stimulus is known as a Johansson, point light or biological motion display.

A number of important observations have emerged from the human behavioural biological motion perception literature. First, the perceptual effect of observing an individual walking or running is severely compromised when the display is inverted (Dittrich 1993; Pavlova and Sokolov 2000). Second, while

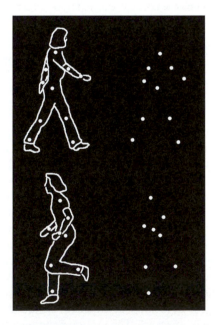

Fig. 1.1 An example of a biological motion stimulus. (Adapted from Johansson (1973), with permission from *Percept. Psychophys.*)

biological motion representing locomotory movements is recognized the most efficiently, social and instrumental actions can also be recognized from these impoverished displays (Dittrich 1993). Third, biological motion can be perceived even within masks of dots (Perrett *et al.* 1990*a*; Thornton *et al.* 1998). Fourth, the gender of the walker (and even the identity of specific individuals) can be recognized from pattern of gait and idiosyncratic body movements in these impoverished displays (Cutting and Kozlowski 1977; Kozlowski and Cutting 1977). Fifth, there is a bias to perceive forward locomotion, at the expense of misinterpreting the underlying form in time-reversed biological motion films (Pavlova *et al.* 2002). Finally, observers can discern various emotional expressions from viewing Johansson faces (Bassili 1978).

In very low light conditions many animals are efficient at catching prey or evading predators. In such conditions the patterns of articulation (typical of biological motion) may be more discernible than the form of stationary animals. Indeed, in behavioural experiments it is evident that point light displays are sufficient for cats to discriminate the pattern of locomotion of conspecifics (Blake 1993). In an ingenious behavioural study in cats, a forced choice task where selection of a biological motion display (of a cat walking or running) was rewarded with food resulting in the animals performing significantly above chance. A series of foil stimuli showing dots changing their spatial location provided a set of tight controls in this experiment (Blake 1993).

Evidence for the existence of specialized brain systems that analyse biological motion (and the motion of humans and non-humans) comes from neuropsychological lesion studies. Dissociations between the ability to perceive biological motion and other types of motion have been demonstrated. Several patients who are to all intents and purposes 'motion blind' can discriminate biological motion stimuli (Vaina *et al.* 1990; McLeod *et al.* 1996). The opposite pattern, i.e. an inability to perceive biological motion yet have relatively normal motion perception in general, has also been reported (Schenk and Zihl 1997).

1.3 Biological motion perception in non-humans

One brain region known as the STP area in the cortex surrounding the STS has been the subject of considerable scrutiny ever since cells selective for the sight of faces were characterized in this region in monkeys (Perrett *et al.* 1982; Desimone 1991). This STS brain region is known to be a convergence point for the dorsal and ventral visual streams. The STP area derives its input from the MST area in the dorsal pathway and the anterior inferior-temporal area in the ventral pathway (Boussaoud *et al.* 1990; Felleman and Van Essen 1991). The cortex of the STS has connections with the amygdala (Aggleton *et al.* 1980) and also with the orbitofrontal cortex (Barbas 1988), regions implicated in the processing of stimuli of social and emotional significance in both human and non-human primates (reviewed in Baron-Cohen 1995; Brothers 1997; Adolphs 1999).

In addition to having face-specific cells, the cortex of the STS has other complex response properties. It has emerged that visual information about the shape and posture of the fingers, hands, arms, legs and torso all impact on STS cell tuning in addition to facial details such as the shape of the mouth and direction of gaze (Desimone *et al.* 1984; Wachsmuth *et al.* 1994; Perrett *et al.* 1984, 1985*a*; Jellema *et al.* 2000). Motion information presumed to arrive from the dorsal stream projections arrives in the STS some 20 ms ahead of form information from the ventral stream (Fig. 2.2*a*), but despite this asynchrony, STS processing overcomes the 'binding problem' and only form and motion arising from the same biological object are integrated within 100 ms of the moving form becoming visible (Oram and Perrett 1996). Indeed, STS cell integration of form and motion is widespread and there are numerous cell types specializing in the processing of different types of face, limb and whole body motion (Perrett *et al.* 1985*b*; Carey *et al.* 1997; Jellema *et al.* 2000, 2002; Jellema and Perrett 2002).

While most STS cells derive sensitivity to body movement by combining signals about the net translation or rotation of the body with the face and body form visible at any moment in time, a smaller proportion (20%) of cells are able to respond selectively to the form of the body defined through patterns of articulation in point light displays (Perrett *et al.* 1990*a*,*b*; Oram and Perrett 1994, 1996; Fig. 1.1). These cells tuned to biological motion are selective for

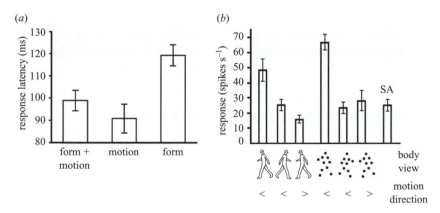

Fig. 1.2 Some response properties of primate STP area neurons elicited by biological motion stimuli. (Adapted from Oram and Perrett (1994, 1996), with permission.) (*a*) Average response latencies for neurons with different response properties. (*b*) An example of a neuron that does not differentiate between real human motion and biological motion. Also, the strongest response is in the motion direction compatible with direction of the body.

the sight of the same action visible in full light and when depicted in point light displays.

Cells responding to whole body motion exhibit selectivity for direction of motion and view of the body: most respond preferentially to compatible motion with the body moving forward in the direction it faces, though some are tuned to backward locomotion with the body moving in the opposite direction to the way it faces (Perrett *et al.* 1985*b*, 1989; Oram and Perrett 1996; Fig. 2.2*b*). This cellular tuning bias for forward locomotion may underlie the forward bias found in perceptual interpretation of locomotion depicted in point light displays (Pavlova *et al.* 2002).

Responses to purposeful hand object actions such as reaching for, picking, tearing and manipulating objects have also been characterized in the STS (Perrett *et al.* 1989, 1990*c*; Jellema *et al.* 2000). These STS cells are sensitive to the form of the hand performing the action, and are unresponsive to the sight of tools manipulating objects in the same manner as hands. Furthermore, the cells code the spatio-temporal interaction between the agent performing the action and the object of the action. For example, cells tuned to hands manipulating an object cease to respond if the hands and object move appropriately but are spatially separated. This selectivity ensures that the cells are more responsive in situations where the agent's motion is causally related to the object's motion. The STS cell populations coding body and hand actions appear to be exclusively visual, although information from the motor system does affect other STS cell populations (Hietanen and Perrett 1996) and modulates STS activity in humans (Iacoboni *et al.* 2001; Nishitani and Hari 2001).

Information defined by the visual characterization of actions in the STS appears to be relayed via parietal systems (Gallese *et al.* 2002) to frontal motor planning systems. In frontal and parietal areas a neural system has recently been found to respond selectively both during the execution of hand actions, and (like STS cells) during the observation of corresponding actions performed by others. The frontal region of primate cortex had long been known to be somatotopically organized for the representation and control of movements of the mouth and arm (Rizzolatti *et al.* 1988). Neurons within area F5 of the monkey premotor cortex have now been labelled 'mirror' neurons, because they discharge when monkeys perform or observe the same hand actions (di Pellegrino *et al.* 1992; Rizzolatti *et al.* 1996*a*,*b*; Gallese *et al.* 1996). An F5 cell selective for the action of grasping would respond for example when the monkey grasps an object in sight or in the dark (thereby demonstrating motoric properties). The visual properties of such an F5 cell are strikingly similar to those described in the STS: both F5 and STS cells will respond when the monkey observes the experimenter reaching and grasping an object, but not to the sight of the experimenter's hand motion alone or the sight of the object alone. These conjoint properties have led Rizzolatti *et al.* (1996*a*,*b*) and Gallese *et al.* (1996) to postulate that the F5 neurons form a system for matching observation and executing actions for the grasping, manipulation and placement of objects.

Because the cells additionally respond selectively to the sound of actions (Kohler *et al*. 2002), the mirror system may provide a supra-modal conceptual representation of actions and their consequences in the world. Crucially the properties of the frontal mirror system indicate that we may understand actions performed by others because we can match the actions we sense through vision (and audition) to our ability to produce the same actions ourselves.

The actions of others are not always fully visible, for example someone may become hidden from our sight as they move behind a tree, or their hands may not remain fully in view as they reach to retrieve an object. The similarity of STS and F5 systems in processing of actions has become more apparent in experiments investigating the nature of processing during these moments when actions are partially or totally occluded from sight. Within the STS it is now apparent that specific cell populations are activated when the presence of a hidden person can be inferred from the preceding visual events (i.e. they were witnessed passing out of sight behind a screen and have not yet been witnessed re-emerging into sight, so they are likely to remain behind the screen; Baker *et al*. 2001). In an analogous manner, F5 cells may respond to the sight of the experimenter reaching to grasp an object. The same cells are active when the experimenter places an object behind a screen and then reaches as if to grasp it (even though the object and hand are hidden from view (Umilta *et al*. 2002)). The sight of equivalent reaching when there is no reason to believe an object is hidden from sight fails to activate the F5 cells. Thus F5 and STS cells code the sight of actions on the basis of what is currently visible and on the basis of the recent perceptual history (Jellema and Perrett 2002; Jellema *et al*. 2002).

The manner in which temporal STS and frontal F5 systems interact is not fully clear, but appears to involve intermediate processing steps mediated by parietal areas (Nishitani and Hari 2000, 2001; Gallese *et al*. 2002). While STS and F5 cells have similar visual properties they may subserve distinct functions; the frontal system perhaps serves to control the behaviour of the self particularly in dealing with objects (Rizzolatti *et al*. 1996*a*,*b*), whereas the STS system is specialized for the detection and recognition of the behaviour of others (Perrett *et al*. 1990*c*; Mistlin and Perrett 1990; Hietanen and Perrett 1996).

1.4 Human neuroimaging and electrophysiological studies of biological motion perception

The first suggestion that humans may possess specialized biological motion perception mechanisms came from a point light display depicting a moving body designed to investigate the response properties of medial temporal/V5, a region of occipito-temporal cortex known to respond to motion. In this fMRI study activation was observed in MT/V5 as well as areas of superior temporal cortex. This was regarded at that time as surprising, as the activation appeared to lie in brain regions traditionally regarded as participating in auditory speech processing (Howard *et al*. 1996). Localization of primary auditory cortex was not performed in this visual stimulation study. In a PET study published in the same year Johansson displays of body motion (depicting a person dancing), hand motion (depicting a hand reaching for a glass and bringing it to a mouth), object motion (depicting a three-dimensional structure rotating and pitching) and control conditions, consisting of either random dot motion or a static display of randomly placed dots, were shown to a group of healthy subjects (Bonda *et al*. 1996). The human motion conditions selectively activated the inferior parietal region and the STS. Specifically, the body motion condition selectively activated the right posterior STS, whereas the hand motion condition activated the left intraparietal sulcus and the posterior STS (Bonda *et al*. 1996). In a more recent fMRI study, a Johansson display depicting a walker was used and the activation contrasted to control conditions that included a dot display with non-random motion and a gender discrimination task with real images of faces (Vaina *et al*. 2001). Biological motion differentially activated a large number of dorsal and ventral regions, most notably the lateral occipital complex, but the STS was not preferentially activated in this study.

Grossman and colleagues found that biological motion stimuli depicting jumping, kicking, running and throwing movements produced more right STS activation than control motion irrespective of the visual field in which the biological motion display was presented. Conversely, the control motion, including scrambled biological motion displays, activated MT/MST areas and the lateral-occipital complex (Grossman *et al*. 2000). Moreover, the STS region could also be activated by *imagining* Johansson stimuli, although the size of the activation was small (Grossman *et al*. 2000). While the most robust STS activation was elicited by viewing upright Johansson displays, a smaller STS activation signal was also seen to viewing inverted Johansson displays.

While biological motion clearly activates the STS region in humans, the function of the region may be more general in performing a visual analysis of bodies based on either the characteristic patterns of articulation that comprise biological motion or information about bodies that can be derived from static images (Downing *et al*. 2001); hence the term 'extrastriate body area' has been applied to one cortical region within the STS complex.

1.5 Biological motion perception versus human motion perception

As in non-human primates, responsiveness to Johansson-like displays of facial motion is present in STS regions that also respond to real images of facial motion, e.g. nonlinguistic mouth movements (Puce *et al*. 2003), although the per cent magnetic resonance signal change to the Johansson-like face was smaller than that observed to the natural facial images. In parallel to the neuroimaging data, direct measures of neural activity in humans, in the form of scalp ERPs, are elicited to Johansson-like and real images of faces (Thompson *et al.* 2002*b*), with a prominent negativity occurring at around 170 ms post-motion onset (N170) over the bilateral temporal scalp. This activity is significantly greater than that seen to motion controls.

Over the latter half of the 1990s, a series of PET and fMRI studies examining activation to viewing the motion and actions of others have pointed to the existence of cortical networks that preferentially process certain attributes of these high-level visual displays (reviewed by Allison *et al.* 2000; Blakemore and Decety 2001). Fig. 1.3 displays activation observed in these studies, lying along the posterior extent of the STS and its ascending limb in inferior parietal cortex in response to observing movements of the body, hands, eye and mouth. Activation in these regions can also be elicited to imagining the motion of others (Grossman *et al.* 2000), and additionally to viewing static images of implied motion (Kourtzi and Kanwisher 2000).

Interestingly, differences in activation patterns can occur when subjects view compatible versus incompatible motion of the head or body (Thompson *et al.* 2002*a*). Specifically, the bilateral posterior lateral temporal cortex is active when viewing compatible motion. By contrast, viewing incompatible motion activates the right posterior lateral temporal cortex, left anterior temporal cortex, left temporoparietal junction and left precentral gyrus. This extended network of activation might be due to the novelty or salience of the incongruent body and head motion stimuli (Downar *et al.* 2002). The differential experience with compatible and incompatible motion may explain STS cell sensitivity to the compatibility of motion direction and body view during the locomotion described above.

What is unique about the motion of animate beings? Animals and humans possess articulated joints, enabling the movement of body parts without having to maintain a constant spatial relationship in space relative to each other. This results in the ability to produce a limitless set of movements. Man-made objects, such as utensils and tools, in general do not have this capability. Beauchamp *et al.* (2002) investigated the differences in brain activation to these different types of high-level motion stimuli. Interestingly, observing human motion stimuli activated the STS and observing the motion of tools/utensils activated cortex ventral to the STS, on the MTG. In another fMRI experiment in this same study, stimuli depicting articulated and non-articulated human motion were presented. The STS responded to the articulated human motion and the MTG to non-articulated motion, indicating that these high-order processing mechanisms process selectively the higher-order motion type (Beauchamp *et al.* 2002).

Grezes *et al.* (2001) also reported activation differences between observing rigid and non-rigid motion. Specifically, they observed an anterior–posterior gradient of activation in the STS regions, with non-rigid motion producing

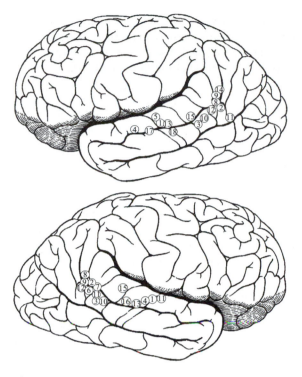

mouth

① Calvert *et al.* lip reading (STG)

② Calvert *et al.* lip reading (AG)

③ Puce *et al.* mouth movement

④ Puce & Allison mouth movement

body

⑤ Howard *et al.* body movement

⑥ Bonda *et al.* body movement

⑦ Senior *et al.* body movement

⑧ Kourtzi & Kanwisher
        body movement

⑨ Grossman *et al.* body movement

eyes

⑩ Puce *et al.* eye gaze

⑪ Wicker *et al.* eye gaze

⑫ Hoffman & Haxby eye gaze

hand

⑬ Neville *et al.* ASL

⑭ Bonda *et al.* hand action

⑮ Grezes *et al.* hand action

⑯ Grezes *et al.* hand movement

⑰ Grafton *et al.* hand grasp

⑱ Rizzolatti *et al.* hand grasp

Fig. 1.3 Centres of activation to viewing the face, hand and body movements of others obtained from a series of PET and fMRI studies. (Adapted from Allison *et al.* (2000), with permission.)

the most anterior activation. Additionally, they observed activation in left intraparietal cortex to non-rigid biological motion (Grezes *et al.* 2001). The magnitude of the activation in the STS to biological motion, and indeed in other cortical regions, can be coloured by the task requirements and the attention that the observer places on the 'human' quality of the motion

(Vaina *et al.* 2001). Additionally, attention to the displayed emotion enhances fMRI activation in the STS, whereas increased activation to facial attributes *per se*, such as identity or isolated features, increased activation in all known face-sensitive cortical regions (Narumoto *et al.* 2001).

(a) Social cognition

The limbic system, in conjunction with the orbitofrontal cortex and the STS, is thought to form a network that is involved in social cognition (Baron-Cohen 1995; Brothers 1997; Adolphs 1999). One important aspect of social cognition is the identification of the direction of another's attention from their direction of gaze or head view (Perrett *et al.* 1985*a*, 1992; Kleinke 1986; Allison *et al.* 2000; Emery 2000). Indeed, the existence of an eye direction detector has been postulated in this hierarchical system of social cognition, which at its top level allows us to 'mindread' and infer the intentions of others (Baron-Cohen 1995; Baron-Cohen *et al.* 1997). While there is evidence for cell populations coding for eye and attention direction within STS (Perrett *et al.* 1985*a*, 1992), the populations are not anatomically grouped in such a way that scalp evoked potentials are necessarily linked to a given eye direction (Bentin *et al.* 1996; Eimer 1998; Taylor *et al.* 2001). Our attention and behaviour can be modified when confronted with a face with averted gaze. A peripheral target stimulus is detected by normal subjects more efficiently when it lies in the direction of gaze of a central stimulus face (Friesen and Kingstone 1998; Driver *et al.* 1999; Hietanen 1999, 2002; Langton and Bruce 2000). Moreover, patients with unilateral neglect are less likely to extinguish a contralesional target stimulus when it lies in the gaze path of a stimulus face (Vuilleumier 2002). Following the attention direction of someone's gaze may be such an over-learned response that it needs little conscious awareness.

(b) Gaze perception

Neuroimaging studies involving gaze perception indicate that there is an active cortical network involving occipito-temporal cortex (fusiform gyrus, inferior temporal gyrus, parietal lobule and bilateral middle temporal gyri) when subjects passively view gaze aversion movements (Wicker *et al.* 1998). One prominently active region to viewing eye movements (gaze aversion and also eyes looking at the observer) is the cortex around the STS, particularly in the right hemisphere, and this same region is active also to viewing opening and closing movements of the mouth (Puce *et al.* 1998). Thus, as is evident from the single cell responses, the STS region contains neural populations representing multiple aspects of the appearance of the face (including gaze) and body and their motion; the STS should not be considered exclusively an 'eye detector' or 'eye processor'. The STS is more activated during judgements of gaze direction than during judgements of identity, whereas the fusiform and inferior occipito-temporal activation is stronger during judgements of identity than gaze direction (Hoffman and Haxby 2000). Intracranial ERP recordings from these structures indicate that the STS responds to facial motion, whereas the ventral-temporal cortex responds more strongly to static facial images (Puce and Allison 1999). This is not surprising if one considers that eye gaze direction changes are transient and their detection might require motion processing systems, whereas identity judgements can be made independently of facial movements. Indeed, the processing of dynamic information about facial expression and the processing of static information about facial identity appear neuropsychologically dissociable (Campbell 1992; Humphreys *et al*. 1993).

(c) Lip reading

Lip reading, an important function for both hearing and deaf individuals, can be neuropsychologically dissociated from face recognition (Campbell *et al*. 1986), in a somewhat similar manner to gaze perception. Normal lip reading uses cortex of the STG in addition to other brain regions such as the angular gyrus, posterior cingulate, medial frontal cortex and frontal pole (Calvert *et al*. 1997). The STG and surrounding cortex activate bilaterally when subjects view face actions that could be interpreted as speech (Puce *et al*. 1998; Campbell *et al*. 2001), while some regions of the posterior right STS activate for the sight of speech and non-speech mouth movements (Campbell *et al*. 2001). Centres of activation to visual speech appear to overlap those associated with hearing speech (Calvert *et al*. 1997), indicating that these regions receive multimodal inputs during speech analysis (Kawashima *et al*. 1999; Calvert *et al*. 2000). Further evidence for this multimodal integration is a phenomenon known as the McGurk effect (McGurk and MacDonald 1976), where what observers hear when listening to speech sounds is altered by simultaneously viewing mouth movements appropriate to a different speech utterance. Indeed, magnetoencephalographic recordings of neural activity to speech stimuli show sensitivity to auditory–visual mismatch (Sams *et al*. 1991) with activity 200 ms post-stimulus augmented when the visual speech does not correspond to the accompanying auditory speech.

(d) The mirror neuron system and action observation/execution

The existence of a mirror neuron system in humans has been investigated during the manipulation of objects (Rizzolatti *et al*. 1996*a,b*; Binkofski *et al*. 1999*a,b*). The activation in fronto-central regions, seen when subjects observe and/or execute grasping behaviours, is accompanied by activity in the parietal cortex and STS (Jeannerod *et al*. 1995; Iacoboni *et al*. 1999, 2001; Rizzolatti *et al*. 2001; Gallese *et al*. 2002), paralleling the mirror neuron system in non-human primates.

Additionally, the secondary somatosensory cortex, SII, located in the temporal operculum is postulated to analyse the intrinsic properties of the graspable object while activation observed in the cortex in the intraparietal sulcus was thought to be related to kineasthetic processes (Binkofski *et al.* 1999*b*), although strictly speaking it is not part of the mirror neuron system.

The neuroimaging data mesh well with reported disturbances in executing grasping movements in the neuropsychological lesion literature. For example, Jeannerod and colleagues have reported a case with bilateral posterior parietal lesions of vascular origin where there was no difficulty in reaching toward the location of the object; however, a profound deficit in executing the anticipatory grasping movement with the fingers occurred to nondescript objects (cylindrical dowels). Interestingly, there was no deficit in grasping behaviour when well-known recognizable objects were used in the same test (Jeannerod *et al.* 1994). Mental imagery of hand and finger movements was found to be impaired in patients with unilateral parietal lesions, who had difficulties in producing movements with their hands and fingers (Sirigu *et al.* 1996). It has been reported that patients with unilateral parietal lesions have more difficulty in imitating gestures involving their own bodies relative to movements involving external objects, particularly if the lesion is in the left hemisphere (Halsband *et al.* 2001).

The human STS in its posterior extent has been found to be active not only to the hand and body movements of others (see Fig. 1.3; Allison *et al.* 2000), but also to faces (Puce *et al.* 1998). Interestingly, ERP recordings indicate that neural activity can differentiate between types of facial movements (Puce *et al.* 2000). Viewing mouth opening movements produces larger N170 responses relative to viewing mouth closing movements. A similar N170 response gradient is seen for observing eyes averting their gaze away from the observer relative to eyes focusing their gaze on the observer. Augmented neural responses to eye aversion movements may be a powerful signal that the observer is no longer the focus of another's attention. Similarly, larger N170s to mouth opening movements might be important for recognizing the beginning of an utterance (Puce *et al.* 2000). With recording electrodes sited in the STS of epilepsy surgery patients, selective responses to mouth opening have been elicited (see Allison *et al.* 2000, box 1). No responses were observed to mouth closing movements or eye deviations, indicating that these regions might be responsive during lip reading (or the sight of gestures and emotional expressions in which the mouth opens, e.g. during eating and surprise). The Talairach coordinates of these electrode positions are comparable to sites of fMRI activation in lip reading (Calvert *et al.* 1997).

If eye aversion movements are given a context, late ERPs that differ as a function of the social significance of the aversion movement can be elicited (Fig. 1.4; A. Cooper and A. Puce, unpublished data). This was demonstrated in a visual task where two permanently gaze-averted flanker faces were presented with a central face that changed its gaze direction. The central face could look in the same direction as both flanker faces, setting up an apparently common focus of attention off to the side ('group attention'). Alternatively, if the central face looked away from the observer in the opposite direction to the

(*a*)

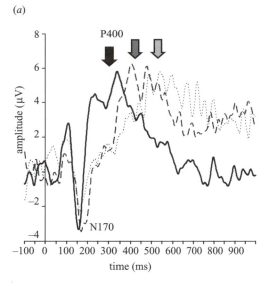

(*b*)

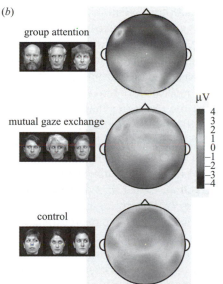

group attention

mutual gaze exchange

μV

control

Fig. 1.4 ERPs elicited to a social attention task. (*a*) ERP waveforms elicited to three conditions: solid line, group attention; dashed line, mutual gaze exchange; dotted line, control. The arrows indicate a late peak of ERP activity that follows the N170 ERP (P400), which changes its latency as a function of viewing condition. (*b*) Voltage maps for the three viewing conditions generated at the peak of P400 activity for the group attention condition (black arrow in (*a*)). The group attention condition shows fronto-temporal positivity, whereas the other two conditions show small posterior positivities. See Plate 1 of the Plate Section, at the centre of this book.

other two faces, a mutual gaze exchange between the central face and one of
the flankers became apparent ('mutual gaze exchange'). Finally, the central
face could look away from the observer and the other two flanker faces by looking up ('control'). An N170 ERP to the gaze aversion of the central face was
elicited, and its characteristics did not change as a function of condition
(see also Puce *et al.* 2000). A later positive ERP, elicited between 300 and 500 ms
post-motion onset (P400) was seen to differentiate in latency as a function of
viewing condition: group attention produced the shortest latency response,
followed by the mutual gaze exchange condition and then the control condition.

Our non-verbal and verbal facial movements usually do occur in an affective
context, and preliminary ERP data indicate that our brains are very sensitive to
these gesture–affect blends. If facial movements (either non-verbal or verbal)
are combined with different types of affect, temporal scalp N170 peak latency
and the amplitude of later ERP activity can be altered as a function of affect
type (Wheaton *et al.* 2002*b*). If gesture–affect combinations are incongruous,
as shown by increased reaction time to classify affect in behavioural data, late
ERP activity from 300 to 975 ms post-motion onset is modulated as a function
of not only affect or gesture but also their combination (Wheaton *et al.* 2002*a*).
These preliminary data indicate that the processing of inconsistencies in
others' behaviour can be detected physiologically.

ERPs, in the form of N170 negativities occurring over bilateral temporal
scalp regions, have been elicited not only to facial movements but also to hand
and body movements (Wheaton *et al.* 2001). The N170 activity was larger for
observing hand clenching movements relative to hand opening movements. In
addition, ERP activity was also observed to hand and body motion over the central scalp. Interestingly, ERP activity was larger to observing a body stepping
forward than to a body stepping back (paralleling the cellular bias for forward
or compatible direction of locomotion; Perrett *et al.* 1985*b*; Oram and Perrett
1994). Taken together, the ERP differentiation in the hand and body movements
might indicate a stronger neural signal for potentially threatening movements
(Wheaton *et al.* 2001). When fMRI activation to these movement types is compared, there is a robust signal within the temporoparietal cortex to all of these
motion types (Wheaton *et al.* 2002*c*). Fig. 1.5 summarizes the main findings
from the ERP studies (Puce *et al.* 2000; Wheaton *et al.* 2001; Thompson *et al.*
2002*b*), and indicates that processing between movement types begins before
200 ms post-motion onset not only in the posterior temporal cortex but also in
the frontocentral regions, which would be expected from the distribution of
action processing evident in fMRI and cell recording.

*(e) Gesture and action processing: Implications for disorders of
social communication*

The processing of non-verbally presented messages, in the form of face and
hand gestures, is crucial for social primates to be able to interact with one

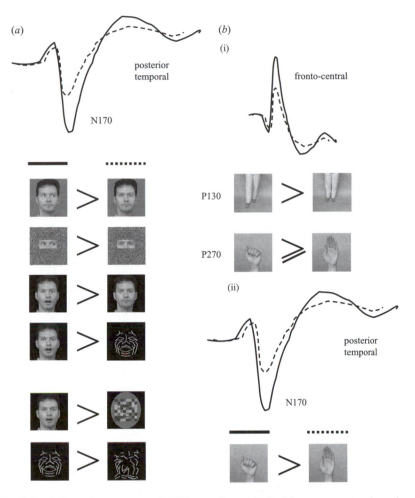

Fig. 1.5 Schematic summary of ERP waveforms elicited in response to observing human motion. (*a*) Posterior temporal N170 (solid line) to conditions listed in the left column is larger relative to N170 (dashed line) elicited to conditions listed in the right column. *b*(i) Frontocentral ERPs show larger P130 and P270 components across body and hand motion conditions shown in the left and right columns (solid versus dashed line). *b*(ii) Posterior temporal N170 (solid line) is larger to hand closure relative to hand opening (dashed line).

another—and there are considerable similarities in the high-level biological motion processing systems in human and non-human primates. The importance of comprehending actions of others may also be evident when such comprehension is impaired in clinical conditions. Disorders such as autism, Asperger syndrome, and schizophrenia are characterized by the inability to form or maintain social relationships. This can be difficult if the sufferer cannot process incoming social messages communicated by the bodily and facial actions of others, or sends inappropriate social reactions to such signals (e.g. Williams *et al.* 2001). Further neuroimaging and neurophysiological studies of healthy subjects and those with impairments of human motion processing may shed light on the interactions between the various components of these high-level biological motion processing systems.

A.P.'s research has been supported by the National Health and Medical Research Council (Australia) and the Australia Research Council.

References

Adolphs, R. (1999). Social cognition and the human brain. *Trends Cogn. Sci.* **3**, 469–79.

Aggleton, J. P., Burton, M. J. and Passingham, R. E. (1980). Cortical and subcortical afferents to the amygdala of the rhesus monkey (*Macaca mulatta*). *Brain Res.* **190**, 347–68.

Allison, T., Puce, A. and McCarthy, G. (2000). Social perception from visual cues: role of the STS region. *Trends Cogn. Sci.* **4**, 267–78.

Baker, C. I., Keysers, C., Jellema, T., Wicker, B. and Perrett, D. I. (2001). Neuronal representation of disappearing and hidden objects in temporal cortex of the macaque. *Exp. Brain Res.* **140**, 375–81.

Barbas, H. (1988). Anatomic organization of basoventral and mediodorsal visual recipient prefrontal regions in the rhesus monkey. *J. Comp. Neurol.* **276**, 313–42.

Baron-Cohen, S. (1995). *Mindblindness: an essay on autism and theory of mind.* Cambridge, MA: MIT Press.

Baron-Cohen, S., Wheelwright, S. and Joliffe, T. (1997). Is there a 'language of the eyes'? Evidence from normal adults, and adults with autism or Asperger syndrome. *Vis. Cogn.* **4**, 311–31.

Bassili, J. N. (1978). Facial motion in the perception of faces and of emotional expression. *J. Exp. Psychol. Hum. Percept. Perf.* **4**, 373–9.

Beauchamp, M. S., Lee, K. E., Haxby, J. V. and Martin, A. (2002). Parallel visual motion processing streams for manipulable objects and human movements. *Neuron* **34**, 149–59.

Bentin, S., Allison, T., Puce, A., Perez, A. and McCarthy, G. (1996). Electrophysiological studies of face perception in humans. *J. Cogn. Neurosci.* **8**, 551–65.

Binkofski, F., Buccino, G., Posse, S., Seitz, R. J., Rizzolatti, G. and Freund, H. J. (1999*a*). A fronto-parietal circuit for object manipulation in man: evidence from an fMRI study. *Eur. J. Neurosci.* **11**, 3276–86.

Binkofski, F., Buccino, G., Stephan, K. M., Rizzolatti, G., Seitz, R. J. and Freund, H. J. (1999*b*). A parieto-premotor network for object manipulation: evidence from neuroimaging. *Exp. Brain Res.* **128**, 210–13.

Blake, R. (1993). Cats perceive biological motion. *Psychol. Sci.* **4**, 54–7.

Blakemore, S.-J. and Decety, J. (2001). From the perception of action to the understanding of intention. *Nature Rev. Neurosci.* **2**, 561–7.

Bonda, E., Petrides, M., Ostry, D. and Evans, A. (1996). Specific involvement of human parietal systems and the amygdala in the perception of biological motion. *J. Neurosci.* **16**, 3737–44.

Boussaoud, D., Ungerleider, L. G. and Desimone, R. (1990). Pathways for motion analysis: cortical connections of the medial superior temporal and fundus of the superior temporal visual areas in the macaque. *J. Comp. Neurol.* **296**, 462–495.

Brothers, L. (1997). *Friday's footprint: how society shapes the human mind*. New York: Oxford University Press.

Calvert, G. A., Bullmore, E. T., Brammer, M. J., Campbell, R., Williams, S. C., McGuire, P. K., *et al.* (1997). Activation of auditory cortex during silent lipreading. *Science* **276**, 593–5.

Calvert, G. A., Campbell, R. and Brammer, M. J. (2000). Evidence from functional magnetic resonance imaging of crossmodal binding in the human heteromodal cortex. *Curr. Biol.* **10**, 649–657.

Campbell, R. (1992). The neuropsychology of lipreading. *Phil. Trans. R. Soc. Lond.* B **335**, 39–45.

Campbell, R., Landis, T. and Regard, M. (1986). Face recognition and lipreading. *Brain* **109**, 509–521.

Campbell, R., MacSweeney, M., Surguladze, S., Calvert, G., McGuire, P., Suckling, J., *et al.* (2001). Cortical substrates for the perception of face actions: an fMRI study of the specificity of activation for seen speech and for meaningless lower-face acts (gurning). *Brain Res. Cogn. Brain Res.* **12**, 233–43.

Carey, D. P., Perrett, D. I. and Oram, M. W. (1997). Recognizing, understanding and reproducing action. In *Handbook of neuropsychology*, vol. 11. *Action and cognition* (ed. M. Jeannerod), pp. 111–29. Amsterdam: Elsevier.

Cutting, J. E. and Kozlowski, L. T. (1977). Recognizing friends by their walk: gait perception without familiarity cues. *Bull. Psychonomic. Soc.* **9**, 353–6.

Desimone, R. (1991). Face-selective cells in the temporal cortex of monkeys. *J. Cogn. Neurosci.* **3**, 1–8.

Desimone, R., Albright, T. D., Gross, C. G. and Bruce, C. (1984). Stimulus-selective properties of inferior temporal neurons in the macaque. *J. Neurosci.* **4**, 2051–62.

di Pellegrino, G., Fadiga, L., Fogassi, V., Gallese, V. and Rizzolatti, G. (1992). Understanding motor events: a neurophysiological study. *Exp. Brain Res.* **91**, 176–80.

Dittrich, W. H. (1993). Action categories and the perception of biological motion. *Perception* **22**, 15–22.

Downar, J., Crawley, A. P., Mikulis, D. J. and Davis, K. D. (2002). A cortical network sensitive to stimulus salience in a neutral behavioral context across multiple sensory modalities. *J. Neurophysiol.* **87**, 615–20.

Downing, P. E., Jiang, Y. H., Shuman, M. and Kanwisher, N. (2001). A cortical area selective for visual processing of the human body. *Science* **293**, 2470–3.

Driver, J., Davis, G., Ricciardelli, P., Kidd, P., Maxwell, E. and Baron-Cohen, S. (1999). Gaze perception triggers reflexive visuospatial orienting. *Vis. Cogn.* **6**, 509–40.

Eimer, M. (1998). Does the face-specific N170 component reflect the activity of a specialized eye processor? *Neuroreport* **9**, 2945–8.

Emery, N. J. (2000). The eyes have it: the neuroethology, function and evolution of social gaze. *Neurosci. Biobehav. Rev.* **24**, 581–604.

Felleman, D. J. and Van Essen, D. C. (1991). Distributed hierarchical processing in the primate cerebral cortex. *Cerebr. Cortex* **1**, 1–47.

Friesen, C. K. and Kingstone, A. (1998). The eyes have it! Reflexive orienting is triggered by nonpredictive gaze. *Psychol. Bull. Rev.* **5**, 490–5.

Gallese, V., Fadiga, L., Fogassi, L. and Rizzolatti, G. (1996). Action recognition in the premotor cortex. *Brain* **119**, 593–609.

Gallese, V., Fadiga, L., Fogassi, L. and Rizzolatti, G. (2002). Action representation and the inferior parietal lobule. *Attention Perform.* **19**, 247–66.

Grezes, J., Fonlupt, P., Bertenthal, B., Delon-Martin, C., Segebarth, C. and Decety, J. (2001). Does perception of biological motion rely on specific brain regions? *Neuroimage* **13**, 775–85.

Grossman, E., Donnelly, M., Price, R., Pickens, D., Morgan, V., Neighbor, G. *et al.* (2000). Brain areas involved in perception of biological motion. *J. Cogn. Neurosci.* **12**, 711–20.

Halsband, U., Schmitt, J., Weyers, M., Binkofski, F., Grützner, G. and Freund, H. J. (2001). Recognition and imitation of pantomimed motor acts after unilateral parietal and premotor lesions: a perspective on apraxia. *Neuropsychologia* **39**, 200–16.

Hietanen, J. K. (1999). Does your gaze direction and head orientation shift my visual attention? *Neuroreport* **10**, 3443–7.

Hietanen, J. K. (2002). Social attention orienting integrates visual information from head and body orientation. *Psychol. Res.* **66**, 174–9.

Hietanen, J. K. and Perrett, D. I. (1996). Motion sensitive cells in the macaque superior temporal polysensory area: response discrimination between self- and externally generated pattern motion. *Behav. Brain Res.* **76**, 155–67.

Hoffman, E. A. and Haxby, J. V. (2000). Distinct representations of eye gaze and identity in the distributed human neural system for face perception. *Nature Neurosci.* **3**, 80–4.

Howard, R. J., Brammer, M., Wright, I., Woodruff, P. W., Bullmore, E. T. and Zeki, S. (1996). A direct demonstration of functional specialization within motion-related visual and auditory cortex of the human brain. *Curr. Biol.* **6**, 1015–19.

Humphreys, G. W., Donnelly, N. and Riddoch, M. J. (1993). Expression is computed separately from facial identity, and it is computed separately for moving and static faces: neuropsychological evidence. *Neuropsychologia* **31**, 173–81.

Iacoboni, M., Woods, R. P., Brass, M., Bekkering, H., Mazziotta, J. C. and Rizzolatti, G. (1999). Cortical mechanisms of human imitation. *Science* **286**, 2526–8.

Iacoboni, M., Koski, L. M., Brass, M., Bekkering, H., Woods, R. P., Dubeau, M. C., Mazziotta, J. C. and Rizzolatti, G. (2001). Reafferent copies of imitated actions in the right superior temporal cortex. *Proc. Natl Acad. Sci. USA* **98**, 13 995–9.

Jeannerod, M., Decety, J. and Michel, F. (1994). Impairment of grasping movements following a bilateral posterior parietal lesion. *Neuropsychologia* **32**, 369–80.

Jeannerod, M., Arbib, M. A., Rizzolatti, G. and Sakata, H. (1995). Grasping objects: the cortical mechanisms of visuomotor transformation. *Trends Neurosci.* **18**, 314–20.

Jellema, T. and Perrett, D. I. (2002). Coding of visible and hidden actions. *Attention Perform.* **19**, 356–80.

Jellema, T., Baker, C. I., Wicker, B. and Perrett, D. I. (2000). Neural representation for the perception of the intentionality of hand actions. *Brain Cogn.* **44**, 280–302.

Jellema, T., Oram, M. W., Baker, C. I. and Perrett, D. I. (2002). Cell populations in the banks of the superior temporal sulcus of the macaque and imitation. In *The imitative mind: development, evolution, and brain bases* (ed. A. Meltzoff and W. Prinz), pp. 267–90. Cambridge: Cambridge University Press.

Johansson, G. (1973). Visual perception of biological motion and a model of its analysis. *Percept. Psychophys.* **14**, 202–11.

Kawashima, R., Imaizumi, S., Mori, K., Okada, K., Goto, R., Kiritani, S., *et al.* (1999). Selective visual and auditory attention toward utterances: a PET study. *Neuroimage* **10**, 209–15.

Kleinke, C. L. (1986). Gaze and eye contact: a research review. *Psychol. Bull.* **100**, 78–100.

Kohler, E., Keysers, C., Umilta, M. A., Fogassi, L., Gallese, V. and Rizzolatti, G. (2002). Hearing sounds, understanding actions: action representation in mirror neurons. *Science* **297**, 846–8.

Kourtzi, Z. and Kanwisher, N. (2000). Activation in human MT/MST by static images with implied motion. *J. Cogn. Neurosci.* **12**, 48–55.

Kozlowski, L. T. and Cutting, J. E. (1977). Recognizing the sex of a walker from a dynamic point-light display. *Percept. Psychophys.* **21**, 575–80.

Langton, S. R. H. and Bruce, V. (2000). You must see the point: automatic processing of cues to the direction of social attention. *J. Exp. Psychol. Hum. Percep. Perf.* **26**, 747–57.

McGurk, H. and MacDonald, J. (1976). Hearing lips and seeing voices. *Nature* **264**, 746–8.

McLeod, P., Dittrich, W., Driver, J., Perrett, D. I. and Zihl, J. (1996). Preserved and impaired detection of structure from motion in a 'motion-blind' patient. *Vis. Cogn.* **3**, 363–91.

Mistlin, A. J. and Perrett, D. I. (1990). Visual and somatosensory processing in the macaque temporal cortex: the role of 'expectation'. *Exp. Brain Res.* **82**, 437–50.

Narumoto, J., Okada, T., Sadato, N., Fukui, K. and Yonekura, Y. (2001). Attention to emotion modulates fMRI activity in human right superior temporal sulcus. *Cogn. Brain Res.* **12**, 225–31.

Nishitani, N. and Hari, R. (2000). Temporal dynamics of cortical representation for action. *Proc. Natl Acad. Sci. USA* **97**, 913–18.

Nishitani, N. and Hari, R. (2001). Sign language and mirror neuron system. *Neuroimage* **12**(6), S452.

Oram, M. W. and Perrett, D. I. (1994). Responses of anterior superior temporal polysensory (STPa) neurons to 'biological motion' stimuli. *J. Cogn. Neurosci.* **6**, 99–116.

Oram, M. W. and Perrett, D. I. (1996). Integration of form and motion in the anterior superior temporal polysensory area (STPa) of the macaque monkey. *J. Neurophysiol.* **76**, 109–29.

Pavlova, M. and Sokolov, A. (2000). Orientation specificity in biological motion perception. *Percept. Psychophys.* **62**, 889–99.

Pavlova, M., Krägeloh-Mann, I., Birbaumer, N. and Sokolov, A. (2002). Biological motion shown backwards: the apparent-facing effect. *Perception* **31**, 435–443.

Perrett, D. I., Rolls, E. T. and Caan, W. (1982). Visual neurons responsive to faces in the monkey temporal cortex. *Exp. Brain Res.* **47**, 329–42.

Perrett, D. I., Smith, P. A. J., Potter, D. D., Mistlin, A. J., Head, A. S., Milner, A. D. *et al.* (1984). Neurones responsive to faces in the temporal cortex: studies of functional organization, sensitivity to identity and relation to perception. *Hum. Neurobiol.* **3**, 197–208.

Perrett, D. I., Smith, P. A. J., Potter, D. D., Mistlin, A. J., Head, A. S., Milner, A. D. *et al.* (1985*a*). Visual cells in the temporal cortex sensitive to face view and gaze direction. *Proc. R. Soc. Lond.* B **223**, 293–317.

Perrett, D. I., Smith, P. A. J., Mistlin, A. J., Chitty, A. J., Head, A. S., Potter, D. D., *et al.* (1985*b*). Visual analysis of body movements by neurones in the temporal cortex of the macaque monkey: a preliminary report. *Behav. Brain Res.* **16**, 153–70.

Perrett, D. I., Harries, M. H., Bevan, R., Thomas, S., Benson, P. J., Mistlin, A. J., *et al.* (1989). Frameworks of analysis for the neural representation of animate objects and actions. *J. Exp. Biol.* **146**, 87–113.

Perrett, D. I., Harries, M. H., Benson, P. J., Chitty, A. J. and Mistlin, A. J. (1990a). Retrieval of structure from rigid and biological motion; an analysis of the visual response of neurons in the macaque temporal cortex. In *AI and the eye* (ed. T. Troscianko and A. Blake), pp. 181–201. Chichester, UK: Wiley.

Perrett, D. I., Harries, M., Chitty, A. J. and Mistlin, A. J. (1990b). Three stages in the classification of body movements by visual neurones. In *Images and understanding* (ed. H. B. Barlow, C. Blakemore and M. Weston-Smith), pp. 94–108. Cambridge: Cambridge University Press.

Perrett, D. I., Mistlin, A. J., Harries, M. H. and Chitty, A. J. (1990c). Understanding the visual appearance and consequence of hand actions. In *Vision and action: the control of grasping* (ed. M. A. Goodale), pp. 163–180. Norwood, NJ: Ablex Publishing.

Perrett, D. I., Hietanen, J. K., Oram, M. W. and Benson, P. J. (1992). Organization and functions of cells responsive to faces in the temporal cortex. *Phil. Trans. R. Soc. Lond.* B **335**, 23–30.

Puce, A. and Allison, T. (1999). Differential processing of mobile and static faces by temporal cortex. *Neuroimage* **9**(6), S801.

Puce, A., Allison, T., Bentin, S., Gore, J. C. and McCarthy, G. (1998). Temporal cortex activation in humans viewing eye and mouth movements. *J. Neurosci.* **18**, 2188–99.

Puce, A., Smith, A. and Allison, T. (2000). ERPs evoked by viewing moving eyes and mouths. *Cogn. Neuropsychol.* **17**, 221–39.

Puce, A., Syngeniotis, A., Thompson, J. C., Abbott, D. F., Wheaton, K. J. and Castiello, U. (2003). The human temporal lobe integrates facial form and motion: evidence from FMRI and ERP studies. *Neuroimage* **19**, 861–9.

Rizzolatti, G., Camarda, R., Fogassi, L., Gentilucci, M., Luppino, G. and Matelli, M. (1988). Functional organization of inferior area 6 in the macaque monkey. II. Area F5 and the control of distal movements. *Exp. Brain Res.* **71**, 491–507.

Rizzolatti, G., Fadiga, L., Gallese, V. and Fogassi, L. (1996a). Premotor cortex and the recognition of motor actions. *Brain Res. Cogn. Brain Res.* **3**, 131–41.

Rizzolatti, G., Fadiga, L., Matelli, M., Bettinardi, V., Paulesu, E., Perani, D. *et al.* (1996b). Localization of grasp representations in humans by PET. 1. Observation versus execution. *Exp. Brain Res.* **111**, 246–52.

Rizzolatti, G., Fogassi, L. and Gallese, V. (2001). Neurophysiological mechanisms underlying the understanding and imitation of action. *Nature Rev. Neurosci.* **2**, 661–70.

Sams, M., Aulanko, R., Hämäläinen, M., Hari, R., Lounasmaa, O. V., Lu, S. T. *et al.* (1991). Seeing speech: visual information from lip movements modifies activity in the human auditory cortex. *Neurosci. Lett.* **127**, 141–45.

Schenk, T. and Zihl, J. (1997). Visual motion perception after brain damage: II. Deficits in form-from-motion perception. *Neuropsychologia* **35**, 1299–310.

Sirigu, A., Duhamel, J. R., Cohen, L., Pillon, B., Dubois, B. and Agid, Y. (1996). The mental representation of hand movements after parietal cortex damage. *Science* **273**, 1564–8.

Taylor, M. J., Edmonds, G. E., McCarthy, G. and Allison, T. (2001). Eyes first! Eye processing develops before face processing in children. *Neuroreport* **12**, 1671–6.

Thompson, J. C., Wheaton, K., Berkovic, S. F., Jackson, G. and Puce, A. (2002a). Hemodynamic responses in humans to the perception of compatible and incompatible body motion. In *The fMRI Experience IV Proc.* NIH, Maryland, 2002, 93.

Thompson, J. C., Wheaton, K., Castiello, U. and Puce, A. (2002*b*). ERPs differentiate between facial motion and motion in general. Abstract no. 14221. Academic Press OHBM Annual Scientific Meeting 2002.

Thornton, I. M., Pinto, J. and Shiffrar, M. (1998). The visual perception of human locomotion. *Cogn. Neuropsychol.* **15**, 535–2.

Umilta, M. A., Kohler, E., Gallese, V., Fogassi, L., Fadiga, L., Keysers, C., *et al.* (2001). I know what you are doing: a neurophysiological study. *Neuron* **31**, 155–65.

Vaina, L. M., LeMay, M., Bienfang, D. C., Choi, A. Y. and Nakayama, K. (1990). Intact 'biological motion' and 'structure from motion' perception in a patient with impaired motion mechanisms: a case study. *Vis. Neurosci.* **5**, 353–69.

Vaina, L. M., Solomon, J., Chowdhury, S., Sinha, P. and Belliveau, J. W. (2001). Functional neuroanatomy of biological motion perception in humans. *Proc. Natl Acad. Sci. USA* **98**, 11 656–61.

Vuilleumier, P. (2002). Perceived gaze direction in faces and spatial attention: a study in patients with parietal damage and unilateral neglect. *Neuropsychologia* **40**, 1013–26.

Wachsmuth, E., Oram, M. W. and Perrett, D. I. (1994). Recognition of objects and their component parts: responses of single units in the temporal cortex of the macaque. *Cerebr. Cortex* **4**, 509–22.

Wheaton, K. J., Pipingas, A., Silberstein, R. and Puce, A. (2001). Neuronal responses elicited to viewing the actions of others. *Vis. Neurosci.* **18**, 401–6.

Wheaton, K. J., Aranda, G. and Puce, A. (2002*a*). ERPs elicited to combined emotional and gestural movements of the face as a function of congruency. Abstract no. 14186. Academic Press OHBM Annual Scientific Meeting 2002.

Wheaton K. J., Aranda, G. and Puce, A. (2002*b*). Affective modulation of gestural and visual speech stimuli: an ERP study. Abstract no. 14215. Academic Press OHBM Annual Scientific Meeting 2002.

Wheaton, K. J., Thompson, J. C., Berkovic, S. F., Jackson, G. and Puce, A. (2002*c*). Brain regions responsive to the perception of human motion. *The fMRI Experience IV Proc.* NIH, Maryland 2002, p. 103.

Wicker, B., Michel, F., Henaff, M.-A. and Decety, J. (1998). Brain regions involved in the perception of gaze: a PET study. *Neuroimage* **8**, 221–7.

Williams, J. H., Whiten, A., Suddendorf, T. and Perrett, D. I. (2001). Imitation, mirror neurons and autism. *Neurosci. Biobehav. Rev.* **25**, 287–95.

Glossary

ERP: event-related potential
fMRI: functional magnetic resonance imaging
MST: medial superior temporal
MTG: mid-temporal gyrus
PET: positron emission tomography
STG: superior temporal gyrus
STP: superior temporal polysensory
STS: superior temporal sulcus

2

Teleological and referential understanding of action in infancy

Gergely Csibra

There are two fundamentally different ways to attribute intentional mental states to others upon observing their actions. Actions can be interpreted as *goal-directed*, which warrants ascribing intentions, desires and beliefs appropriate to the observed actions, to the agents. Recent studies suggest that young infants also tend to interpret certain actions in terms of goals, and their reasoning about these actions is based on a sophisticated teleological representation. Several theorists proposed that infants rely on motion cues, such as self-initiated movement, in selecting goal-directed agents. Our experiments revealed that, although infants are more likely to attribute goals to self-propelled than to non-self-propelled agents, they do not need direct evidence about the source of motion for interpreting actions in teleological terms. The second mode of action-based mental state attribution interprets actions as *referential*, and allows ascription of attentional states, referential intents, communicative messages, etc., to the agents. Young infants also display evidence of interpreting actions in referential terms (for example, when following others' gaze or pointing gesture) and are very sensitive to the communicative situations in which these actions occur. For example, young infants prefer faces with eye-contact and objects that react to them contingently, and these are the very situations that later elicit gaze following. Whether or not these early abilities amount to a 'theory of mind' is a matter of debate among infant researchers. Nevertheless, they represent skills that are vital for understanding social agents and engaging in social interactions.

Keywords: infancy; referential action; goal-directed action; teleology; theory of mind

2.1 Introduction

People cannot help but interpret each other's actions in terms of hidden mental states like beliefs, desires, etc. The attribution of these intentional mental states helps them to explain observed, and predict future, behaviour of others, and also enables them to influence what social partners will do. According to philosophers (e.g. Dennett 1987), the distinctive aspect of intentional mental states is their 'aboutness'—they are 'about' certain states of the world. There are two fundamentally different ways to interpret actions as indicating mental states that are about something. First, we can interpret an observed behaviour as a *goal-directed action*. A goal-directed action is 'about' the end state of that action; it is performed in order to make the end state occur. If you see someone drilling a corkscrew into the cork of a bottle of wine, you will know what this action is about: an open bottle of wine. Because goal-directed actions are seen to be determined by their end state, this kind of action interpretation is essentially *teleological*. Teleological interpretation of an action enables us to attach a goal to the action (an open bottle), but it also allows us to attribute to the agent desires (e.g. a desire to drink wine), beliefs (e.g. a belief that there is wine in the bottle) and possibly further mental states as well. The second way to reveal what an action is about is to interpret it as a *referential action*. A referential action is about the state of the world that it highlights. If you see someone pointing to a car, you will know what this action is about: it is about the car. Interpretation of an action as referential emphasizes some aspect of the world as connected to the agent, and allows attribution of referential intentions (drawing your attention to the car), communicative messages (e.g. 'this is the car I was talking about'), and other mental states to the agent.

During the past decade, several studies have been published that attempted to see whether young, preverbal infants are engaged in these kinds of action interpretations and whether they attribute intentional mental states to others. The answer to these questions bears relevance to the debates on the origins and the nature of the human 'theory of mind' and may also help us to understand developmental disorders that are characterized by deficits in social cognition. This paper reviews some of the evidence relevant to these questions. I shall argue that this body of evidence unambiguously shows that infants younger than 1 year of age employ both kinds of action interpretation and do this in a more and more sophisticated way as they approach their first birthday. At the same time, I shall also argue that neither of these action interpretation systems is necessarily mentalistic; both can function without attribution of representational mental states. In other words, goals can be attached to actions without understanding desires, and referents can be identified without figuring out the meaning of the underlying communicative act. I propose that these two action interpretation systems operate independently in early infancy. The independence of these cognitive mechanisms is supported by various facts: they rely on different types of computations, they are triggered by different stimulus conditions, and they can be dissociated in animal behaviours and developmental disorders. Crucially, there is no evidence for transfer between these action interpretation systems (for example attribution of goals on the basis of referential actions) in infants at, or below, 1 year of age. I suggest that the combining of these action interpretation systems into a higher-order mentalistic representation of actions takes place during the second year of life.

2.2 Teleological understanding of actions

Understanding goals requires connecting actions not to their antecedents but to their consequents. Some studies suggest that infants as young as six months of age are sensitive to the end state of observed events. Woodward (1998), for example, repeatedly presented infants with an action in which a hand reached towards and grasped one of two toys. When the infants had been habituated to this event, she swapped the toys and the hand either grasped the same toy in the new location, or the other toy in the same location. Looking times for these two events were markedly different: infants looked longer at the hand grasping the 'new' toy at the 'old' location, as if they expected the hand to reach towards the same toy. This result shows that infants are more likely to associate a grasping hand with the grasped object than with its location, which is useful for interpreting the grasping action as directed to the goal of acquiring a specific object. Nothing in this experiment, however, demonstrates that infants do not simply discriminate between end states. It does not show that they relate actions to end states in an 'in-order-to' clause: the hand performed the reaching and grasping sequence *in order to* acquire a certain object.

An action is goal directed if it is performed not for itself but to achieve an end; in other words, if it is an instrumental action. Whether an action is instrumental in relation to an end state or not can be intuitively tested by considering if we would expect it to be performed when it is not needed for goal achievement. Pulling out a cork from a wine bottle, for example, can be an instrumental action to access the wine, but only when the bottle is not empty. Even when the bottle is not empty, we would not expect to see this action if all the glasses were filled with wine. As this example suggests, interpreting something as an instrumental action that has been performed to achieve, and gets its meaning from, a particular goal state requires consideration of many things— not just the action and its end state but also the environment in which it occurs. We have demonstrated that nine-month-old infants are already capable of doing this trick and, depending on the environment, interpret observed actions as goal directed.

These studies (Gergely *et al.* 1995; Csibra *et al.* 1999) presented infants with computer animations. Since the seminal work by Heider and Simmel (1944) several experiments provided evidence that high-level, sophisticated social interpretation of actions does not require featural identification of agents (for a review see Scholl and Tremoulet 2000). Triangles and circles moving on a two-dimensional surface are readily interpreted as if they were people engaged in various kinds of social interactions. One explanation of this phenomenon is that during development the motion patterns of human behaviour are abstracted away from their usual context and from human features, and when these patterns are recognized in artificially created animations, we tend to project further human attributes to those abstract figures. An alternative explanation, which I defend here, suggests that certain motion patterns that allow interpretation of the behaviour of the abstract figures as goal-directed actions will always attract such an interpretation and this tendency does not depend on extensive experience with human behaviour. This explanation predicts that young infants will as readily attribute goals to animated figures as they do to human agents.

Our experiments repeatedly presented infants with a simple animation (Fig. 2.1) in which a ball approached and contacted another ball by jumping over an obstacle. In this event, the jumping action can be interpreted as an instrumental action because it is necessary to achieve the end state (the spatial position beside the other ball). Whether or not the infants arrived at the same interpretation was tested by showing them two modified versions of the event and measuring their looking time. In the test events, we removed the obstacle, which changed the relevant aspects of the environment in a way that made the jumping action unnecessary for goal achievement. One of these events (old action) displayed the same jumping approach, which, however, was no longer necessary and was therefore inefficient, while the other event (new action) displayed a straight-line approach to the same position, which was an efficient action in the new situation. If infants interpreted the original event as a goal-directed action, they should find the new instrumental action more compatible with their interpretation and should respond with longer looking at the old, inefficient action.

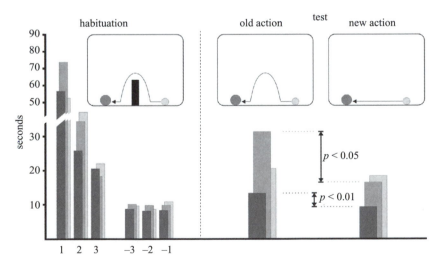

Fig. 2.1   The experimental events and the looking time results in Gergely *et al.* (1995) and Csibra *et al.* (1999). Light grey bars, six-month-old infants; medium grey bars, nine-month-old infants; dark grey bars, 12-month-old infants.

This is exactly what we found in 9- and 12-month-old infants (see figure 1). Further control studies were performed to verify whether these looking time differences were indeed attributable to the interpretation of the habituation event. The control studies involved the same test events but they were preceded by a habituation event, which differed only slightly from the original habituation event but did not show a proper instrumental action. In this event the 'obstacle' was positioned not in between the two balls but behind the moving ball (see Fig. 2.2). In this environment the jumping action cannot be considered to be an instrumental action, and the infants were not expected to attribute the end position as the goal of the moving ball's action. Their looking times confirmed this prediction.

How can we explain infants' early emerging ability to attribute goals to animated shapes? We have proposed (Gergely and Csibra 1997; Csibra *et al.* 2003) that, watching these animations on a computer screen, infants adopt a *teleological stance*. The teleological stance is akin to the *intentional stance* of Dennett (1987) in that it represents an interpretational strategy that seeks to construe an event in terms of goals (see Keil (1995) for a different version of the teleological stance). It is, however, different from the intentional stance in that it does not attribute mental states to the agents (I will return to the relation between these two stances later). Note that the teleological stance (and the intentional stance) is not an explicit inferential system but a bias: a tendency to construe events in accord with a certain formal structure. Construing an action as goal-directed implies, as we have seen, relating at least three different aspects of the observed event to each other: the behaviour, its physical context

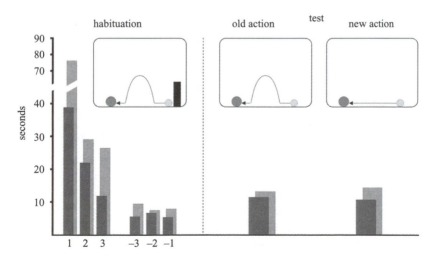

Fig. 2.2 The control events and the looking time results in Gergely *et al.* (1995) and Csibra *et al.* (1999). Medium grey bars, nine-month-old infants; dark grey bars, 12-month-old infants.

and the end state (see Fig. 2.3). These three elements will create a well-formed *teleological representation* of the event if, and only if, the behaviour is an efficient action towards the end state in the given physical environment. The habituation event in our study (Fig. 2.1) met this criterion (jumping over the obstacle was the most efficient action towards the end position in that environment) while the habituation event in the control study (Fig. 2.2) did not (jumping over nothing was not an efficient action towards the end position in that environment). Thus, the habituation event represented in Fig. 2.1 allowed goal attribution, while the habituation event represented in Fig. 2.2 did not, and this difference was reflected in the differential patterns of looking time by infants.

As Fig. 2.3 suggests, goal attribution and efficiency evaluation are inseparable in the teleological stance. But perhaps this is only true for behaviours of abstract figures, and infants may be willing to attribute goals to inefficient actions as well, if they are performed by real human beings. Recent studies suggest that this is not the case. Woodward and Sommerville (2000), for example, presented infants with two transparent boxes that contained two different toys. They habituated 12-month-old infants to an action in which a hand first touched one of the boxes, then opened it and grasped the toy inside. After habituation, the toys were swapped between the boxes. During the test event the hand either touched the same box as before (which, however, now contained the other toy) or it touched the other box (which contained the same toy that had been previously grasped). Infants looked longer at the former action, indicating that they did not expect the hand to perform the familiar action seen before, as that was no longer necessary, and in fact would have been an inefficient way to obtain the goal object (i.e. the toy that had been grasped during habituation). In a control study Woodward and Sommerville habituated the infants to the same hand actions (first touching the box, then grasping the toy) with the exception that the toys were not inside but in front of the boxes; hence, opening the box could not have been considered as an efficient instrumental action for grasping the toy. In this condition, the infants did not develop any specific expectation about which box the hand should touch when the toys were swapped and, in fact, they even looked slightly longer when the

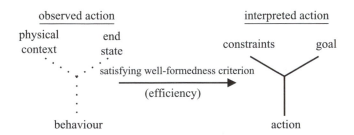

Fig. 2.3   The teleological representation for actions.

hand touched the other box. Note that, just as in our study described above, the only difference between the two conditions was the efficiency of the action: opening the box is an efficient instrumental action if, and only if, the target object is in the box.

A more recent study has also demonstrated that infants do care about efficiency when they interpret actions in terms of goals. Onishi's (2001) studies also confirmed that actions (removing obstacles) that make a target object accessible to a hand are interpreted as goal-directed by 10-month-old infants, but the same actions do not lead to goal attribution if they are not justified by the relative positions of the obstacles and the target object. Furthermore, evaluating the efficiency of actions is not restricted to looking-time context either. Gergely *et al.* (2002) provided evidence that infants modulate their imitative behaviour according to the justifiability of the goal-directed actions performed by a model. These authors replicated the well-known demonstration of Meltzoff (1988) that 14-month-old infants tend to imitate a behaviour that they have never seen before and would not perform spontaneously. In Meltzoff's study, infants watch a model leaning forward and touching an object on a table with his head, causing it to light up. A week later, when they are brought back to the laboratory, the majority of the infants perform the same action. In an additional condition, however, Gergely *et al.* slightly modified the model's behaviour. Before touching the object with her forehead, the experimenter covered her shoulder with a blanket, which then she held onto tightly with her hands—then she performed the same action. Or was it the same action? Touching the object with her head was a perfectly reasonable action in a situation where the actor's hands were unavailable, while in the other situation, where she kept her hands free, it just seemed unjustifiable. If infants are not sensitive to this difference, they should imitate the head-action equally. In fact, only a minority of them imitated the head-action in the 'hands occupied' version, which suggests that they interpreted this action as an instrumental action that one does not have to copy if he or she is free from the constraints that affected the model. In other words, they could attempt to achieve the same effect in the most efficient manner that was available to them: by touching the object with their hands. Infants do care about efficiency of perceived actions.

We have seen that nine-month-old infants will attribute the end state as the goal of the action if it is an efficient instrumental action, but people do not have to observe a complete action to attribute a goal to it. We can figure out what the goal of an action could be by considering what end state that action would be instrumental to. Pulling out the cork from a bottle is most likely to be carried out in order for the agent be able to access the content of the bottle. When we make these kinds of inferences, we have information about the agent's behaviour and the physical environment in which it takes place. We then adopt the teleological stance, and try to fill out the missing third element (the end state) of the teleological representation in order to satisfy the well-formedness criterion of efficiency (see Fig. 2.3). Can infants do the same trick?

Meltzoff (1995) let 18-month-old infants watch a model who performed apparently failed actions on novel objects. When these babies had a chance to imitate the model, they did not copy the failure but performed the complete intended action that led to the goal state that one could have inferred from the model's behaviour. This is a clear demonstration that 18-month-olds do not have to see the goal realized in order to be able to attribute it to an action. Twelve-month-old infants, however, fail in this task (Bellagamba and Tomasello 1999), suggesting that they may not be able to extract the goal from the observation of failed attempts. It is possible, though, that this test requires too much from babies: they not only have to attribute an unseen goal to the agent, they also have to ignore the observed end state of the action and replace it with an inferred one. In other words, Meltzoff's task requires a kind of counterfactual reasoning that may exceed 12-month-old infants' capabilities even if they were able to figure out goals for unfinished actions.

To avoid the complications inherent in the Meltzoff (1995) study, we created a computer animation that allows teleological interpretation of an action even though the goal is never seen achieved (Csibra *et al.* 2003). The animation shows a simple chase event in which a bigger ball follows a smaller one (see Fig. 2.4, habituation event). When the small one passes through a narrow gap between two barriers, the big ball takes a detour around the barriers and then continues its path in the direction where the small one left the screen. The goal of the big ball can easily be identified: catching the small ball. Note, however, that this goal is never seen achieved and can only be inferred from the evaluation of the big ball's behaviour. We performed two different tests on two

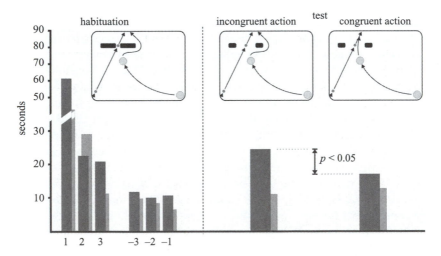

Fig. 2.4 Evidence for attribution of an unseen goal in 12-month-old infants. Medium grey bars, nine-month-old infants; dark grey bars, 12-month-old infants. (Data from Csibra *et al.* (2003), experiment 1.)

different groups of 12-month-old infants to check whether they interpret the unfinished chase event as a goal-directed action. In the first test (Fig. 2.4), we changed the physical environment by enlarging the gap between the barriers and presented two actions: the big ball either adjusted its path to the new constraints and followed the small ball through the gap (congruent action), or took the same detour as before, which, however, was no longer an efficient action towards the same goal (incongruent action). In the second test (Fig. 2.5), we opened up the previously hidden part of the scene where the balls had left and confronted the infants with two different endings for the story: the small ball halted and the big ball either stopped next to it (congruent goal) or changed its path, travelled past the small one, and left the scene (incongruent goal). Seeing an incongruent action or an incongruent goal resulted in longer looking times than seeing the corresponding congruent action or congruent goal events, indicating that 12-month-old infants took the teleological stance and were able to figure out the unseen goal of an agent. This result was recently replicated by Wagner and Carey (2002).

The teleological representational schema for actions (Fig. 2.3) allows a further type of inference as well. So far we have seen that, knowing the goal and the physical constraints, infants can predict new actions, and, knowing the physical constraints and the actions, they can attribute goals. A third type of inference that one can logically derive from this representational format would allow figuring out some invisible physical constraints on the basis of the observed action and its end state. This inference would be drawn on the same basis as the previous inferences: filling in the missing element (in this case, the physical constraints) of the schema with something that makes it a well-formed

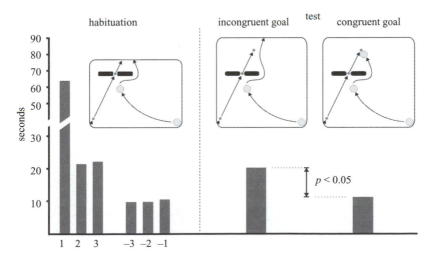

Fig. 2.5 Evidence for attribution of an unseen goal in 12-month-old infants. (Data from Csibra *et al.* (2003), experiment 1A.)

representation, i.e. with something that satisfies the efficiency principle. To
elaborate our example, if someone takes a corkscrew and starts drilling it into
a bottle, we will spontaneously assume that there is a cork in the bottle,
because otherwise this action would not make any sense, i.e. it could not be
interpreted as an efficient action towards the known goal (accessing the wine
in the bottle).

To test whether infants make similar inferences, we presented them with
a computer-animated event (Csibra *et al.* 2003), which was similar to those
we used in our earlier studies (see Fig. 2.1): a ball approached another ball by
a jumping action. The event here, however, differed from the original studies
in two respects: we made the animation three dimensional, and occluded the
part of the space that the ball jumped over (Fig. 2.6). In the test phase, the
occluder was removed and it either revealed an object or an empty space. If
infants justify the observed jumping action by inferring the presence of an
obstacle behind the occluder, seeing the obstacle would confirm, while seeing
the empty space would violate, their expectation, which should be reflected by
longer looking time in the latter case. This is exactly what we found. Twelve-
month-old infants inferred the presence of an obstacle on the sole basis of
the behaviour of the ball. Note that the absence of the obstacle does not
violate any physical knowledge; it does not *have to be* there. But its absence
violates our expectation that the object approaches its goal efficiently and
questions the interpretation that the action is performed *in order to* achieve an
end, i.e. that it is a goal-directed action.

All these results indicate that, at least by their first birthday, if not earlier,
infants rely on a quite sophisticated teleological representational system when

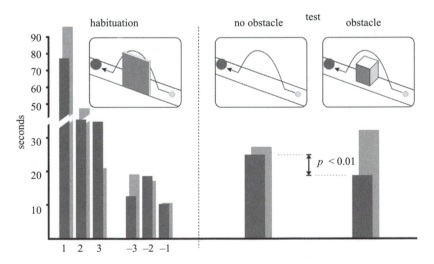

Fig. 2.6 Evidence for the inference of an invisible action constraint in 12-month-old
infants. Medium grey bars, nine-month-old infants; dark grey bars, 12-month-old
infants. (Data from Csibra *et al.* (2003), experiment 2.)

they interpret behaviours, and they use this system productively to figure out invisible aspects of actions (Csibra *et al.* 2003). Does this conclusion entail that they use a 'theory of mind', i.e. do they attribute representational mental states, such as intentions, desires and beliefs to the agents? Infants may, indeed, interpret the observed behaviours in mentalistic terms, but this is not a necessary implication of these results. No doubt, one could account for these findings by assuming that the infants interpreted the observed event as 'the ball wanted to touch the other ball, believed that the obstacle was impenetrable and decided to jump over it'. In this interpretation, the elements of the teleological schema are projected into the agent's mind as contents of his/her mental states: goals become desires, constraints become beliefs, and actions become intentions (Fig. 2.7). Note, however, that, within the particular context of action interpretation, there is no benefit gained from the computationally more demanding mental state attribution—one can predict exactly the same actions from goals and physical constraints as from contents of desires (i.e. goals) and contents of beliefs (i.e. physical constraints). The additional benefit of relying on mental states comes from situations where the mental states are attributed independently of the actual action and are used in action predictions ('he opens the bottle but he does not like wine, so he wants to offer it to someone else'). But none of the studies I have reviewed above required such inferences and therefore they did not provide conclusive evidence for mental state attribution. In fact, we have argued earlier (Csibra and Gergely 1998) that a non-mentalistic, purely teleological action interpretation system (the teleological stance) developmentally precedes the later emerging mature theory of mind (the intentional stance).

A further question arises from the fact that interpreting an action as goal-directed is not a causal inference but a result of a specific *stance* (whether it is teleological or intentional). What makes infants decide that an observed behaviour is to be interpreted from this stance, i.e. it is to be evaluated in terms of its efficiency? We all take the intentional stance when dealing with fellow human beings, but we also apply mentalistic terms to animals, to natural phenomena, and even to machines (see Dennett 1987), and neither Heider and Simmel's (1944) triangles nor our jumping balls had any animate, let alone human, features. A plausible assumption is therefore that we (and infants) rely on

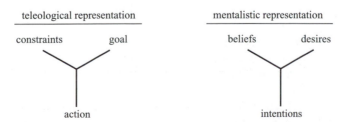

Fig. 2.7   The teleological and mentalistic action explanations.

behavioural, rather than featural, cues to identify agents that are possibly engaged in goal-directed actions. The most direct hypothesis about these cues was put forward by David Premack (1990). According to him, infants will treat as intentional (hence goal-directed) any agent that appears to be self-propelled. This idea has been incorporated into several theories of infant development (Mandler 1992; Baron-Cohen 1994; Carey and Spelke 1994; Leslie 1994) and was originally one of the hypotheses that inspired our studies (Gergely *et al*. 1995). Surprisingly, however, not much research was devoted to verifying this hypothesis. Some studies (e.g. Kaufman 1998) suggest that infants make a distinction between self-propelled and externally driven objects from an early age and develop different kinds of expectations towards the two classes of objects (Luo and Baillargeon 2002). Our recent studies indicate that 12-month-old infants are more likely to attribute goals to animated agents that appear to move by themselves than to agents that are launched by other objects (Gergely and Csibra 2003). This indicates that self-motion does indeed work as a cue for goal-directedness.

But this is not the whole story. Infants in our study were more reluctant to attribute goals to externally propelled objects but still tended to take the tele-ological stance towards them as long as their behaviour appeared efficient. Even when we removed all cues of self-motion and animacy but left enough information to evaluate the efficiency of goal approach (Csibra *et al*. 1999), 9- and 12-month-old infants were willing to attribute a goal to the observed action. These results suggest that, although self-propulsion works as cue, it is not obligatory and there may also be other cues for goal-directedness. Such cues can be derived from the efficiency principle itself. The principle requires, for example, that behaviours directed to the same goal be adjusted in relation to the relevant aspects of the environment in which they occur. Consequently, the perception of behavioural adjustment that is a function of situational constraints may serve as the triggering condition for analysing the behaviour as goal directed.

The left side of Table 2.1 summarizes the proposed specifics of the cognitive system that allows infants to interpret actions as goal-directed.

2.3 Referential understanding of actions

Understanding an action as referential requires linking the actor's behaviour to specific objects or to specific aspects of the environment. These actions, such as pointing to or looking at an object, normally occur in communicative con-texts, direct the observer's attention to that object, and may help to secure a referent for other communicative signals, such as verbal utterances.

Studies on early language acquisition indicate that there is a special context where referential understanding of actions is indispensable. Young children have been shown to be specifically sensitive to where someone is looking or

Table 2.1   The main characteristics of the two-action interpretation systems.

	goal-directed action	referential action
about	a future state	a current state
criteria of application	self-propelled agent; contingent adjustment; biological motion	communicative situations
initial principle	efficiency	(eye contact, contingent reactivity) directionality
mature principle	rationality	relevance
representation	constraints goal	agent

constraints   goal
\\   /
  \\ /
   Y
   |
 action

agent
↓
action
↓
referent

pointing at when uttering a new word and interpret the word and the observed action as referring to the same thing (Baldwin 1993; Tomasello 1999; Bloom 2000). In other words, they use referential interpretation of non-verbal actions to disambiguate the new word's referent. This is a clear demonstration that 18-month-old infants can understand actions in referential terms. Unfortunately, linguistic tests are difficult to administer before 18 months of age so they are not feasible for testing the understanding of referential actions in younger infants.

To find earlier referential contexts that do not rely on word learning, Louis Moses and his colleagues turned to another phenomenon, known as 'social referencing' (Moses *et al.* 2001). When infants are confronted with a new situation or with a novel object, they tend to check their parents' or other adults' face before approaching it, and modulate their behaviour accordingly (Campos and Stenberg 1981). For example, they cross a visual cliff, if their mother is smiling at the other side, but refrain from crawling over if she looks worried (Sorce *et al.* 1985). Moses and his colleagues tested whether this modulation of behaviour is specific to the object that the adult was looking at when she expressed a certain emotion. They arranged situations where an experimenter and the infant were focusing on either the same or different objects, and then the experimenter expressed either a positive or a negative affect both verbally and by facial expressions. In response to this, infants always looked at the adult's face and checked their line of regard. If infants understand the adult's emotional expressions in referential terms, they should modulate their behaviour towards the object that the experimenter was looking at with that emotion, even when their own attention was engaged by another object. And this is precisely what they found. Twelve-month-old infants explored the target object longer when it had been associated with positive affect, even when it was not in their own attentional focus. This is a clear evidence for referential understanding of looking.

This referential understanding of looking behaviour is assisted by infants' tendency to follow the gaze of other human beings. If you make eye contact with a 12-month-old infant and then conspicuously look at some other object in the environment, she will follow your gaze and many times she will rest her gaze on the same object. This behaviour, which is often called 'joint attention', emerges during the second half of the first year and its accuracy develops rapidly (Butterworth and Jarrett 1991).

But sensitivity to the gaze direction of others can be demonstrated even earlier in laboratory situations. If three- to six-month-old infants are presented with a target object on one side of a computer screen, they are more inclined to orient towards it if they perceive a gaze-shift on a face to the same direction just milliseconds earlier (Hood *et al.* 1998). This phenomenon has been shown to be partly explainable by sensitivity to motion cues provided by the perceived shift of pupil position (Farroni *et al.* 2000), but this does not account for all aspects of the results. Recent studies revealed that pupil motion cues are effective in eliciting shifts of attention in infants if, and only if, they are preceded by a period of eye contact (Farroni *et al.* 2003). Motion cues do not elicit attentional shifts if the perceived gaze of the face on the computer screen is moving from the side to the centre (i.e. from an averted to an eye-contact position), or when the face is presented upside down. This makes sense because, at least in humans, making eye contact is the simplest way of establishing a communicative situation, and referential actions usually occur in communicative contexts.

An interesting hypothesis that one can draw from these results is that referential understanding of actions is assisted by infants' sensitivity to two kinds of cues: those that indicate a communicative situation and those that indicate spatial directions. The combination of these two tendencies ('look for communicative situations and, if you find one, follow the direction') may ensure that infants will find the referent of a communicative act in most cases. Again, the sensitivity to communicative situations does not imply an understanding of communication. Rather, it represents a bias in processing the information available in the infant's environment. This hypothesis provided us with the prediction that even the youngest infants must be sensitive to the best cue for a communicative situation, i.e. eye contact. We tested this hypothesis with newborns in a simple preferential looking paradigm (Farroni *et al.* 2002). Seventeen 1–5-day-old newborns were shown two faces: one that looked straight at them (direct gaze) and one that looked away (averted gaze). All but two of them looked longer at and all of them looked more times towards the face with the direct gaze (Fig. 2.8). This early, and most probably innate, preference for eye contact can be interpreted in various theoretical frameworks that were developed to explain early sensitivity to social cues. It fits well into the eye-direction detection mechanism hypothesized by Baron-Cohen (1994) and it can also be adapted into Morton and Johnson's (1991) 'CONSPEC' mechanism, which orients babies to faces. The fact that faces with direct gaze engage four-month-old infants' brain circuits that are associated with face

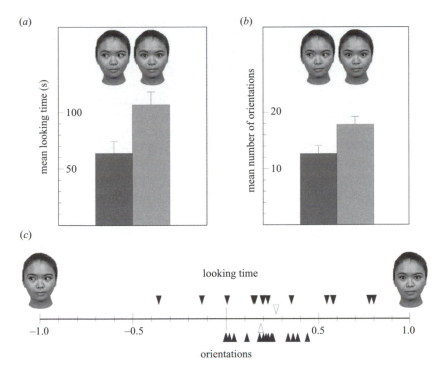

Fig. 2.8 Newborn babies look longer at (*a*), and more times towards (*b*), faces with direct eye gaze. (*c*) Individual preference scores also show a bias towards direct eye gaze both in looking times and number of orientations. (Data from Farroni *et al.* (2002).)

perception stronger than do faces with averted gaze (Farroni *et al.* 2002) is more consistent with the latter theory. But whatever the exact mechanism is, the fact that newborns are sensitive not just to faces (Johnson *et al.* 1991) and eyes (Batki *et al.* 2000) but also to eye contact gives them a kick-start towards understanding referential actions.

However, eye contact is not the only method for establishing a communicative situation. Contingent responses from a source may also indicate that the source is communicating with you. John Watson argued 30 years ago that very young infants' well-known sensitivity for objects that respond to their own actions with high but imperfect contingency is not simply a preparedness for operant conditioning but a way to find social partners in the world (Watson 1972). Susan Johnson and colleagues have demonstrated that 12-month-old infants will follow the 'gaze' of a non-human object if it reacts to the children's actions and vocalizations contingently (Johnson *et al.* 1998; see also Chapter 10 this volume). This is a very clear example of interpreting a behaviour as a referential action when the only cue for treating the object's behaviour meaningfully is the communicative situation established by contingent reactivity.

And contingent reactivity can indicate a communicative context for 10-month-old infants even when it comes from a clearly mechanical object, like a robot (Movellan and Watson 2002).

This example suggests that early understanding of referential actions evident in 'gaze following' phenomena originates not from a rich comprehension of the link between a mental state of an agent and its referent but from a blind tracking of motion cues in communicative contexts. In other words, referential interpretation of actions, just like teleological interpretation of actions, represents not a knowledge but a 'stance'. Taking this 'referential stance' triggers a search for referents on the basis of directional cues and should be initially restricted to well-defined communicative contexts. This interpretation of early capacities explains several aspects of the results in this field. Although infants tend to follow the gaze of others, initially they will not find the object looked at by the other person (Butterworth and Jarrett 1991). Even when nine-month-old infants follow pointing gestures, they would not necessarily associate the pointing action with the pointed object (Woodward and Guajardo 2002). It is not before they are 16 months of age that they tie directional motion cues to the line of regard of others correctly, for example, when they follow head turns that they observe from behind (Muir and Lee 2002; see also Johnson 2003).

What purpose does this rudimentary understanding of referential actions serve, if it does not specify what the actor's intentions have been behind his/her actions, i.e. if it does not provide mental state attribution? The answer seems obvious: referential understanding of actions might have evolved to support children's word learning. If infants interpret linguistic utterances and non-verbal communicative actions, like looking or pointing, in referential terms, then they can assume that simultaneous references by the same person will refer to the same object. If nonarbitrary referential relationships, like the spatial relationships inherent in looking and pointing, help them find a referent, it may also help them establish arbitrary referential relationships, like the one between words and objects. (The study by Moses *et al.* (2001) that is mentioned above shows how this works in a non-linguistic context.) This role of action interpretation in word learning is well documented (Baldwin 1993; Tomasello 1999; Bloom 2000) but it is usually assumed that this interpretation must yield a mental state (i.e. the referential intention of the speaker), to which both the verbal and non-verbal actions can be mapped. This is, however, not required; direct mapping between words and non-verbally referred objects can also function as a bootstrapping mechanism into word learning. Recently, Sperber and Wilson (2002) have also proposed that the early processing of communicative signals may not be based on general-purpose mind-reading mechanisms but relies on a sub-module which evolved to support fast comprehension of ostensive stimuli. Understanding of referential intentions does indeed play an important role in language acquisition from 18 to 24 months of age. Nevertheless, the development of this essential cognitive skill suggests that an understanding of referential intentions is not a precondition for, but the product of, understanding referential actions. This hypothesis is parallel with the one I proposed for teleological action understanding. Just as the notion of pre-existing goals (i.e. desires) is derived developmentally from teleological understanding of actions, and not the other way around, I propose that the notion of pre-existing 'meaning' (i.e. the communicative message) is derived developmentally from referential understanding of actions, and not the other way around.

It is not yet clear how this development is achieved. However, early understanding of referential actions, at least in one respect, seems to be very similar to the principle that governs mature human communication, the relevance principle (Sperber and Wilson 1986). The application of both the relevance principle and the referential interpretation of actions depends only on the recognition of a communicative context, and both work as a presumption that cannot be violated. The specifics of the referential action interpretation system are summarized in Table 2.1.

2.4 Teleological versus referential understanding of actions

The evidence reviewed so far suggests that 12-month-old or even younger infants readily interpret action as goal-directed or referential. What is the relationship between these two types of action understanding? Some researchers of infants tend to treat these two kinds of action interpretation as equivalent (e.g. Phillips *et al*. 2002; Woodward and Guajardo 2002), calling them both 'object-directed actions'. This is because in the majority of experiments with infants the agent's goal is to seize an object or the referred state of affairs is an object. I think, however, that 'object-directedness' is a misleading term because it relies on a surface similarity between these particular cases of action interpretation (namely, that both refer to a relationship between an agent and a distal object) and conceals the fact that they rely on different kinds of action understanding. Indeed, a comparison of the specifics of these two systems (see Table 2.1) suggests that there is not much common in them: they are triggered by different cues, apply different representations and computations, serve different functions, and are likely to be implemented in separate mechanisms.

One may argue, however, that the distinction between these systems is artificial; after all, both represent intentional actions and the difference between them is simply determined by the content of the actual intention. In other words, they may be subsystems of a single 'theory of mind' mechanism (Leslie 1994). Nevertheless, it is not only formal arguments that support the claim that these two kinds of action interpretation reflect two distinct cognitive mechanisms. Various kinds of dissociations confirm that these action interpretation systems can operate independently without the help of a higher-level theory of mind. The first of these dissociations occurs in the animal kingdom.

Chimpanzees, for example, seem to be able to attribute goals to observed actions (Uller and Nichols 2000), and can be trained to follow gaze alterations (Tomasello *et al.* 2001; Okamoto *et al.* 2002). They also understand what other individuals can see (Call 2001). However, there is no evidence that they conceive representational mental states at all (Call and Tomasello 1999), and indeed, their understanding of seeing does not reflect an understanding of reference (Povinelli *et al.* 1999). A second dissociation can be seen in autism, a developmental disorder characterized by severe difficulties in attributing mental states to others (Frith 2001). However, people with autism can attribute goals to animated shapes the same way as typical children (Abell *et al.* 2000; Castelli *et al.* 2002), suggesting that their teleological action interpretation system is intact. At the same time, their main difficulties seem to be rooted in a non-functioning referential interpretational system: they do not make eye contact (Phillips *et al.* 1992), fail to understand eye gaze (Baron-Cohen 1994), and as a result their acquisition of language is seriously delayed and impaired. These dissociations could hardly occur if the two action interpretation systems discussed in this paper were simply different manifestations of the same mechanism (for a more detailed discussion of these dissociations see Gergely (2002)).

A third type of dissociation is provided by the studies of human infants themselves. If a single, mentalistic action interpretation system existed, which could attribute intentions by both teleological and referential interpretation of actions, it would provide a link between these mechanisms, as it does in older children and adults. We can use a referential act (e.g. pointing) to figure out the likely goal of another person (e.g. obtaining the referred object); and can use a goal-directed act (e.g. searching) to figure out the referent of a word (Tomasello and Barton 1994). There is no evidence, however, that young infants would be able to make such inferences. Thus, I hypothesize that these two action interpretation systems initially represent separate mechanisms which will be integrated into a higher-order, mentalistic action interpretation during the second year of life.

Indeed, a suitable test for whether and when infants attribute mental states to others would be a demonstration of a transfer between these systems. At what age do infants pass this test? A recent study claimed to demonstrate such a transfer, i.e. goal prediction on the basis of looking behaviour, at 12 and 14 months of age. Phillips *et al.* (2002) habituated infants to a person looking at one of two objects with a positive emotion. In the test phase, infants displayed longer looking time when the person held in her hands the other object than when she held the same object. Phillips *et al.* concluded that infants were able to predict a goal-directed action (grabbing an object) from the referential relation (looking) between the person and one of the objects. Note, however, that no instrumental action was presented to the infants in these studies. They may have inferred that a certain action (grabbing the object) must have taken place between looking and holding behind the closed curtain, but they did not have to do that. All they needed to do was match two referential actions (looking, and holding *plus* looking) with their referent and notice the change of the referred object. In other words, they could have detected the incompatibility between habituation and test events without goal attribution and action prediction, i.e. entirely within the referential action interpretation system.

Other laboratories (e.g. Sodian and Thörmer 2000) have also been trying to establish the age when a link between teleological and referential understanding of actions can be demonstrated. Further research is needed to establish not just the timing but also the mechanism of the integration between these systems, as this step represents a major milestone in the development of a mature theory of mind.

I thank Teresa Farroni, György Gergely, Mark Johnson, and an anonymous reviewer for their helpful comments on an earlier version of this paper. The author was supported by the UK Medical Research Council (programme grant G9715587).

References

Abell, F., Happé, F. and Frith, U. (2000). Do triangles play tricks? Attribution of mental states to animated shapes in normal and abnormal development. *Cogn. Dev.* **15**, 1–16.

Baldwin, D. A. (1993). Early referential understanding: infants' ability to recognize referential acts for what they are. *Devl Psychol.* **29**, 832–43.

Baron-Cohen, S. (1994). How to build a baby that can read minds: cognitive mechanisms in mind reading. *Cah. Psychol. Cogn./Curr. Psychol. Cogn.* **13**, 513–52.

Batki, A., Baron-Cohen, S., Wheelwright, S., Connellan, J. and Ahluwalia, J. (2000). Is there an innate gaze module? Evidence from human neonates. *Infant Behav. Dev.* **23**, 223–9.

Bellagamba, F. and Tomasello, M. (1999). Re-enacting intended acts: comparing 12- and 18-month-olds. *Infant Behav. Dev.* **22**, 277–82.

Bloom, P. (2000). *How children learn the meanings of words*. Cambridge, MA: MIT Press.

Butterworth, G. and Jarrett, N. (1991). What minds have in common is space: spatial mechanisms serving joint visual attention in infancy. *Br. J. Devl. Psychol.* **9**, 55–72.

Call, J. (2001). Chimpanzee social cognition. *Trends Cogn. Sci.* **5**, 388–93.

Call, J. and Tomasello, M. (1999). A non-verbal false belief task: the performance of children and great apes. *Child Dev.* **70**, 381–95.

Campos, J. J. and Stenberg, C. R. (1981). Perception, appraisal, and emotion: the onset of social referencing. In *Infant social cognition* (ed. M. Lamb and L. Sherrod), pp. 273–314. Hillsdale, NJ: Lawrence Erlbaum Associates.

Carey, S. and Spelke, E. (1994). Domain-specific knowledge and conceptual change. In *Mapping the mind: domain specificity in cognition and culture* (ed. L. Hirschfeld and S. Gelman), pp. 169–200. New York: Cambridge University Press.

Castelli, F., Frith, C., Happé, F. and Frith, U. (2002). Autism, Asperger syndrome and brain mechanisms for the attribution of mental states to animated shapes. *Brain* **125**, 1839–49.

Csibra, G. and Gergely, G. (1998). The teleological origins of mentalistic action explanations: a developmental hypothesis. *Devl Sci.* **1**, 255–9.

Csibra, G., Gergely, G., Bíró, S., Koós, O. and Brockbank, M. (1999). Goal attribution without agency cues: the perception of 'pure reason' in infancy. *Cognition* **72**, 237–67.

Csibra, G., Bíró, S., Koós, O. and Gergely, G. (2003). One-year-old infants use teleological representations of actions productively. *Cogn. Sci.* **27**, 111–33.

Dennett, D. C. (1987). *The intentional stance*. Cambridge, MA: MIT Press.

Farroni, T., Johnson, M. H., Brockbank, M. and Simion, F. (2000). Infants' use of gaze direction to cue attention: the importance of perceived motion. *Visual Cogn.* **7**, 705–18.

Farroni, T., Csibra, G., Simion, F. and Johnson, M. F. (2002). Eye-contact detection in humans from birth. *Proc. Natl Acad. Sci. USA* **99**, 9602–5.

Farroni, T., Mansfield, E. M., Lai, C. and Johnson, M. H. (2003). Infants perceiving and acting on the eyes: tests of an evolutionary hypothesis. *J. Exp. Child Psychol.*, in press.

Frith, U. (2001). Mind blindness and the brain in autism. *Neuron* **32**, 969–79.

Gergely, G. (2002). The development of understanding self and agency. In *Blackwell's handbook of childhood cognitive development* (ed. U. Goswami), pp. 26–46. Oxford: Blackwell.

Gergely, G. and Csibra, G. (1997). Teleological reasoning in infancy: the infant's naive theory of rational action. A reply to Premack and Premack. *Cognition* **63**, 227–33.

Gergely, G. and Csibra, G. (2003). Perception of autonomous motion and goal attribution by one-year-old infants. (In preparation.)

Gergely, G., Nádasdy, Z., Csibra, G. and Bíró, S. (1995). Taking the intentional stance at 12 months of age. *Cognition* **56**, 165–93.

Gergely, G., Bekkering, H. and Király, I. (2002). Rational imitation in preverbal infants. *Nature* **415**, 755.

Heider, F. and Simmel, S. (1944). An experimental study of apparent behavior. *Am. J. Psychol.* **57**, 243–59.

Hood, B. M., Willen, J. D. and Driver, J. (1998). Adult's eyes trigger shifts of visual attention in infants. *Psychol. Sci.* **9**, 131–4.

Johnson, M. H., Dziurawiec, S., Ellis, H. and Morton, J. (1991). Newborns' preferential tracking of face-like stimuli and its subsequent decline. *Cognition* **40**, 1–19.

Johnson, S. C., Slaughter, V. and Carey, S. (1998). Whose gaze will infants follow? The elicitation of gaze-following in 12-month-olds. *Devl Sci.* **1**, 233–8.

Kaufman, L. E. (1998). Five-month-old infants distinguish between inert and self-moving inanimate objects. In *11th Biannual Int. Conf. on Infant Stud.*, April 1998, Atlanta, GA.

Keil, F. C. (1995). The growth of causal understanding of natural kinds. In *Causal cognition: a multidisciplinary debate* (ed. D. Sperber, D. Premack and A. J. Premack), pp. 234–62. Oxford: Oxford University Press.

Leslie, A. M. (1994). ToMM, ToBy and Agency: core architecture and domain specificity. In *Mapping the mind: domain specificity in cognition and culture* (ed. L. Hirschfeld and S. Gelman), pp. 119–48. New York: Cambridge University Press.

Luo, Y. and Baillargeon, R. (2002). Does a self-moving box possess an 'internal force' and 'mind'? In *13th Biennial Int. Conf. on Infant Stud.*, April 2002, Toronto, Ontario, Canada.

Mandler, J. M. (1992). How to build a baby. II. Conceptual primitives. *Psychol. Rev.* **99**, 587–604.

Meltzoff, A. N. (1988). Infant imitation after a 1-week delay: long-term memory for novel acts and multiple stimuli. *Devl. Psychol.* **24**, 470–6.

Meltzoff, A. N. (1995). Understanding the intentions of others: re-enactment of intended acts by 18-month-old children. *Devl. Psychol.* **31**, 838–50.

Morton, J. and Johnson, M. H. (1991). CONSPEC and CONLERN: a two-process theory of infant face recognition. *Psychol. Rev.* **98**, 164–81.

Moses, L. J., Baldwin, D. A., Rosicky, J. G. and Tidball, G. (2001). Evidence for referential understanding in the emotions domain at twelve and eighteen months. *Child Dev.* **72**, 718–35.

Movellan, J. R. and Watson, J. S. (2002). The development of gaze following as a Bayesian systems identification problem. UCSD Machine Perception Laboratory Technical Reports 2002.01.

Muir, D. and Lee, K. (2002). Invisible gaze following: perspective taking at 12 months of age. In *13th Biennial Int. Conf. on Infant Stud.*, April 2002, Toronto, Ontario, Canada.

Okamoto, S., Tomonaga, M., Ishii, K., Kawai, N., Tanaka, M. and Matsuzawa, T. (2002). An infant chimpanzee (*Pan troglodytes*) follows human gaze. *Anim. Cogn.* **5**, 107–14.

Onishi, K. H. (2001). Ten-month-old infants understand that a goal object can be obtained in multiple ways. In *The Soc. Res. Child Dev.*, Minneapolis, April 2001.

Phillips, A. T., Wellman, H. M. and Spelke, E. S. (2002). Infants' ability to connect gaze and emotional expression to intentional action. *Cognition* **85**, 53–78.

Phillips, W., Baron-Cohen, S. and Rutter, M. (1992). The role of eye contact in goal detection: evidence from normal infants and children with autism or mental handicap. *Dev. Psychopathol.* **4**, 375–83.

Povinelli, D. J., Bierschwale, D. T. and Cech, C. G. (1999). Comprehension of seeing as a referential act in young children, but not juvenile chimpanzees. *Br. J. Devl Psychol.* **17**, 37–60.

Premack, D. (1990). The infant's theory of self-propelled objects. *Cognition* **36**, 1–16.

Scholl, B. J. and Tremoulet, P. D. (2000). Perceptual causality and animacy. *Trends Cogn. Sci.* **4**, 299–309.

Sodian, B. and Thörmer, C. (2000). Understanding the epistemic aspects of seeing. Precursors in infancy? In *12th Biennial Int. Conf. on Infant Stud.*, July 2000, Brighton, UK.

Sorce, J., Emde, R. N., Campos, J. J. and Klinnert, M. (1985). Maternal emotional signaling: its effect on the visual cliff behavior in 1-year-olds. *Devl. Psychol.* **21**, 195–200.

Sperber, D. and Wilson, D. (1986). *Relevance: communication and cognition.* Oxford: Blackwell.

Sperber, D. and Wilson, D. (2002). Pragmatics, modularity and mond-reading. *Mind Lang.* **17**, 3–23.

Tomasello, M. (1999). *The cultural origins of human cognition.* Cambridge, MA: Harvard University Press.

Tomasello, M. and Barton, M. E. (1994). Learning words in nonostensive contexts. *Devl. Psychol.* **30**, 639–50.

Tomasello, M., Hare, B. and Fogleman, T. (2001). The ontogeny of gaze following in chimpanzees, *Pan troglodytes*, and rhesus macaques, *Macaca mulatta. Anim. Behav.* **61**, 335–43.

Uller, C. and Nichols, S. (2000). Goal attribution in chimpanzees. *Cognition* **76**, B27–B34.

Wagner, L. and Carey, S. (2002). Coming to conclusions: 12-month-old infants form expectations about probable endings of motion events. In *13th Biennial Int. Conf. on Infant Stud.*, April 2002, Toronto, Ontario, Canada.

Watson, J. S. (1972). Smiling, cooing, and 'the game'. *Merril Palmer Q.* **18**, 323–39.

Woodward, A. L. (1998). Infants selectively encode the goal object of an actor's reach. *Cognition* **69**, 1–34.

Woodward, A. L. and Guajardo, J. J. (2002). Infants' understanding of the point gesture as an object-directed action. *Cogn. Dev.* **17**, 1061–84.

Woodward, A. L. and Sommerville, J. A. (2000). Twelve-month-old infants interpret action in context. *Psychol. Sci.* **11**, 73–7.

3

Development and neurophysiology of mentalizing

Uta Frith and Christopher D. Frith

The mentalizing (theory of mind) system of the brain is probably in operation from around 18 months of age, allowing implicit attribution of intentions and other mental states. Between the ages of 4 and 6 years explicit mentalizing becomes possible, and from this age children are able to explain the misleading reasons that have given rise to a false belief. Neuroimaging studies of mentalizing have so far only been carried out in adults. They reveal a system with three components consistently activated during both implicit and explicit mentalizing tasks: medial prefrontal cortex (MPFC), temporal poles and posterior superior temporal sulcus (STS). The functions of these components can be elucidated, to some extent, from their role in other tasks used in neuroimaging studies. Thus, the MPFC region is probably the basis of the decoupling mechanism that distinguishes mental state representations from physical state representations; the STS region is probably the basis of the detection of agency, and the temporal poles might be involved in access to social knowledge in the form of scripts. The activation of these components in concert appears to be critical to mentalizing.

Keywords: mentalizing; theory of mind; medial prefrontal cortex; anterior cingulated cortex; temporal poles; superior temporal sulcus

3.1 Development of mentalizing

In 1978 a paper by Premack and Woodruff appeared with the provocative title 'Does the chimpanzee have a "theory of mind"?' (Premack and Woodruff 1978). The phrase 'theory of mind' was not to be taken literally of course, and certainly it did not imply the possession of an explicit philosophical theory about the contents of the mind. Instead, it crystallized the question of whether the mind of the chimpanzee works like the human mind, in that it makes the implicit assumption that the behaviour of others is determined by their desires, attitudes and beliefs. These are not states of the world, but states of the mind. Over the years, alternatives for the term 'theory of mind', such as 'ToM', 'mentalizing' and 'intentional stance', have also come into use. We will mainly use the term 'mentalizing'.

Premack and Woodruff in their seminal paper reported studies that tested the possibility that chimpanzees are implicitly aware that different individuals can have different thoughts and use this ability to predict their behaviour.

One of the more striking outcomes of this social insight would be the ability to deceive others and to understand deception. The results of the experiments were equivocal and subsequent studies have remained tantalizing (Byrne and Whiten 1988; Heyes 1998; Povinelli and Bering 2002). While some studies reported an incipient but not very robust theory of mind in the chimpanzee and other great apes, the verdict fell the other way for monkeys: they do not show any evidence of the ability to attribute mental states (Cheney and Seyfarth 1990).

In contrast to the uncertainty about mentalizing in other species, the development of a fluent mentalizing ability, with far-reaching consequences for social insight, is undoubtedly a human accomplishment. How does this ability develop? When do children first show evidence of mentalizing? Evidence might come from explicit mental state language ('I *think* my brother is *pretending* to be a ghost'), but mentalizing might also be implicit in behaviour (far from being frightened, the child removes the sheet to reveal her brother underneath). In his commentary on Premack and Woodruff's paper, Dennett (1978) proposed a stringent test for the presence of theory of mind, the prediction of another person's behaviour on the basis of this person's false belief. A true belief would not do, as in this case it would be impossible to decide unequivocally whether the other person behaves in accordance with reality or in accordance with his or her own belief about reality. So, if the child runs towards the curtain when another person is hiding there, this may be because the other person is indeed there, or because the child believes the other person to be there. A new experimental paradigm was needed, and this was created by Heinz Wimmer and Josef Perner (1983). This paradigm opened the door to a new era in the study of social cognition. It goes like this: Maxi has some chocolate and puts it into a blue cupboard. Maxi goes out. Now his mother comes in and moves the chocolate to a green cupboard. Maxi comes back to get his chocolate. Where will Maxi look for the chocolate? The answer is of course: Maxi will look in the blue cupboard, because this is where he falsely believes the chocolate to be. Control questions checked that the child understood the sequence of events: where is the chocolate really? Do you remember where Maxi put the chocolate in the beginning?

A series of subsequent studies established that children of around 4 years of age, but no younger, begin to understand this scenario and can verbally explain it when asked. At age 5 years over 90%, and at age 6 years all children, could understand the task (Baron-Cohen *et al.* 1985; Perner *et al.* 1987). Other researchers used variants of this task with essentially similar results. Studies were also carried out in other cultures indicating the universality of this clear developmental phenomenon (Avis and Harris 1991).

(a) From age 5 years

Perner and Wimmer (1985) devised a more difficult task that required the attribution of a belief about another person's belief, a so-called second-order task. Here, Mary believes that John believes that something is the case. Children from the age of around 5 or 6 years effortlessly understand this task (Sullivan *et al*. 1994). Even more complex scenarios are used in suspense stories with detectives and spies where people carry around secrets and resort to bluff, and double bluff if necessary. These plots are popular from late childhood onwards and do not seem to require much mental effort. Of course to know about the full range of mentalizing situations and to use this knowledge to predict other people's behaviour, experience is necessary. There are many shades of social insight and social competence in adults. The successful Machiavellian individual probably has to practice for many years, and benefits from the study of suitable handbooks. Niccolo Machiavelli's (1469–1527) treatise on political acumen in *The Prince* is still unsurpassed.

(b) From age 3 years

But what happens before the age of five? Do young children not act as if they knew that other people had thoughts and that thoughts are different from physical states? Of course they do. A number of experimental paradigms suitable for younger ages have been invented to demonstrate this. Three-year-olds certainly know the difference between physical and mental entities. For instance, Wellman and Estes (1986) told children that one character had a biscuit and another was thinking about a biscuit. Children had no trouble saying which biscuit could be touched.

From 3 years of age or earlier children use words which refer to mental states, 'I *thought* it was an alligator. Now I *know* it's a crocodile', is an example quoted by Shatz *et al*. (1983) from a 3-year-old. Examples of mental state words in use by many 2-year-olds are *want, wish* and *pretend*.

The false-belief scenario with Maxi and the chocolate, which at first glance is quite complicated, has been transformed into a little play that can be watched by young children aged 3 years. In this way, Clements and Perner (1994, 2001) were able to show that when Maxi comes back to look for his chocolate, 3-year-olds reliably look first at the door near the blue cupboard, where he initially put the chocolate rather than the door near the green cupboard. Nevertheless, when asked the test question, the same children point towards the green cupboard, and give the wrong answer.

Three-year-olds also have an incipient understanding of the difference between knowing, thinking and guessing. Masangkay *et al*. (1974) and Flavell *et al*. (1981) showed that children aged 3 years, but not younger ones, could tell that if there were different pictures on each side of a card, the person sitting opposite would see a different picture when the card was held up. Hogrefe *et al*. (1986) showed that 3-year-olds realize that only the person who has looked inside a box knows what is inside it, but not another person, who did not look inside. However, such understanding is evident even earlier in the right communicative context. In the context of requesting an object, 2-year-olds show themselves to be sensitive to the knowledge state of a parent. They actively direct their mother's attention to the location of an object, if, unbeknown to her, the object had been moved (O'Neill 1996). Four-year-olds are less dependent on this context and can give reasons why seeing leads to knowing, and not seeing to not knowing (e.g. O'Neill and Gopnik 1991; Povinelli and deBlois 1992). Remarkably, when tested in implicit form, infants from as young as 18 months of age appear to have a practical understanding of this logic (Poulin-Dubois *et al.* 2003). The infants in this study were surprised, and looked longer, if a woman pointed to the wrong place after she had observed where another person hid an object. By contrast, they were not surprised and, did not look longer, when she had been unable to observe the hiding place.

(c) From 18 months of age

The age of 18 months (or thereabouts) is, in many respects, a developmental watershed, which marks the end of infancy. Thus, beginning at around this time, language learning takes off rapidly. This may be because from that time onwards word learning is facilitated by the ability to track a speaker's intention when he or she utters a word (Baldwin and Moses 1996; Bloom 2000). The child knows when the mother is naming an object for the benefit of the child rather than saying words that have nothing to do with the object the child is holding at the time. Without making this distinction the child would learn accidental sound and object associations. In fact such errors are rare. This age is also significant for the onset of pretend play. As Leslie (1987) cogently argued, the understanding of pretence is an unequivocal manifestation of the ability to mentalize. Leslie's well-known example is the mother playfully picking up a banana and pretending to telephone. The child laughs and does not get confused about the property of telephones and bananas. To prevent such confusion the child must have the ability to represent the attitude the mother takes to the banana. This has to be different from the representation of the banana's real life use. A possible cognitive mechanism suggested by Leslie was termed 'decoupling'. This term vividly conveys the need to keep separate representations of real events from representations of thoughts that no longer need to refer to such events.

The examples of pretend play and rapid language acquisition involve the joint attention of two people. Mother and child jointly attend to the object being named or to the object that is the target of pretence. When is joint attention first documented? The answer depends on whether strict or lenient criteria are used. The minimum requirement for joint attention is that both infant and adult look together at a third object. But this may be accidental or contrived. A more stringent requirement is that one person's attention towards the object is deliberately drawn there by the other person, starting with a direct gaze. From approximately 12 months of age infants tend to look automatically at a target that an adult is looking at (Butterworth and Jarrett 1991). However, this achievement is not as impressive as it seems, as this only happens when the target is already within the infant's point of view. It is not until approximately 18 months that the infant reliably turns towards a goal that an adult is pointing to or gazing at, when this goal is not already in the line of vision (Butterworth 1991; Caron *et al.* 1997). Using the most stringent criterion one might therefore date joint attention from 18 months, even though joint looking and gaze following can be observed much earlier. Strictly defined joint attention indicates an implicit awareness of the fact that different people can pay attention to different things at the same time, and of the fact that their attention can be 'directed' to coincide with one's own interests. The development of joint attention between 14 and 24 months has been shown to have an orderly progression by Carpenter *et al.* (1998) and to be correlated with other significant developments in social competence. Reliable imitation of intentional actions performed by others, regardless of whether these actions reach their goal, also emerges at approximately 18 months, as demonstrated in a classic study by Meltzoff (1995).

At this stage, infants also seem to respond to a novel toy by taking into account their mother's emotional expression: they will not approach it if she signals fear (Repacholi 1998). Children at this age understand eye gaze as a communicative tool. They know that a person cannot see through an obstacle and they try to remove the hands if their mother covers her eyes when they want to show her a picture (Lempers *et al.* 1977)

At earlier ages, examples of mentalizing have rarely been reported, and this may indicate that the index behaviour is less robust at younger ages. One highly interesting study by Onishi and Baillargeon (2002) suggests that appropriate methods using length of looking time, can reveal an implicit form of false-belief understanding in children aged 15.5 months.

(d) From 12 months of age

There are some achievements from the age of 12 months (or thereabouts) that may well be vital milestones on the road to the development of mentalizing and suggest a dawning awareness of mental states such as intentions and desires. Perhaps the most impressive achievement is that from the age of 1 year onwards, infants can respond to an object as an intentional agent, purely on the basis of its interactive behaviour with another person (see Chapter 10, this volume).

Some of the most important tools for communication outside language come from looking and pointing gestures. They allow even infants to predict the action of agents. Woodward *et al.* (2001) showed that from 12 months of age but not before, there is a primitive understanding that gaze involves a relation between a person and the object of her gaze.

From approximately 12 months of age infants use information about an adult's gaze direction and positive emotional expression to predict that the adult will reach for the object (Phillips *et al*. 2002). This indicates an early ability to appreciate that a person may have different goals and that these goals may have different meanings. Sodian and Thoermer (2003) demonstrated that infants expect agents to grasp the object that they look at, rather than another object that is also present. However, if a pointing gesture was used as a cue for grasping instead of gaze, infants were less surprised if the agent grasped the other object instead.

(e) From nine months of age

Gergely *et al*. (1995; see also Chapter 2, this volume) obtained evidence from an ingenious experiment concerning infants' ability to reason about goals. They call it the principle of rationality: infants aged between 9 and 12 months expect agents to approach a goal in the most economic way. They are surprised if an agent does not do so, but jumps instead over an invisible hurdle. This demonstrates that they can separately represent goals of agents and the means used to reach the goal. The ability to represent goals and the ability to reason 'rationally' are likely to be an important prerequisite of the ability to represent intentions.

(f) From six months of age

Infants at about this age are surprised if an object moves on its own, but not if a person does (Spelke *et al*. 1995). This suggests that they can distinguish animate agents by the fact that they are self-propelled. By this definition a self-propelled agent need not be a biological creature, but can be a mechanical toy or even a car. The importance of agents is not that they are biological entities but that they may move unpredictably 'of their own will'. The representation of the action of agents is likely to be an essential requirement for the representation of the intention of agents.

Woodward (1998) showed that infants expected a human hand to reach towards the same goal objects when its location had been changed rather than for a different object that would have been easy to reach. By contrast, the infants did not show this differentiated expectation when no human hand was used, but instead a mechanical rod. The distinction between biological and mechanical movement is probably another prerequisite for the understanding of intentions. As we shall see in Section 3.4*b*, in adults, specific regions in the STS of the brain are active in response to these different types of movement. That the difference is detected at such an early age suggests that these regions mature early and that learning must be ultra-fast.

(g) From three months of age

The range of behaviours that can be observed in the early months of life is quite limited, and this limits the sources of evidence. However, it is clear that infants only a few weeks old smile more and vocalize more towards people than towards objects (Legerstee 1992). This could well suggest an innate preference for social stimuli.

Not only eye movements but also other forms of biological motion seem to have a privileged status in attracting infants' attention at an extremely early age. They track objects with self-propelled movement (Crichton and Lange Kuettner 1999). They also show more interest in the kinematic patterns of point-light displays of a person walking than of random movement (Bertenthal *et al.* 1984).

The ability to react reflexively to movement of gaze as a priming cue for one's own eye movement is likely to be innate as it can already be observed at three months of age (Hood *et al.* 1998). This is different from the voluntary following of the general direction of an adult's gaze, which is not accomplished until around 12–18 months of age. The same observable action, gaze following, is guided by different mechanisms and thus can mean very different things. It is unlikely that the early gaze reflex evident at age three months rests on the same neural substrate as the type of sophisticated gaze following seen at age 18 months that implies the ability to mentalize.

3.2 Conclusions

Evidence of mentalizing becomes abundant only from around 18 months of age. Accomplishments at, and just before, 12 months of age are nevertheless astounding in their own right. They suggest that the infant can represent separately agents, goals and means of getting to the goal. Representing the visible goals of agents, however, is not the same as representing the invisible intentions in agents. It is unclear whether, and how, this early ability relates to the later understanding of intentions. Intentions, after all, can result in actions that may be thwarted or never fulfilled. So far, clear evidence for understanding intentions is only available from 18-month-olds, at the same time as they begin to understand other mental states.

One remarkable fact about the studies reviewed is that they suggest universal developmental stages, applicable to all children, notwithstanding individual differences in the speed of development. For this reason it is possible to identify abnormal development in those children who appear to have a faulty mentalizing mechanism. This is suggested to be the case in autism (Baron-Cohen *et al.* 1985).

Perhaps it is difficult to find evidence for the intentional stance in the first year of life because there are limits set by the experience that is available to young infants, but there are also limits set by the state of maturation of the brain. The presence of developmental abnormalities in brain function that affect mentalizing would not be readily discovered at this young age. Would enhanced experience at this stage be helpful? Possibly, but even if experience is available, innate mechanisms may not be mature enough to take advantage of it. Cognitive mechanisms may go through a number of developmental stages, and this could well be the case for the mentalizing system.

Tentatively, we can conclude that an implicit version of the intentional stance emerges first, concerned with desires, goals and intentions. This is usually dated at around 18 months. At 18–24 months there is a convergence of several important developmental milestones, including a true understanding of joint attention, deliberate imitation and the ability to track a speaker's intention while learning words. There is also evidence for the ability to understand knowing and seeing at an implicit level, and possibly even an implicit understanding of false belief.

In summary, we can probably assume that the understanding of many mental states (wanting, intending, knowing, pretending and believing) is already available in implicit form to 2-year-olds and governs their behaviour as well as their understanding of other people's behaviour. We would therefore expect that if functional brain imaging were done in children aged 2 years (for example, while watching an agent performing actions that do not reach their goal versus a robot performing mechanical goaldirected actions), the mentalizing system of the brain (see Section 3.4) would already be in operation. Conversely, in children with autism, the presumed fault in this system should show up at this age too.

We can also conclude that another major leap in the development of mentalizing occurs between the ages of 4 and 6 years. It is only from 6 years of age onwards that we can safely attribute to a normally developing child a full and explicit awareness of mental states and their role in the explanation and prediction of other people's behaviour. What explains this significant change? Different theories are currently debated. One assumes that the change is extraneous to mentalizing but has to do with the executive components of false-belief tasks (e.g. Russell 1996). Another theory postulates that only the older child can apply the full ability to simulate another person's mental states, moving freely from their own to another's perspective (Harris 1991). A third proposal is that the child behaves like a theorist who, from time to time, is compelled by the facts to change his concepts about the physical and social world (Gopnik and Wellman 1994). While all these theories might help to explain changes in task performance, an even more parsimonious theory is that the mentalizing mechanism itself makes another leap in development at around 4 years of age. If it were possible to make visible the mentalizing system in the brain during implicit watching of a false-belief scenario before and after the observed changes in explicit task performance, this question might be answered.

(a) What role for early components of social cognition in mentalizing?

While other primitive neural mechanisms may facilitate social learning, we do not know whether they contribute directly to the social insight that is facilitated by the intentional stance. It is possible that strong connections between the brain regions that subserve these mechanisms, strengthened through learning, eventually give rise to the ability to mentalize. It is also possible that an additional neural mechanism is needed for the development of this ability, which is, after all, of late origin in terms of evolution.

We can only speculate about the role of early-appearing components of social cognition in mentalizing. There are three such functions, which might be particularly relevant. First, there is the preference for social stimuli. Evidence from behavioural and electrophysiological studies suggests that even newborn infants are responsive to human faces and preferentially orient towards stimuli that resemble faces. In adults the fusiform gyrus and STS are thought to subserve this function (Chao *et al.* 1999; Allison *et al.* 2000). In newborn babies, however, these cortical areas are not yet mature, and subcortical regions are probably involved (Johnson and Morton 1991), Second, an agency detection mechanism might be the basis of the sensitivity of three-month-olds to biological motion and eye movement. This mechanism in adults is thought to be sub-served by the STS. Third, there may be a mechanism that enables an understanding of the meaning of actions, a differentiation of the goals of actions and the means to reach them. Mirror neurons, situated in the ventral part of the lateral premotor cortex, might be involved in such a mechanism (Rizzolatti *et al.* 2002).

Might these potentially innate components (a preference for conspecifics, a predisposition to detect agency and a predisposition to understand actions), contribute to the development of mentalizing? They might be necessary prerequisites. However, by themselves they are not sufficient for the development of mentalizing. This follows from the assumption that they are shared with a great many other species, most of which do not possess a trace of mentalizing ability. As we shall see in the review of neuroimaging studies (section 3.4), the neural components of the mentalizing system comprise some of the putative prerequisites that developmental studies have demonstrated. However, the mentalizing system comprises additional components whose function in development is as yet unknown. We speculate that only when all these components are connected together in the brain are both necessary and sufficient conditions for mentalizing present. One of the reasons that we cannot make more precise links from the detailed and ingenious behavioural studies with infants and young children to neuroimaging studies with adults is our lack of knowledge of the developing human brain either in terms of structure or function.

The role of learning and experience in the development of mentalizing still needs to be investigated. Different individuals have different experiences and this is likely to be reflected in their mentalizing competence. So far, studies have rarely focused on individual differences, and thus our knowledge is currently very limited. Wellman *et al.* (2000) report that the first achievement of explicit false-belief understanding can vary from between 2 years 6 months to 6 years. Some evidence exists that the presence of older siblings facilitates the understanding of false beliefs (after age 4 years) (Ruffman *et al.* 1998), and it is widely believed that girls achieve the developmental milestones of mentalizing somewhat earlier than boys. While crosscultural studies do not suggest marked differences in early achievements, it is obvious that cultural differences could play a large, if not dominant, role in the development of the content of an adult theory of mind (Lillard 1998).

3.3 Neuroimaging studies of mentalizing

Neuroimaging provides another kind of evidence about the nature and components of the ability to mentalize. All the studies carried out so far have concerned adults rather than children. Most studies have been modelled on the story of Maxi and the chocolate. For example, while being scanned the volunteer reads a series of very short stories in which the behaviour of the protagonist is determined by his or her false belief about the situation. An example is the 'burglar story' from a set of stories testing mentalizing ability (Happé 1994).

'A burglar who has just robbed a shop is making his getaway. As he is running home, a policeman on his beat sees him drop his glove. He doesn't know the man is a burglar, he just wants to tell him he dropped his glove. But when the policeman shouts out to the burglar, "Hey, you! Stop!" The burglar turns round, sees the policeman, and gives himself up. He puts his hands up and admits that he did the break-in at the local shop'.

Subsequently the volunteer is asked to explain the burglar's behaviour. An appropriate answer would be that the burglar falsely believes that the policeman knows he has just robbed the shop. Reading and understanding such stories engages many processes in addition to mentalizing and so control stories, matched for difficulty, are necessary. Such stories also involve people, but the critical events are explained in terms of physical causality.

'A burglar is about to break in to a jewellers' shop. He skilfully picks the lock on the shop door. Carefully he crawls under the electronic detector beam. If he breaks this beam it will set off the alarm. Quietly he opens the door of the storeroom and sees the gems glittering. As he reaches out, however, he steps on something soft. He hears a screech and something small and furry runs out past him towards the shop door. Immediately the alarm sounds'.

In this example, the appropriate answer to the question, 'Why did the alarm go off?' would be because some animal had triggered it.

3.4 A neural system for mentalizing

In the first study to use such stories (Fletcher *et al.* 1995) a comparison of mentalizing with physical stories revealed activity in the MPFC, posterior cingulate and right posterior STS. In comparison with a low-level baseline of unlinked sentences, activity was also seen in the temporal poles, bilaterally. The MPFC seemed to be particularly linked to mentalizing since it was the only area that was not also activated by the physical stories. Two subsequent fMRI studies used the same stories and obtained very similar results (Gallagher *et al.* 2000; Vogeley *et al.* 2001). Activity was seen in the MPFC, temporal poles and STS when reading mentalizing stories compared with physical stories, although in Vogeley *et al.* the STS activity was most marked in a novel condition in which the volunteer imagined herself as the protagonist in a mentalizing story.

Two studies have presented mentalizing scenarios using drawings rather than words. Brunet *et al.* (2000) presented cartoon strips in which the sequence could only be understood in terms of the goals and intentions of the protagonist. Gallagher *et al.* (2000) used cartoons without captions in which the jokes involved false beliefs. Again in both these studies activity was observed in the MPFC, temporal poles and STS.

Goel *et al.* (1995) used a very different task to engage mentalizing. Volunteers were shown objects and had to indicate whether or not Christopher Columbus would have known what each object was used for. Such a decision involves inferring something about the knowledge and beliefs of someone who lived 500 years ago. In comparison to various control tasks activity was again seen in MPFC, temporal pole and STS.

Berthoz *et al.* (2002) have reported a study of social norm transgression that also involved mentalizing. Volunteers read short vignettes in which social transgressions occurred. These could be accidental or deliberate. An example of an accidental transgression is as follows; 'Joanna is invited for a Japanese dinner at her friend's house. She has a bite of the first course, chokes and spits out the food while she is choking'. Volunteers were asked to try and imagine how the character in the story would feel. In comparison with matched stories in which no transgression occurred, both deliberate and accidental transgressions elicited activity in the MPFC, temporal poles and STS. Activity was also seen in areas responding to aversive emotional expressions such as anger.

An implicit mentalizing task which activated all three of these areas was based on the observation by Heider and Simmel (1944) that people will attribute intentions and desires to moving geometric shapes if these movements are of sufficient complexity. Castelli *et al.* (2000), using positron emission tomography, presented an animated sequence in which two triangles interacted with each other. The more the observers attributed mental states to the triangles the greater the activity in the MPFC, temporal pole and STS. Schultz *et al.* (2003)

used a similar task and, using fMRI, observed activations in the same regions. In both these studies where mentalizing was elicited by the movements of abstract shapes, the activity in the temporal pole extended into the amygdala and activity was also seen in the fusiform gyrus.

All these studies, except possibly those using passive viewing of animations, have involved explicit mentalizing since the subjects were asked to describe the mental states of other people or make decisions based on the mental states of other people. In addition, in all these studies, mentalizing was elicited by the material presented. The approach is analogous to studies in which the colour area in the visual system is identified by comparing the activity elicited by stimuli with and without colour (Zeki *et al.* 1991). An alternative approach is to keep the stimulus material constant and change the attitude of the volunteer. For example, the same visual stimulus is presented, but the volunteer is required to attend to colour in one condition and to motion in another (Corbetta 1993). Two studies have used this approach to identify brain areas associated with mentalizing. McCabe *et al.* (2001) scanned volunteers while they played an economic game with another person. In this game mutual cooperation between players increases the amount of money that can be won. In the comparison task the volunteers believed they were playing with a computer that used fixed rules. Gallagher *et al.* (2002) scanned volunteers while they played the game 'Stone–Paper–Scissors'. This is a competitive game in which success depends upon predicting what the other player will do next. In this study the comparison condition was also created by telling the volunteers that they were playing against a computer. In fact, the sequence of the opponent's moves was the same in both conditions.

In these studies the volunteers were not explicitly instructed to mentalize while performing their task. However, an intensive debriefing of the volunteers in the study of 'Stone–Paper–Scissors' confirmed that they had engaged in mentalizing while playing against a person. They described guessing and second guessing their opponent's responses and felt that they could understand and 'go along with' what their opponent was doing. Playing against a computer felt distinctly different. The volunteers considered that the computer was in principle very predictable, but the rules it used might be difficult to detect. They also felt that the computer might be too fast for them to keep up with.

Both studies revealed activity in the MPFC when the volunteers believed that they were interacting with another person. But this was the only area that was more active in this condition than in the condition where they believed they were playing against a computer. This dissociation between the MPFC and the other regions suggests that the posterior regions are more concerned with the nature of the sensory signals that elicit mentalizing, whereas MPFC activity reflects the attitude taken towards those signals. In order to explore the precise role of the various areas in the mentalizing network we shall now consider studies that activate some or all of these areas, but which were not explicitly designed to engage mentalizing.

In this review we have restricted ourselves to those imaging studies that declare mentalizing as an experimental variable and that have used appropriate controls and statistical analysis. Furthermore, throughout our review we have relied on those studies that report their results in Tailarach space. Without such standardized indicators of the location of changes of activity in the critical conditions, a comparison with other studies is not possible.

(a) Temporal pole

Five different mentalizing tasks as used in 10 studies have elicited activity in the temporal poles bilaterally, with somewhat greater effects on the left (Fig. 3.1). This region of the anterior temporal lobe is a site for the potential convergence of all sensory modalities and also limbic inputs (Moran *et al.* 1987). As shown in Fig. 3.2, this region is frequently activated in studies of language and semantics, although in these cases the activity is restricted to the left temporal pole. In particular, this region is activated when sentences are compared with unrelated word strings (Bottini *et al.* 1994; Vandenberghe *et al.* 2002), when narratives are compared with nonsense (Mazoyer *et al.* 1993) or with unrelated sentence strings (Fletcher *et al.* 1995), and when highly

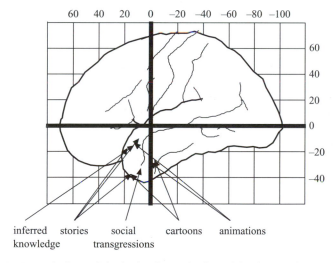

Fig. 3.1 Lateral view of the brain shown in the Talairach coordinate system. Peak activations in the temporal pole are shown for five different tasks used in 10 studies of mentalizing. Where activation was bilateral the two sides have been combined. Inferred knowledge: Goel *et al.* (1995); stories: Fletcher *et al.* (1995), Gallagher *et al.* (2000), Vogeley *et al.* (2001), Ferstl and von Cramon (2002); social transgressions: Berthoz *et al.* (2002); cartoons: Brunet *et al.* (2000), Gallagher *et al.* (2000); animations: Castelli *et al.* (2000), Schultz *et al.* (2003).

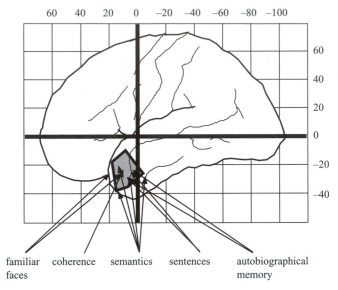

Fig. 3.2 Lateral view of the brain shown in the Talairach coordinate system. The shaded area shows the region activated by the studies of mentalizing shown in detail in Fig. 3.1. Peak activations are shown for 11 studies of other processes that activate adjacent regions of the temporal poles. Familiar faces and voices: Nakamura *et al.* (2000, 2001); coherence: Maguire *et al.* (1999); semantics: Vandenberge *et al.* (1996), Noppeney and Price (2002*a,b*); sentences: Bottini *et al.* (1994), Vandenberghe *et al.* (2002); autobiographical memory: Fink *et al.* (1996), Maguire and Mummery (1999), Maguire *et al.* (2000).

coherent narratives are compared with less coherent narratives (Maguire *et al.* 1999). The same region is also activated when volunteers make semantic decisions (e.g. Which is more similar to cow? Horse or bear? (Vandenberghe *et al.* 1996; see also Noppeney and Price 2002*a,b*)). In addition, this area is activated during memory retrieval. This is particularly the case during retrieval from autobiographical memory (Fink *et al.* 1996; Maguire and Mummery 1999; Maguire *et al.* 2000), during the incidental retrieval of emotional context in single-word recognition (Maratos *et al.* 2001) and during the recognition of familiar faces, scenes and voices (Nakamura *et al.* 2000, 2001).

We tentatively conclude that this region is concerned with generating, on the basis of past experience, a wider semantic and emotional context for the material currently being processed. This function would aid the interpretation of stories and pictures whether or not they involve mentalizing. One component of the wider semantic context is sometimes referred to as a 'script' (Schank and Abelson 1977). Scripts are built up through experience and record the particular goals and activities that take place in a particular setting at a particular time. A much used example is the 'restaurant script' which leads us to expect that we will first get the menu, then order, taste the wine, and so on. Identifying which script is most appropriate to a situation will be of considerable help in predicting what people are going to do. The temporal poles, especially on the left, may well be concerned with the retrieval of scripts. Patients with semantic dementia show atrophy in the anterior temporal lobes, especially on the left (Chan *et al.* 2001). As this atrophy progresses, these patients lose knowledge of all but the simplest and most concrete scripts (Funnell 2001).

Scripts provide a useful framework within which mentalizing can be applied. Events rarely conform exactly to the established script and mentalizing is needed to understand the deviations.

(b) Posterior STS

Mentalizing tasks elicit activity in the posterior STS (temporo-parietal junction extending towards the angular gyrus) bilaterally with somewhat greater effect on the right (see Fig. 3.3). The same 10 studies as shown in figure 1 are represented in this diagram. Fig. 3.4 shows activations of this region by 19 other studies, mostly concerned with living agents and biological motion. The posterior STS is also a multimodal convergence zone with connections to the limbic system (Barnes and Pandya 1992). It is well known that this region is activated when volunteers observe biological motion (see Allison *et al.* 2000;

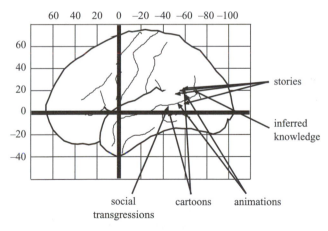

Fig. 3.3 Lateral view of the brain shown in the Talairach coordinate system. Peak activations in the posterior STS are shown for 10 studies of mentalizing. Where activation was bilateral the two sides have been combined. Stories: Fletcher *et al.* (1995), Gallagher *et al.* (2000), Vogeley *et al.* (2001), Ferstl and von Cramon (2002); inferred knowledge: Goel *et al.* (1995); animations: Castelli *et al.* (2000), Schultz *et al.* (2003); cartoons: Brunet *et al.* (2000), Gallagher *et al.* (2000); social transgressions: Berthoz *et al.* (2002).

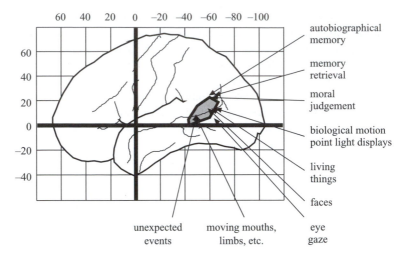

Fig. 3.4 Lateral view of the brain shown in the Talairach coordinate system. The shaded area shows the region activated by studies of mentalizing shown in detail in Fig, 3.3 Peak activations are shown for 19 studies of other processes that activate adjacent regions of the STS. Autobiographical memory: Vandenberge *et al.* (1996), Maguire and Mummery (1999), Maguire *et al.* (2000); memory retrieval: Maratos *et al.* (2001), Lee *et al.* (2002); moral judgement: Greene *et al.* (2001); biological motion, point light displays: Bonda *et al.* (1996), Grossman *et al.* (2000), Grèzes *et al.* (2001); living things: Price *et al.* (1997), Chao *et al.* (1999); static faces: Chao *et al.* (1999); eye gaze: Wicker *et al.* (1998), Hoffman and Haxby (2000); biological motion, mouths, eyes, hands: Puce *et al.* (1998), Grezes *et al.* (1998), Calvert *et al.* (2000), Campbell *et al.* (2001); unexpected events: Downar *et al.* (2000), Corbetta *et al.* (2000).

Chapter 1 this volume). Activation is seen during presentation of moving bodies and parts of bodies (Grezes *et al.* 1998; Puce *et al.* 1998; Campbell *et al.* 2001), while hearing speech and seeing speaking mouths (Calvert *et al.* 2000), and during presentations of action reduced to moving points of light (Bonda *et al.* 1996; Grossman *et al.* 2000; Grezes *et al.* 2001). The location of the maximum response to biological motion is around 10 mm superior and anterior to V5, which responds to visual motion in general (Zeki *et al.* 1991). However, this region of the STS is also activated by static images of faces and animals (e.g. Chao *et al.* 1999) especially when attending to eye gaze (Wicker *et al.* 1998; Hoffman and Haxby 2000), by names of animals (e.g. Chao *et al.* 1999), and by making semantic decisions about living things (e.g. Price *et al.* 1997). These observations suggest that this region is activated when observing the behaviour of living things and also when retrieving information about the behaviour of living things. An adjacent area closer to the angular gyrus is also activated by retrieval from semantic memory (e.g. Vandenberghe *et al.* 1996; Maratos *et al.* 2001; Lee *et al.* 2002) and from autobiographical memory (e.g. Maguire and Mummery 1999; Maguire *et al.* 2000). Whether this activity is specific to retrieval of memories about living things is not yet known.

An interesting set of parallel observations have been made about the area of fusiform gyrus that was activated in the two studies that elicited mentalizing using animations (Castelli *et al.* 2000; Schultz *et al.* 2003). This is also an area that seems to be concerned with knowledge about living things such as faces and animals (Chao *et al.* 1999). Presumably the knowledge in this region in the ventral stream primarily concerns the appearance of living things, their form and colour, rather than their patterns of behaviour. For example, this region is more active than the STS when volunteers make decisions about the identity of faces (Hoffman and Haxby 2000).

There is, however, another kind of event that elicits activity in the STS and does not specifically involve living things. An unexpected change of stimulation in any modality elicits activity in the same location as biological motion (Corbetta *et al.* 2000; Downar *et al.* 2000). Furthermore, learning to follow complex but predictable patterns of movement activates this region (Maquet *et al.* 2003). These results suggest that this region is not specifically concerned with the behaviour of living things, but with complex behaviour whatever its source. Nevertheless, we suggest that sudden changes of stimulation and complex patterns of movement are far more likely to be associated with living things than with mechanical or physical systems.

Knowledge about complex behaviour and, in particular, the ability to predict the next move in a sequence of behaviour is extremely valuable in any social interaction and could underlie some of the precursors of mentalizing, like gaze following and joint attention. Indeed it is known that activity in the STS increases when volunteers are asked to attend to gaze direction (Hoffman and Haxby 2000). The mentalizing system goes one step further and uses the observed patterns of behaviour to perceive the mental states that underlie this behaviour.

(c) MPFC

All 12 mentalizing tasks available to this review have elicited activity in the MPFC, with the interactive gameplaying tasks (McCabe *et al.* 2001; Gallagher *et al.* 2002) activating this region only (see Fig. 3.5). The medial prefrontal region activated by these studies is the most anterior part of the paracingulate cortex, where it lies anterior to the genu of the corpus callosum and the ACC proper. The MPFC has direct connections to the temporal pole and to the STS (Bachevalier *et al.* 1997). The paracingulate cortex (BA 32) is often considered to be part of the ACC that incorporates the cytoarchitectonically defined Brodmann areas 24, 25 and 33. The ACC is an ancient structure that has been broadly defined by Broca as belonging to the limbic lobe (Bush *et al.* 2000).

However, the existence of an unusual type of projection neuron (spindle cell) found in the sub-areas of the ACC 24a, 24b and 24c in the human, and

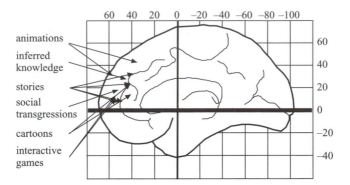

Fig. 3.5 Medial view of the brain shown in the Talairach coordinate system. Peak activations are shown for the 10 studies of mentalizing shown in Fig. 3.1 and Fig. 3.3. In addition, two studies using a sixth mentalizing task (interactive games) are included which only activated the MPFC. Animations: Castelli *et al.* (2000), Schultz *et al.* (2003); inferred knowledge: Goel *et al.* (1995); stories: Fletcher *et al.* (1995), Gallagher *et al.* (2000), Vogeley *et al.* (2001), Ferstl and von Cramon (2002); social transgressions: Berthoz *et al.* (2002); cartoons: Brunet *et al.* (2000), Gallagher *et al.* (2000); interactive games: McCabe *et al.* (2001), Gallagher *et al.* (2002).

some other higher primates (pongids and hominids) but not monkeys, is evidence that the ACC has undergone changes in recent evolution (Nimchinsky *et al.* 1999). Furthermore, in humans these cells are not present at birth, but first appear at approximately four months of age (Allman *et al.* 2001). However, BA 32 has been described as cytoarchitectonically a cingulo-frontal transition area (Devinsky *et al.* 1995) and therefore anatomically (and speculatively functionally) distinct from the ACC proper. It remains to be seen whether the recent evolutionary changes observed in the ACC are relevant to the more anterior region of medial frontal lobe where activations associated with mentalizing are observed. Recent anatomical changes in this region would be consistent with the observation that mentalizing has never been observed in monkeys (Cheney and Seyfarth 1990) and can only be found in a most rudimentary form in great apes (Byrne and Whiten 1988; Povinelli and Preuss 1995; Heyes 1998).

Evidence from anatomy and from functional studies shows that the ACC can be divided into distinct areas with different functions, as indicated in Fig. 3.6. In terms of the nomenclature of Picard and Strick (1996) the mentalizing region overlaps with, but is mostly anterior to, the rCZa. In terms of the functional nomenclature of Bush *et al.* (2000) the mentalizing region overlaps with the emotional division of the ACC.

(i) Executive processes
One plausible characterization of mentalizing tasks is that they involve complex problem solving of the type required by executive tasks, but this idea is

not supported by imaging studies. Many kinds of executive tasks are known to activate the ACC. Duncan and Owen (2000) have performed a careful meta-analysis of such tasks showing that increasing the difficulty in a wide range of tasks activates the same region of the ACC whatever the nature of the task. However, all but one of the 26 peak activations that they list lie posterior to the mentalizing region, being centred instead in the rCZp. The mean coordinates derived from the meta-analysis of Stroop-like tasks from Barch *et al.* (2001) also lie in this division of the ACC (see Fig. 3.6). Independent confirmation of this distinction between executive tasks and theory of mind tasks comes from studies of patients with lesions. Patients can be found who perform executive tasks very badly, while still performing mentalizing tasks well (Varley *et al.* 2001) and vice versa (Fine *et al.* 2001). Rowe *et al.* (2001)

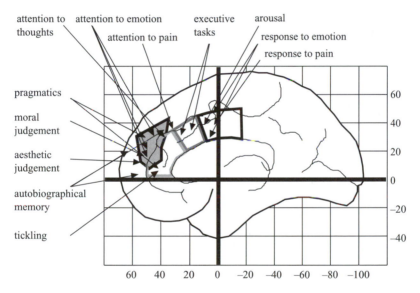

Fig. 3.6 Medial view of the brain shown in the Talairach coordinate system. The shaded area shows the region activated by studies of mentalizing shown in detail in figure 5. Peak activations are shown for 19 studies of other processes that activate the ACC and adjacent MPFC. Approximate divisions of the ACC are shown. From right to left: cCZ, rCZ, rCZa. Arousal: Critchley *et al.* (2000, 2001); response to emotion: Lane *et al.* (1998), Gusnard *et al.* (2001); response to pain: Rainville *et al.* (1999), Petrovic and Ingvar (2002); executive tasks: Duncan and Owen (2000), Barch *et al.* (2001); attention to emotion: Lane *et al.* (1997), Gusnard *et al.* (2001); attention to pain: Rainville *et al.* (1999), Petrovic and Ingvar (2002); attention to thoughts: McGuire *et al.* (1996); pragmatics: Bottini *et al.* (1994), Ferstl and von Cramon (2002); moral judgement: Greene *et al.* (2001); aesthetic judgement: Zysset *et al.* (2002); autobiographical memory: Maguire and Mummery (1999), Maguire *et al.* (2000); tickling: Blakemore *et al.* (1998).

observed that patients with frontal-lobe lesions performed badly on mentalizing tasks and executive tasks. However, within this group poor performance on one type of task was not related to poor performance on the other type of task.

(ii) Representing emotion

The recent meta-analysis of Phan *et al.* (2002) shows that tasks involving emotion can elicit activity in most regions of the ACC including the mentalizing region. What is the difference between the kinds of emotional task that activate the different divisions of the ACC? Lane (2000) highlights an important distinction between having an emotional experience and attending to an emotional experience. Lane *et al.* (1998) studied the effects of having an emotional experience by comparing responses to emotional experiences (happiness, sadness and disgust) with those to neutral experiences. The contrast revealed activity in the ACC, but in a posterior part at the border of the rostral cingulate zone and the cCZ. In another study, Lane *et al.* (1997) investigated the effects of attending to an emotion. Volunteers were shown emotionally arousing scenes. In one condition they indicated whether the scene was indoors or outdoors, while in the other condition they indicated the emotion aroused in them by the picture. When volunteers attended to their emotional experience, activity was seen in the mentalizing region, just anterior to the rCZa. The same distinction was observed by Gusnard *et al.* (2001) in a replication of Lane *et al.* (1997). Volunteers were shown pleasant, unpleasant or neutral scenes and were asked to indicate either their emotional response or whether the scenes were indoors or outdoors. Emotionally laden scenes elicited activity in the posterior ACC (cCZ at the border with supplementary motor area) whatever the task, while attention to emotion increased activity in the mentalizing region.

Petrovic and Ingvar (2002) have pointed out that a very similar distinction can be found in the study of pain. As stimuli become increasingly noxious, increases in activity are seen in the cCZ. However, the *perception* of pain does not relate directly to the nature of the stimulus, but can be altered by cognitive manipulations such as hypnotic suggestion, distraction or placebo analgesia. Variations in the perception of pain are related to activity in the rCZa overlapping with the mentalizing region. These studies of emotion and pain suggest that first-order representations of these states are located in the cCZ where correlates of arousal and stress are also observed (Critchley *et al.* 2000). Second-order representations of these states, available for attention and report, are located in the rCZa. We call these representations second order because they do not reflect the physical nature of the stimulus, but the mental attitude to that stimulus. To use the terminology of Leslie (1994), these representations are *decoupled* from the physical world and are no longer subject to normal input–output relations.

This formulation is consistent with our earlier suggestion (Frith and Frith 1999) that the mentalizing region of the MPFC is engaged when we attend to our own mental states as well as the mental states of others. Other situations where attention to mental states of the self activates this region include attention to the irrelevant thoughts that occur during scanning (McGuire *et al.* 1996) and attention to being tickled (Blakemore *et al.* 1998). We would also include two other tasks as examples of attending to the emotional states of the self although this was not necessarily the interpretation given by the authors. Zysset *et al.* (2002) observed activation in the mentalizing area when volunteers evaluated things (for example, answering the question, 'Do you like Leipzig?'). Greene *et al.* (2001) observed activation in the same area when volunteers considered moral dilemmas. We suggest that one component in the answering of such questions involves attending to the emotion aroused by topic (Does the thought of Leipzig make me happy or sad? How distressed would I feel if I had to take this particular course of action?). It is notable that the moral dilemma study of Greene *et al.* also activated the STS component of the mentalizing system, and it may be argued that this task is also a mentalizing task.

(iii) Autobiographical memory
A rather different task that can require representations of the self is autobiographical memory. Tulving (1985) has suggested that there is a form of autobiographical or episodic memory in which we perform 'mental time travel' and relive our past experiences (autonoetic memory). This would be a case of representing a past mental state clearly decoupled from current reality. In a series of studies Eleanor Maguire and her colleagues (Maguire and Mummery 1999; Maguire *et al.* 2000, 2001) have shown that retrieval from autobiographical memory reliably activates the mentalizing region of the MPFC (in addition to medial temporal lobe structures and the STS). Autobiographical memory tasks can often be solved simply on the basis of a feeling of familiarity rather than truly reliving the event and it is usually difficult to relate these different processes to specific brain regions. However, Maguire *et al.* (2001) also studied patient Jon who has considerable memory problems associated with early and severe damage to his hippocampi. Jon spontaneously makes the distinction between past events that he can clearly remember happening and others that he knows a lot about, but does not recall the event occurring. Memories of events where he clearly remembered them happening were associated with greater activity in the MPFC. This effect was independent of his ratings of emotional intensity and valence for the events.

(iv) Pragmatics
The studies we have discussed so far are consistent with our suggestion that the area of MPFC activated in mentalizing tasks is concerned with the representation of the mental states of the self and others decoupled from reality. There is one last set of studies that at first glance cannot be so easily incorporated into this scheme. Ferstl and von Cramon (2002) have shown that a certain kind of language task activates the same region of the MPFC as a simple mentalizing task. In both cases volunteers heard pairs of sentences. Examples

of these sentence pairs include (i) 'Mary's exam was about to begin. Her palms were sweaty'; and (ii) 'The lights have been on since last night. The car doesn't start'. In the mentalizing task volunteers had to think about the motivations and feelings of the people in the sentences of type (i). In the language condition they had to decide whether there was a logical connection between the two sentences of type (ii). In comparison to a control task both conditions elicited activations in the mentalizing region of the MPFC.

Interpreting the two unlinked sentences in these examples depends upon an aspect of language processing often referred to as pragmatics. In many real-life cases the understanding of an utterance cannot be based solely on the meanings of the individual words (semantics) or upon the grammar by which they are connected (syntax). It has been proposed that a successful understanding of an utterance depends upon perceiving the intention of the speaker (Grice 1957). The idea that the purpose of utterances is for the listener to recognize the intention of the speaker has been elaborated by Sperber and Wilson (1995) in their theory of relevance. If this analysis is correct then pragmatics, the understanding of utterances, depends upon mentalizing whether or not this is required by the task instruction. This would apply also to the type (ii) sentences used by Ferstl and van Cramon (2002) where logical connections had to be found. For instance the example above may evoke the idea that 'someone (stupidly or maliciously) left the lights on'.

The need for mentalizing is particularly clear in nonliteral figures of speech such as metaphor and irony. Sperber and Wilson analyse the example in which a mother says to her daughter, 'Your room is a pigsty'. How is the daughter to understand this? Her room is not literally a pigsty, but it shares with pigsties the characteristic of being very messy and untidy. But why didn't the mother simply say, 'Your room is very messy and untidy'? This utterance would accurately describe the state of the room. The value of the metaphor in this example is that it not only conveys the state of the room, but also, as the mother intends, her displeasure at this state. We would therefore expect that metaphors, in comparison to literal statements, would activate the mentalizing area and this expectation has been confirmed in the study of Bottini et al. (1994). Irony (e.g. 'Peter is well read. He's even heard of Shakespeare') is an even more extreme example than metaphor since the listener has to recognize that the speaker intends to convey a meaning opposite to the literal content of the words (i.e. Peter is not at all well read). In such cases the meaning is decoupled from the words. We are not aware of any imaging study, but we would predict that the understanding of sarcasm or irony would activate the mentalizing network.

One aspect of pragmatics that has received little attention to date is the initiation of communication by calling someone's name or by gazing at them intently. These are sometimes referred to as 'ostensive' signals. Such stimuli normally signal the intention to communicate and therefore 'guarantee relevance' in Sperber and Wilson's terminology. The effects of such ostensive signals were examined in a recent neuroimaging study (Kampe et al. 2003).

Subjects were asked to respond to a rare target, while they viewed a series of faces with direct or averted gaze (versus scrambled faces) or listened to voices calling either the subject's own name or another name (versus scrambled voices). The results showed that independent of modality the initiation of communication activated two components of the mentalizing system, the MPFC and temporal poles. This study is consistent with other neuroimaging studies of pragmatics in demonstrating that the relationship between communicative and mentalizing functions is remarkably close.

3.5 Conclusions

We conclude, from the facts available to date, that the region of the MPFC associated with mentalizing tasks is activated whenever people are attending to certain states of the self or others. These states, which are usually referred to as mental states, must be decoupled from reality. To understand the response to pain, whether it is my pain or someone else's pain, I must represent, not the noxiousness of the stimulus, but how I or the other person perceive the pain. Likewise, it is not the unpleasantness of the picture that determines our emotional response to it, but the unpleasantness we feel. Such decoupled representations are also needed for mentalizing. What determines our behaviour is not the state of the world, but our beliefs about the state of the world. Activity in the MPFC is connected with the creation of these decoupled representations of beliefs about the world. In the case of false beliefs there is a discrepancy between the belief and the actual state of the world. However, we are not claiming that activity in the MPFC signals these discrepancies. This would be equivalent to error detection. We are claiming that the MPFC is equally active when true beliefs are involved. This is because beliefs may or may not map onto the actual state of the world. This would also be true for other mental states such as wishes, intentions and pretence. Activity in the MPFC signals that these representations are decoupled from the real world to which they may or may not correspond. Thus, the role of this particular region of the MPFC would be analogous to that of the more posterior region (rCZp) where neuronal activity signals the existence of response conflict or multiple response possibilities rather than errors (Petit *et al*. 1998; Botvinick *et al*. 1999).

Mentalizing is not only about representing our own thoughts, feelings and beliefs as distinct from reality. It is also about representing the mental states of other people. Clearly, other components of the mentalizing system need to supply the content of these thoughts, feelings and beliefs and their relation to people's actions. This knowledge is supplied partly from our knowledge of the world based on past experience applied to the current situation and partly from our observations and predictions about people's current behaviour (STS). Both types of knowledge help to understand the content of mental states and their relation to actions, and may be accessible via temporal poles and the STS.

By identifying the roles of the regions in this way it should be possible to link the various precursors of mentalizing that emerge during the first 4 years of life to specific components of the brain's mature mentalizing system. This will have to await the development of suitable methods for using fMRI techniques to study infants and young children.

The authors are grateful to Sarah Blakemore, Paul Fletcher, Josef Perner and Beate Sodian for their comments on this paper. This work was supported by MRC grant no. G961 7036 to U.F. C.D.F. is supported by the Wellcome Trust.

References

Allison, T., Puce, A. and McCarthy, G. (2000). Social perception from visual cues: role of the STS region. *Trends Cogn. Sci.* **4**, 267–78.

Allman, J. M., Hakeem, A., Erwin, J. M., Nimchinsky, E. and Hof, P. (2001). The anterior cingulate cortex—the evolution of an interface between emotion and cognition. *Unity Know. Converg. Nat. Hum. Sci.* **935**, 107–17.

Avis, J. and Harris, P. L. (1991). Belief–desire reasoning among Baka children—evidence for a universal conception of mind. *Child Dev.* **62**, 460–7.

Bachevalier, J., Meunier, M., Lu, M. X. and Ungerleider, L. G. (1997). Thalamic and temporal cortex input to medial prefrontal cortex in rhesus monkeys. *Exp. Brain Res.* **115**, 430–44.

Baldwin, D. A. and Moses, L. J. (1996). The ontogeny of social information gathering. *Child Dev.* **67**, 1915–39.

Barch, D. M., Braver, T. S., Akbudak, E., Conturo, T., Ollinger, J. and Snyder, A. (2001). Anterior cingulate cortex and response conflict: effects of response modality and processing domain. *Cereb. Cortex* **11**, 837–48.

Barnes, C. L. and Pandya, D. N. (1992). Efferent cortical connections of multimodal cortex of the superior temporal sulcus in the rhesus monkey. *J. Comp. Neurol.* **318**, 222–44.

Baron-Cohen, S., Leslie, A. M. and Frith, U. (1985). Does the autistic child have a theory of mind? *Cognition* **21**, 37–46.

Bertenthal, B. I., Proffitt, D. R. and Cutting, J. E. (1984). Infant sensitivity to figural coherence in biomechanical motions. *J. Exp. Child Psychol.* **37**, 213–30.

Berthoz, S., Armony, J. L., Blair, R. J. R. and Dolan, R. J. (2002). An fMRI study of intentional and unintentional (embarrassing) violations of social norms. *Brain* **125**, 1696–708.

Blakemore, J.-S., Wolpert, D. M. and Frith, C. D. (1998). Central cancellation of self-produced tickle sensation. *Nature Neurosci.* **1**, 635–9.

Bloom, P. (2000). *How children learn the meanings of words*. Cambridge, MA: MIT Press.

Bonda, E., Petrides, M., Ostry, D. and Evans, A. (1996). Specific involvement of human parietal systems and the amygdala in the perception of biological motion. *J. Neurosci.* **16**, 3737–44.

Bottini, G., Corcoran, R., Sterzi, R., Paulesu, E., Schenone, P., Scarpa, P., *et al.* (1994). The role of the right hemisphere in the interpretation of figurative aspects of language: a positron emission tomography activation study. *Brain* **117**, 1241–53.

Botvinick, M., Nystrom, L. E., Fissell, K., Carter, C. S. and Cohen, J. D. (1999). Conflict monitoring versus selection-foraction in anterior cingulate cortex. *Nature* **402**, 179–81.

Brunet, E., Sarfati, Y., Hardy-Bayle, M.-C. and Decety, J. (2000). A PET investigation of the attribution of intentions with a nonverbal task. *NeuroImage* **11**, 157–66.

Bush, G., Luu, P. and Posner, M. I. (2000). Cognitive and emotional influences in anterior cingulate cortex. *Trends Cogn. Sci.* **4**, 215–22.

Butterworth, G. (1991). The ontogeny and phylogeny of joint visual attention. In *Natural theories of mind: evolution, development and simulation of everyday mindreading* (ed. A. Whiten), pp. 223–32. Cambridge, MA: Blackwell.

Butterworth, G. and Jarrett, N. (1991). What minds have in common is space—spatial mechanisms serving joint visual-attention in infancy. *Br. J. Dev. Psychol.* **9**, 55–72.

Byrne, R. W. and Whiten, A. (1988). *Machiavellian intelligence.* Oxford: Clarendon Press.

Calvert, G. A., Campbell, R. and Brammer, M. J. (2000). Evidence from functional magnetic resonance imaging of crossmodal binding in the human heteromodal cortex. *Curr. Biol.* **10**, 649–57.

Campbell, R., MacSweeney, M., Surguladze, S., Calvert, G., McGuire, P., Suckling, J., *et al.* (2001). Cortical substrates for the perception of face actions: an fMRI study of the specificity of activation for seen speech and for meaningless lower-face acts (gurning). *Cogn. Brain Res.* **12**, 233–43.

Caron, A. J., Caron, R., Roberts, J. and Brooks, R. (1997). Infant sensitivity to deviations in dynamic facial–vocal displays: the role of eye regard. *Devl Psychol.* **33**, 802–13.

Carpenter, M., Nagell, K. and Tomasello, M. (1998). Social cognition, joint attention, and communicative competence from 9 to 15 months of age. *Monogr. Soc. Res. Child Dev.* **63**, 176.

Castelli, F., Happé, F., Frith, U. and Frith, C. D. (2000). Movement and mind: a functional imaging study of perception and interpretation of complex intentional movement patterns. *NeuroImage* **12**, 314–25.

Chan, D., Fox, N. C., Scahill, R. I., Crum, W. R., Whitwell, J. L., Leschziner, G., *et al.* (2001). Patterns of temporal lobe atrophy in semantic dementia and Alzheimer's disease. *Ann. Neurol.* **49**, 433–42.

Chao, L. L., Haxby, J. V. and Martin, A. (1999). Attribute-based neural substrates in temporal cortex for perceiving and knowing about objects. *Nature Neurosci.* **2**, 913–19.

Cheney, D. L. and Seyfarth, R. M. (1990). *How monkeys see the world: inside the mind of another species.* Chicago, IL: University of Chicago Press.

Clements, W. A. and Perner, J. (1994). Implicit understanding of belief. *Cogn. Dev.* **9**, 377–95.

Clements, W. A. and Perner, J. (2001). When actions really do speak louder than words, but only explicitly; young children's understanding of false belief in action. *Br. J. Devl Psychol.* **19**, 413–32.

Corbetta, M. (1993). Positron emission tomography as a tool to study human vision and attention. *Proc. Natl Acad. Sci. USA* **90**, 10901–3.

Corbetta, M., Kincade, J. M., Ollinger, J. M., McAvoy, M. P. and Shulman, G. L. (2000). Voluntary orienting is dissociated from target detection in human posterior parietal cortex. *Nature Neurosci.* **3**, 292–7.

Crichton, M. T. and Lange Kuettner, C. (1999). Animacy and propulsion in infancy: tracking, waving and reaching to self-propelled and induced moving objects. *Devl Sci.* **2**, 318–24.

Critchley, H. D., Corfield, D. R., Chandler, M. P., Mathias, C. J. and Dolan, R. J. (2000). Cerebral correlates of autonomic cardiovascular arousal: a functional neuroimaging investigation in humans. *J. Physiol. (Lond.)* **523**, 259–70.

Critchley, H. D., Mathias, C. T. and Dolan, R. J. (2001). Neuroanatomical basis for first- and second-order representations of bodily states. *Nature Neurosci.* **4**, 207–12.

Dennett, D. C. (1978). Beliefs about beliefs. *Behav. Brain Sci.* **1**, 568–70.

Devinsky, O., Morrell, M. J. and Vogt, B. A. (1995). Contributions of anterior cingulate cortex to behavior. *Brain* **118**, 279–306.

Downar, J., Crawley, A. P., Mikulis, D. J. and Davis, K. D. (2000). A multimodal cortical network for the detection of changes in the sensory environment. *Nature Neurosci.* **3**, 277–83.

Duncan, J. and Owen, A. M. (2000). Dissociative methods in the study of frontal lobe function. In *Control of cognitive processes*, vol. XVIII (ed. S. Monsell and J. Driver), pp. 567–76. Cambridge, MA: MIT Press.

Ferstl, E. C. and von Cramon, D. Y. (2002). What does the frontomedian cortex contribute to language processing: coherence or theory of mind? *NeuroImage* **17**, 1599–612.

Fine, C., Lumsden, J. and Blair, R. J. R. (2001). Dissociation between 'theory of mind' and executive functions in a patient with early left amygdala damage. *Brain* **124**, 287–98.

Fink, G. R., Markowitsch, H. J., Reinkemeier, M., Bruckbauer, T., Kessler, J. and Heiss, W. D. (1996). Cerebral representation of one's own past: neural networks involved in autobiographical memory. *J. Neurosci.* **16**, 4275–82.

Flavell, J. H., Everett, B. A., Croft, K. and Flavell, E. R. (1981). Young children's knowledge about visual-perception—further evidence for the level 1–level 2 distinction. *Devl Psychol.* **17**, 99–103.

Fletcher, P. C., Happé, F., Frith, U., Baker, S. C., Dolan, R. J., Frackowiak, R. S. J., *et al.* (1995). Other minds in the brain: a functional imaging study of 'theory of mind' in story comprehension. *Cognition* **44**, 283–96; **57**, 109–28.

Frith, C. D. and Frith, U. (1999). Interacting minds—a biological basis. *Science* **286**, 1692–5.

Funnell, E. (2001). Evidence for scripts in semantic dementia. Implications for theories of semantic memory. *Cogn. Neuropsychol.* **18**, 323–41.

Gallagher, H. L., Happe, F., Brunswick, N., Fletcher, P. C., Frith, U. and Frith, C. D. (2000). Reading the mind in cartoons and stories: an fMRI study of 'theory of mind' in verbal and nonverbal tasks. *Neuropsychologia* **38**, 11–21.

Gallagher, H. L., Jack, A. I., Roepstorff, A. and Frith, C. D. (2002). Imaging the intentional stance. *NeuroImage* **16**, 814–21.

Gergely, G., Knadasdy, Z., Csibra, G. and Biro, S. (1995). Taking the international stance at 12 months of age. *Cognition* **56**, 165–93.

Goel, V., Grafman, J. N. S. and Hallett, M. (1995). Modelling other minds. *NeuroReport* **6**, 1741–6.

Gopnik, A. and Wellman, H. M. (1994). The theory. In *Mapping the mind: domain specificity in cognition and culture* (ed. L. A. Hirschfeld and S. A. Gelman), pp. 257–93. New York: Cambridge University Press.

Greene, J. D., Sommerville, R. B., Nystrom, L. E., Darley, J. M. and Cohen, J. D. (2001). An fMRI investigation of emotional engagement in moral judgment. *Science* **293**, 2105–8.

Grezes, J., Costes, N. and Decety, J. (1998). Top-down effect of strategy on the percption of human biological motion: a PET investigation. *Cogn. Neuropsychol.* **15**, 553–82.

Grezes, J., Fonlupt, P., Bertenthal, B., Delon-Martin, C., Segebarth, C. and Decety, J. (2001). Does perception of biological motion rely on specific brain regions? *NeuroImage* **13**, 775–85.

Grice, H. P. (1957). *Meaning. Phil. Rev.* **66**, 377–88.

Grossman, E., Donnelly, M., Price, R., Pickens, D., Morgan, V., Neighbor, G., *et al.* (2000). Brain areas involved in perception of biological motion. *J. Cogn. Neurosci.* **12**, 711–20.

Gusnard, D. A., Akbudak, E., Shulman, G. L. and Raichle, M. E. (2001). Medial prefrontal cortex and self-referential mental activity: relation to a default mode of brain function. *Proc. Natl Acad. Sci. USA* **98**, 4259–64.

Happé, F. G. E. (1994). An advanced test of theory of mind: understanding of story characters' thoughts and feelings by able autistic, mentally handicapped and normal children and adults. *J. Autism Devl Disord.* **24**, 129–54.

Harris, P. L. (1991). The work of the imagination. In *Natural theories of mind: evolution, development and simulation of everyday mindreading* (ed. A. Whiten), pp. 283–304. Cambridge, MA: Blackwell.

Heider, F. and Simmel, M. (1944). An experimental study of apparent behaviour. *Am. J. Psychol.* **57**, 243–59.

Heyes, C. M. (1998). Theory of mind in nonhuman primates. *Behav. Brain Sci.* **21**, 101–34.

Hoffman, E. A. and Haxby, J. V. (2000). Distinct representations of eye gaze and identity in the distributed human neural system for face perception. *Nature Neurosci.* **3**, 80–4.

Hogrefe, G. J., Wimmer, H. and Perner, J. (1986). Ignorance versus false belief—a developmental lag in attribution of epistemic states. *Child Dev.* **57**, 567–82.

Hood, B. M., Willen, J. D. and Driver, J. (1998). Adult's eyes trigger shifts of visual attention in human infants. *Psychol. Sci.* **9**, 131–4.

Johnson, M. H. and Morton, J. (1991). *Biology and cognitive development: the case of face recognition.* Oxford: Blackwell.

Kampe, K., Frith, C. D. and Frith, U. (2003). 'Hey John': signals conveying communicative intention towards the self activate brain regions associated with mentalizing regardless of modality. *J. Neurosci.* **23**, 5258–63.

Lane, R. D. (2000). Neural correlates of conscious emotional experience. In *Cognitive neuroscience of emotion* (ed. R. D. Lane and L. Nadel), pp. 345–70. New York: Oxford University Press.

Lane, R. D., Fink, G. R., Chua, P. M. and Dolan, R. J. (1997). Neural activation during selective attention to subjective emotional responses. *NeuroReport* **8**, 3969–72.

Lane, R. D., Reiman, E. M., Axelrod, B., Yun, L. S., Holmes, A. and Schwartz, G. E. (1998). Neural correlates of levels of emotional awareness: evidence of an interaction between emotion and attention in the anterior cingulate cortex. *J. Cogn. Neurosci.* **10**, 525–35.

Lee, A. C. H., Robbins, T. W., Graham, K. S. and Owen, A. M. (2002). 'Pray or prey?' Dissociation of semantic memory retrieval from episodic memory processes using positron emission tomography and a novel homophone task. *Neuroimage* **16**, 724–35.

Legerstee, M. (1992). A review of the animate/inanimate distinction in infancy. *Early Dev. Parent.* **1**, 59–67.

Lempers, J. D., Flavell, E. R. and Flavell, J. H. (1977). The development in very young children of tacit knowledge concerning visual perception. *Genet. Psychol. Monogr.* **95**, 3–53.

Leslie, A. M. (1987). Pretence and representation: the origins of 'theory of mind'. *Psychol. Rev.* **94**, 412–26.

Leslie, A. M. (1994). Pretending and believing: issues in the theory of mind TOMM. *Cognition* **50**, 211–38.

Lillard, A. (1998). Ethnopsychologies: cultural variations in theories of mind. *Psychol. Bull.* **123**, 3–32.

McCabe, K., Houser, D., Ryan, L., Smith, V. and Trouard, T. (2001). A functional imaging study of cooperation in two-person reciprocal exchange. *Proc. Natl Acad. Sci. USA* **98**, 11832–5.

McGuire, P. K., Paulesu, E., Frackowiak, R. S. J. and Frith, C. D. (1996). Brain activity during stimulus independent thought. *NeuroReport* **7**, 2095–9.

Maguire, E. A. and Mummery, C. J. (1999). Differential modulation of a common memory retrieval network revealed by positron emission tomography. *Hippocampus* **9**, 54–61.

Maguire, E. A., Frith, C. D. and Morris, R. G. M. (1999). The functional neuroanatomy of comprehension and memory: the importance of prior knowledge. *Brain* **122**, 1839–50.

Maguire, E. A., Mummery, C. J. and Buchel, C. (2000). Patterns of hippocampal–cortical interaction dissociate temporal lobe memory subsystems. *Hippocampus* **10**, 475–82.

Maguire, E. A., Vargha-Khadem, F. and Mishkin, M. (2001). The effects of bilateral hippocampal damage on fMRI regional activations and interactions during memory retrieval. *Brain* **124**, 1156–70.

Maquet, P., Schwartz, S., Passingham, R. and Frith, C. D. (2003). Sleep-related consolidation of a visuo-motor skill: brain mechanisms as assessed by fMRI. *J. Neurosci.* **23**, 1432–40.

Maratos, E. J., Dolan, R. J., Morris, J. S., Henson, R. N. A. and Rugg, M. D. (2001). Neural activity associated with episodic memory for emotional context. *Neuropsychologia* **39**, 910–20.

Masangkay, Z. S., McCluskey, K. A., McIntyre, C. W., Sims-Knight, J., Vaughn, B. E. and Flavell, T. H. (1974). The early development of inferences about the visual percepts of others. *Child Dev* **45**, 357–66.

Mazoyer, B. M., Tzourio, N., Frak, V., Syrota, A., Murayama, N., Levrier, O., *et al.* (1993). The cortical representation of speech. *J. Cogn. Neurosci.* **5**, 467–79.

Meltzoff, A. N. (1995). Understanding the intentions of others—re-enactment of intended acts by 18-month-old children. *Devl Psychol.* **31**, 838–50.

Moran, M. A., Mufson, E. J. and Mesulam, M. M. (1987). Neural inputs into the temporopolar cortex of the rhesus monkey. *J. Comp. Neurol.* **256**, 88–103.

Nakamura, K., Kawashima, R., Sato, N., Nakamura, A., Sugiura, M., Kato, T., *et al.* (2000). Functional delineation of the human occipito- temporal areas related to face and scene processing—a PET study. *Brain* **123**, 1903–12.

Nakamura, K., Kawashima, R., Sugiara, M., Kato, T., Nakamura, A., Hatano, K., *et al.* (2001). Neural substrates for recognition of familiar voices: a PET study. *Neuropsychologia* **39**, 1047–54.

Nimchinsky, E. A., Gilissen, E., Allman, J. M., Perl, D. P., Erwin, J. M. and Hof, P. R. (1999). A neuronal morphologic type unique to humans and great apes. *Proc. Natl Acad. Sci. USA* **96**, 5268–73.

Noppeney, U. and Price, C. J. (2002*a*). A PET study of stimulus and task-induced semantic processing. *NeuroImage* **15**, 927–35.

Noppeney, U. and Price, C. J. (2002*b*). Retrieval of visual, auditory, and abstract semantics. *NeuroImage* **15**, 917–26.

O'Neill, D. (1996). Two-year-old children's sensitivity to a parent's knowledge state when making requests. *Child Dev.* **67**, 659–77.

O'Neill, D. and Gopnik, A. (1991). Young children's ability to identify the sources of their beliefs. *Devl Psychol.* **27**, 390–7.

Onishi, K. H. and Baillargeon, R. (2002). 15-month-old infants' understanding of false belief. *Int. Conf. Infant Studies, Toronto, Canada.*

Perner, J. and Wimmer, H. (1985). 'John thinks that Mary thinks that…': attribution of second-order beliefs by 5- to 10-year-old children. *J. Exp. Child Psychol.* **39**, 437–71.

Perner, J., Leekam, S. R. and Wimmer, H. (1987). 2-year-olds difficulty with false belief—the case for a conceptual deficit. *Br. J. Devl Psychol.* **5**, 125–37.

Petit, L., Courtney, S. M., Ungerleider, L. G. and Haxby, J. V. (1998). Sustained activity in the medial wall during working memory delays. *J. Neurosci.* **18**, 9429–37.

Petrovic, P. and Ingvar, M. (2002). Imaging cognitive modulation of pain processing. *Pain* **95**, 1–5.

Phan, K. L., Wager, T., Taylor, S. F. and Liberzon, I. (2002). Functional neuroanatomy of emotion: a meta-analysis of emotion activation studies in PET and fMRI. *NeuroImage* **16**, 331–48.

Phillips, A. T., Wellman, H. M. and Spelke, E. S. (2002). Infants' ability, to connect gaze and emotional expression to intentional action. *Cognition* **85**, 53–78.

Picard, N. and Strick, P. L. (1996). Motor areas of the medial wall: a review of their location and functional activation. *Cereb. Cortex* **6**, 342–53.

Poulin-Dubois, D., Tilden, J., Sodian, B., Metz, U. and Schöppner, B. (2003). Implicit understanding of the seeing– knowing relation in 14- to 24-month-old children. (Submitted.)

Povinelli, D. J. and Bering, J. M. (2002). The mentality of apes revisited. *Curr. Direct. Psychol. Sci.* **11**, 115–19.

Povinelli, D. J. and deBlois, S. (1992). Young children's (*Homo sapiens*) understanding of knowledge formation in themselves and others. *J. Comp. Psychol.* **106**, 228–38.

Povinelli, D. J. and Preuss, T. M. (1995). Theory of mind: evolutionary history of a cognitive specialization. *Trends Neurosci.* **18**, 418–24.

Premack, D. and Woodruff, G. (1978). Does the chimpanzee have a theory of mind? *Behav. Brain. Sci.* **1**, 515–26.

Price, C. J., Moore, C. J., Humphreys, G. W. and Wise, R. J. S. (1997). Segregating semantic from phonological processes during reading. *J. Cogn. Neurosci.* **9**, 727–33.

Puce, A., Allison, T., Bentin, S., Gore, J. C. and McCarthy, G. (1998). Temporal cortex activation in humans viewing eye and mouth movements. *J. Neurosci.* **18**, 2188–99.

Rainville, P., Hofbauer, R. K., Paus, T., Duncan, G. H., Bushnell, M. C. and Price, D. D. (1999). Cerebral mechanisms of hypnotic induction and suggestion. *J. Cogn. Neurosci.* **11**, 110–25.

Repacholi, B. M. (1998). Infants' use of attentional cues to identify the referent of another person's emotional expression. *Devl Psychol.* **34**, 1017–25.

Rizzolatti, G., Fogassi, L. and Gallese, V. (2002). Motor and cogntiive functions of the ventral premotor cortex. *Curr. Opin. Neurobiol.* **12**, 149–54.

Rowe, A. D., Bullock, P. R., Polkey, C. E. and Morris, R. G. (2001). 'Theory of mind' impairments and their relationship to executive functioning following frontal lobe excisions. *Brain* **124**, 600–16.

Ruffman, T., Perner, J., Naito, M., Parkin, L. and Clements, W. A. (1998). Older (but not younger) siblings facilitate false belief understanding. *Devl Psychol.* **34**, 161–74.

Russell, J. (1996). *Agency: its role in mental development.* Oxford: Erlbaum.

Schank, R. C. and Abelson, R. P. (1977). *Scripts, plans, goals and understanding: an inquiry into human knowledge structures.* Hillsdale, NJ: Erlbaum.

Schultz, R. T., Grelotti, D. J., Klin, A., Kleinman, J., Van der Gaag, C., Marois, R., *et al.* (2003). The role of the fusiform face area in social cognition: implications for the pathobiology of autism. *Phil. Trans. R. Soc. Lond.* B **358**, 415–24. (DOI 10.1098/rstb.2002.1208.)

Shatz, M., Wellman, H. M. and Silber, S. (1983). The acquisition of mental verbs—a systematic investigation of the 1st reference to mental state. *Cognition* **14**, 301–21.

Sodian, B. and Thoermer, C. (2003). Infants' understanding of looking, pointing and reaching as cues to goal-directed action. (Submitted.)

Spelke, E. S., Phillips, A. and Woodward, A. L. (1995). Infants' knowledge of object motion and human action. In *Causal cognition: a multidisciplinary debate. Symp. Fyssen Foundation* (ed. D. Sperber and D. Premack), pp. 44–78. New York: Clarendon Press/Oxford University Press.

Sperber, D. and Wilson, D. (1995). *Relevance: communication and cognition.* Oxford: Blackwell Scientific.

Sullivan, K., Zaitchik, D. and Tagerflusberg, H. (1994). Preschoolers can attribute 2nd-order beliefs. *Devl Psychol.* **30**, 395–402.

Tulving, E. (1985). Memory and consciousness. *Can. Psychol.* **26**, 1–12.

Vandenberghe, R., Price, C., Wise, R., Josephs, O. and Frackowiak, R. S. J. (1996). Functional anatomy of a common semantic system for words and pictures. *Nature* **383**, 254–6.

Vandenberghe, R., Nobre, A. C. and Price, C. J. (2002). The response of left temporal cortex to sentences. *J. Cogn. Neurosci.* **14**, 550–60.

Varley, R., Siegal, M. and Want, S. C. (2001). Severe impairment in grammar does not preclude theory of mind. *Neurocase* **7**, 489–93.

Vogeley, K., Bussfeld, P., Newen, A., Herrmann, S., Happé, F., Falkai, P., *et al.* (2001). Mind reading: neural mechanisms of theory of mind and self-perspective. *NeuroImage* **14**, 170–81.

Wellman, H. M. and Estes, D. (1986). Early understanding of mental entities—a re-examination of childhood realism. *Child Dev.* **57**, 910–23.

Wellman, H. M., Phillips, A. T. and Rodriguez, T. (2000). Young children's understanding of perception, desire, and emotion. *Child Dev.* **71**, 895–912.

Wicker, B., Michel, F., Henaff, M. and Decety, J. (1998). Brain regions involved in the perception of gaze: a PET study. *NeuroImage* **8**, 221–7.

Wimmer, H. and Perner, J. (1983). Beliefs about beliefs—representation and constraining function of wrong beliefs in young children's understanding of deception. *Cognition* **13**, 103–28.

Woodward, A. L. (1998). Infants selectively encode the goal object of an actor's reach. *Cognition* **69**, 1–34.

Woodward, A. L., Sommerville, J. A. and Guajardo, J. J. (2001). How infants make sense of intentional action. In *Intentions and intentionality: foundations of social cognition* (ed. B. F. Malle and L. J. Moses), pp. 149–69. Cambridge, MA: MIT Press.

Zeki, S., Watson, J. D., Lueck, C. J., Friston, K. J., Kennard, C. and Frackowiak, R. S. (1991). A direct demonstration of functional specialization in human visual cortex. *J. Neurosci.* **11**, 641–9.

Zysset, S., Huber, O., Ferstl, E. and von Cramon, D. Y. (2002). The anterior frontomedian cortex and evaluative judgment: an fMRI study. *NeuroImage* **15**, 983–91.

Glossary

ACC: anterior cingulate cortex
cCZ: caudal cingulate zone
fMRI: functional magnetic resonance imaging
rCZp: rostral cingulate zone, posterior part
rCZa: rostral cingulate zone, anterior part
MPFC: medial prefrontal cortex
STS: superior temporal sulcus

4

Mathematical modelling of animate and intentional motion

Jens Rittscher, Andrew Blake, Anthony Hoogs, and Gees Stein

Our aim is to enable a machine to observe and interpret the behaviour of others. Mathematical models are employed to describe certain biological motions. The main challenge is to design models that are both tractable and meaningful. In the first part we will describe how computer vision techniques, in particular visual tracking, can be applied to recognize a small vocabulary of human actions in a constrained scenario. Mainly the problems of viewpoint and scale invariance need to be overcome to formalize a general framework. Hence the second part of the article is devoted to the question whether a particular human action should be captured in a single complex model or whether it is more promising to make extensive use of semantic knowledge and a collection of low-level models that encode certain motion primitives. Scene context plays a crucial role if we intend to give a higher-level interpretation rather than a low-level physical description of the observed motion. A semantic knowledge base is used to establish the scene context. This approach consists of three main components: visual analysis, the mapping from vision to language and the search of the semantic database. A small number of robust visual detectors is used to generate a higher-level description of the scene. The approach together with a number of results is presented in the third part of this article.

Keywords: computer vision; event recognition; visual tracking; video annotation; mapping from vision to language

4.1 Introduction

Rather than understanding the perception of biological motion we intend to construct a machine that is able to recognize certain biological motions. The crucial question before we derive any mathematical model is the choice of which representation to use. We are particularly interested in computationally efficient approaches that facilitate the instantaneous classification of the observed motion. Moving light displays (Johansson 1976) are often used to test our ability to recognize biological motion. The nature of the internal representations the human visual system uses to recognize these sequences is of particular interest to this work. Bülthoff and Bülthoff (2003) designed a number of experiments to determine whether or not the human recognition capability depends on the viewpoint of the scene. Based on the results of these experiments they conclude that the subjects' recognition performance is strongly tied to the familiarity of the viewpoint from which the sequences are captured. The fact that stereo-depth information only marginally improves the recognition performance furthermore indicates that the internal motion models emphasize the 2D trajectory structure of the sequence over its 3D structure.

Hence the guiding principle of this work is to find an appearance-based approach such that it is not necessary to estimate the person's pose in order to classify the type of motion. Therefore we avoid the use of an articulated model such as a stick figure model or a 3D skeleton. The pose estimation itself is central to the problem of human motion capture. Recent advances in computer vision (Deutscher *et al.* 2000; Sidenbladh *et al.* 2000) allow us to solve the pose estimation problem without having any kind of markers attached to their bodies. But in order to resolve ambiguities multiple views are necessary to accurately estimate the pose. In turn we intend to recognize the type of motion based on the apparent motion. In the current context of this article, one interesting point of discussion would be if the appearance-based information alone is sufficient for movement generation as discussed by Schaal *et al.* (this volume, Chapter 9).

Two distinctly different approaches to modelling biological motion are presented in this article. Following the principles of pattern theory (Grenander 1976–1981), or 'analysis by synthesis', the first approach in Section 4.2 uses a generative model to recognize the observed biological motion. Here, the apparent contour of a person is described by an active contour (Kass *et al.* 1987). The deformation of the contour is controlled by a low-dimensional configuration space. The dynamics of the apparent contour is explicitly modelled as a stochastic process. We demonstrate that finely tuned stochastic processes can be used for both the anticipation and the classification of the observed motion.

The type of biological motion is recognized based on the dynamical information alone. No information about the shape of the apparent contour is used. It has been shown elsewhere that the shape information can be used effectively to detect people and estimate their pose. To facilitate the detection of pedestrians from a moving car Gavrila and Philomin (Gavrila and Philomin 1999; Gavrila 2000) represented a large collection of shapes using a hierarchy of templates that are based on edge-maps. The strength of this approach is that it captures the variety of shapes very efficiently. The similarity of two shapes is computed using a metric that is based on the distance transform (Borgefors 1988). The online matching is realized as a simultaneous coarse-to-fine search over the shape hierarchy and transformation parameters. The hierarchy itself is learnt from training examples using a stochastic optimization technique. Although the main application area of this system is the detection of pedestrians, one can now replace the shape contour with a large collection of example shapes in order to track the object. Toyama and Blake (2001) propose a *metric mixture* model which combines exemplars in a metric space with a probabilistic treatment.

A related but different approach is to recognize the type of motion directly from the spatio-temporal features of the image sequence. In Section 4.3 we explain how the spatio-temporal structure of human motion can be encoded in a very low-dimensional vector. Standard pattern recognition techniques are used to classify sequences containing a variety of different motion classes. Using this technique it is no longer necessary to localize the apparent contour. Consequently, the task of tracking the person is simplified.

If we intend to give a higher-level interpretation rather than a low-level physical description of the observed motion the scene context plays a crucial role. For example, in all the images displayed in Fig. 4.1 men raise their arms, but they perform very different activities. This also relates to the question of which biological motions a machine could possibly recognize. Regardless of which feature space and representation is used none of these approaches measure up to the human ability to learn and recognize biological motion. The task of recognizing a simple motion like walking, independently from scale and viewing angle, is an enormously challenging problem. Apart from the ability to recognize canonical biological motions like walking and running regardless of viewpoint, scale and occlusion, humans are also able to generalize concepts and make very fine context-dependent distinctions. For example, once a child is aware of the difference between walking and running it has no trouble making the analogous distinction for animals (Bloom 2000). Whereas the

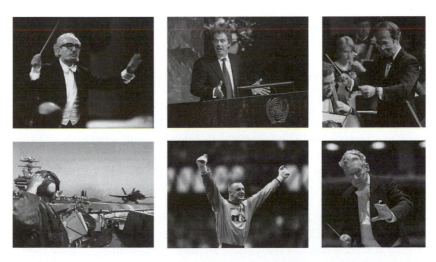

Fig. 4.1 Role of context information. In each of these examples the scene context helps to disambiguate the type of motion. One should notice that there are often very fine and subtle distinctions which allow us to recognize the type of motion.

generalization itself is arguably a very difficult problem, the importance of contextual information is much more apparent.

Once we accept that contextual information is helpful or even crucial, the question of how such knowledge should be represented arises. Such knowledge can be learnt from examples. This particular problem is difficult as we are interested in a very wide variety of scenes. A typical daily news broadcast on television serves as a good example. Hence the challenge of selecting models for motion recognition is to construct a model which is sufficiently abstract that it allows us to recognize events which are different but still related to instances in the training set. A common approach to this problem is the use of probabilistic networks or graphical models (Pearl 1988). Although the field of machine learning is far advanced there are of course limits of the current ability to learn models of very complex systems. An alternative to this approach is the use of a semantic knowledge base. Prior to searching the semantic knowledge base the video is annotated by a set of simple visual descriptors. This information is used to establish the scene context. This context information is then used to give a more specific description of the image sequence. This complex system consists of three different components: the visual analysis, the mapping from vision to language and the search of the semantic database. A description of these components together with a number of results is presented in Section 4.4.

4.2 Dynamical models

The approach of tracking people (Baumberg and Hogg 1994; Blake and Isard 1998) using their apparent contour is mathematically a very rich model which extends naturally to the recognition of certain periodic biological motions. The apparent contour of an object is modelled as a spline contour. The deformation of this contour with respect to a template is controlled by a low-dimensional linear state space, the shape space. The objective of the visual tracking system is the estimation of the state vector X_t based on a set of measurements z_t taken from the current frame of the image sequence at time t. A stochastic filter (Gelb 1979; Lütkepohl 1993) is then employed to estimate the state X_t given the history of the measurements $Z_t = \{z_0, \dots, z_t\}$. A learnt dynamical model is used as a predictor. Under certain assumptions the Kalman filter (Gelb 1979) is the optimal linear filter to estimate the state X_t at time t.

But rather than having a single estimate as in the Kalman filter here the posterior probability $p(X_t|Z_t)$ is propagated over time. The probability density $p(X_t|Z_t)$ is represented in a non-parametric form by a set of K samples $\{X_t^{(i)}\}_i$. Each sample $X_t^{(i)}$ has a likelihood weight π_i associated to it, such that $\Sigma_i \pi_i = 1$. The interpretation of such a particle set is that if the set is *resampled*, meaning that an X is chosen to be one of $X_t^{(n)}$, with probability proportional to its weight $\pi_t^{(n)}$, that X is distributed (approximately) according to the posterior p_t. A condensation or particle filter (Gordon *et al.* 1993; Isard and Blake 1996; Kitagawa 1996) is applied to propagate $p(X_t|Z_t)$ over time. In principle this framework is a generalization of the Kalman filter which also allows the use of nonlinear dynamics in the form of multi-class dynamics.

(a) Multi-class dynamics

Multi-class dynamics are represented by appending to the continuous state vector x_t a discrete state component y_t to make a 'mixed' state $X_t = (x_t, y_t)^{\mathrm{T}}$, where $y_t \, \varepsilon \, \{1, \ldots, Y\}$ is the discrete component of the state, labelling the class of motion. Corresponding to each state $y_t = y$ there is a dynamical model, taken to be a Markov model of order K that specifies $p_i(x_t|x_{t-1} \ldots x_{t-K})$. Each class y has a set (A^y, B^y, d^y) of dynamical parameters, which are learnt from example trajectories (North *et al.* 2000). In addition, and independently, state transitions are governed by the transition matrix for a first-order Markov chain:

$$P(y_t = y'|y_{t-1} = y) = M(y, y').$$

As mentioned earlier, the stochastic process used in the prediction step is the underlying model for the dynamics of the spline contour. To understand why this framework is suited to model certain periodic biological motions a more detailed knowledge of the dynamical process is necessary. A linear-Gaussian Markov model of order K is an ARP (Lütkepohl 1993) defined by

$$x_t \sum_{k=1}^{K} A_k x_{t-k} + d + Bw_t, \tag{2.1}$$

in which each w_t is a vector of N_x independent random $N(0, 1)$ variables and $w_t, w_{t'}$ are independent for $t \neq t'$. Note that the stochastic parameter B is a first-class part of a dynamical model, representing the degree and the shape of uncertainty in motion, allowing the representation of an entire distribution of possible motions for each state y. In continuous time a second-order Markov process is governed by a stochastic differential equation, the Fokker–Plank or Kolmogorov equation (Karatzas and Shreve 1991)

$$m\ddot{x} + c\dot{x} + kx = bw,$$

where w is white noise. When there is no noise present, i.e. $w = 0$, this is an oscillator with mass m, damping constant c and stiffness k. The sample path of such a process in continuous time in one dimension is a damped harmonic oscillation. The damping rate is denoted by β. A multivariate process can be decomposed into damped harmonic oscillations along different directions of the configuration space. An example of a modal analysis of a multivariate

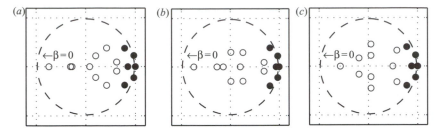

Fig. 4.2 Discrete eigenvalues of motion models learnt from three different walks. Three different walking sequences of one human are tracked. For each sequence a second order ARP is learnt using the maximum-likelihood learning rule. Only the periods in which the walker is in a steady state are used to learn the model. It is crucial to observe that only the first four modes (displayed as black circles) are similar for all three models. From these only the first two nodes are significant since they have a time constant of $\beta^{-1} > 1$ s. All remaining modes have a damping constant of $$\beta^{-1} < 0.2\,\text{s}.$$

process is shown in Fig. 4.2. Depending on the magnitude of the eigenvalue λ each mode can be characterized as unstable, exponentially decaying or harmonic. Harmonic modes with a high damping rate influence the motion only for a very short amount of time, and the least damped modes characterize the motion.

Our experiments indicate that ARPs used for the anticipation of motion (linear, stochastic differential equations and their discrete embodiment as ARPs) are capable of modelling certain repetitive human motions such as running and walking. For example, the modal analysis of three different learnt models for walking presented in Fig. 4.2 indicates that a significant number of modes have a damping constant β^{-1} of less than 0.2 s. They are 'unused'—i.e. discarded by the learning algorithm. Hence there is no need to employ a more complex stochastic process to model the type of motion.

By introducing the class of motion as a discrete variable of the state X_t the particle set which represents the posterior distribution $p(x_t|Z_t)$ enables us not only to track the apparent contour but also to estimate the class of motion at any given time t. Hence we have developed a system where classification feeds back into the perception of motion which means perception and classification are inextricably bound together. In this approach the motion is classified instantaneously and does, for example, in a surveillance application provide the ability to raise an alarm. In case no instantaneous classification is necessary the classification results can be improved by smoothing as shown in North *et al.* (2000). The following experiment demonstrates that an image sequence can now automatically be segmented into subsequences that contain only one type of motion.

(b) Experimental results

Two different motion classes were used for a classification experiment. A *pure jump*, i.e. jumping up and down without lateral arm or leg movement, and a *half star*, which is a 'star jump' without arm movement. In order to illustrate the two motions the contours of the previous time-frames are superimposed onto one frame (Fig. 4.3). A separate set of training sequences that contain only one type of motion was used to learn the motion models. In all the experiments the tracking process is initialized by hand. In order to get a very good model the maximum-likelihood learning rule was used on a sequence of 8 s in length. Note that a combination of these two motions illustrates both types of classification problems: the lateral leg movement makes it easy to decide when the person is in motion class *half star*. The jumping up from the bending down position is, however, very difficult. As can be seen in Fig. 4.4 and Fig. 4.5 we achieve an asymptotic misclassification performance of 10%.

We have demonstrated that a particle filter with mixed states can be used for classifying motions online. In the approach presented by Bregler (1997) the discrete states are used up for modelling atomic motions. In that context a bi-level recursive algorithm (Rabiner and Bing-Hwang 1993) could be tried

(a)   *(b)*

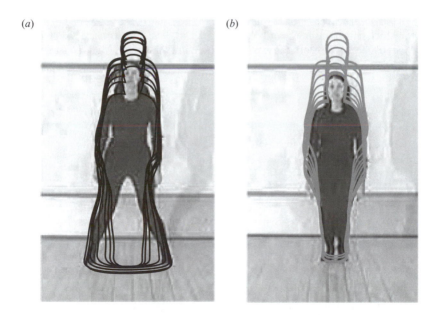

Fig. 4.3 Motion classes used in the experiment. In order to illustrate the motion, contours of previous time-steps are superimposed on one frame. (*a*) Half star: a 'star jump' without arm moment. Notice that both motions begin with an upwards acceleration. Hence it is difficult to discriminate between both motions. (*b*) Pure jump, i.e. jumping up and down without lateral arm or leg movement.

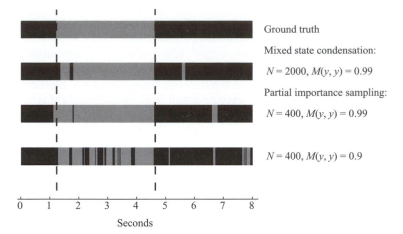

Ground truth

Mixed state condensation:
$N = 2000, M(y, y) = 0.99$

Partial importance sampling:
$N = 400, M(y, y) = 0.99$

$N = 400, M(y, y) = 0.9$

Seconds

Fig. 4.4 Examples of the different segmentations. The motion class pure jump is shown in light grey, half star in black. The top row corresponds to the ground truth obtained by hand segmenting the sequence. A two-state 'condensation' filter without importance sampling is used with $n = 2000$ particles. The third row displays the segmentation obtained using partial importance sampling on the discrete state with $n = 400$ samples. Note that the quality of the segmentations does not get worse when the sample size reduces. The crucial role of the transition matrix is documented in the bottom row. Here, a transition matrix with $M(y, y) = 0.9$ and importance weights with $g(y, y) = 0.8$ are used; hence the expected duration of the motion is no longer correct.

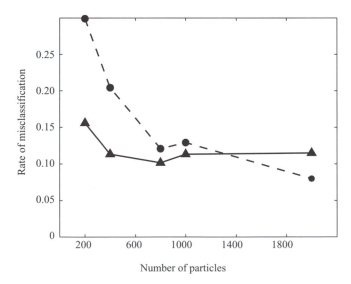

Fig. 4.5 Misclassification graphs. The average error of three tests for each of the three filters on a particular test sequence is displayed for different particle sizes N. Circles and dashed line, mixed state condensation; triangles and solid line, partial importance sampling.

for automatic segmentation. But these algorithms are notoriously computationally expensive. Here, we show that a single autoregressive model is a serious candidate as a model of atomic motions. This leaves the discrete state free for classification. A Markov chain is used to model the state transitions and to apply long-term continuity constraints. It was demonstrated that the Markov chain can be applied more effectively by using partial importance sampling. In general, importance sampling (Hammersley and Handscomb 1964) is a method for variance reduction. The details of this method can be found in Rittscher and Blake (1999). Learning the motion models from a mixed sequence as in North *et al.* (2000) could potentially reduce the asymptotic error rate of 10%. It could well be possible that human intuition imposes a segmentation which is sub-optimal with respect to ARPs. Both motions have a number of similarities so it might be necessary to work with more than two atomic motion models. The motion classes used in this experiment could then correspond to the occurrence of one or two atomic motion models.

But there is one other concern. Tracking complex motions of humans using a contour tracker is very labour intensive. It is especially difficult to initialize the visual tracking process. Although the background of the scene is very simple we failed to track the full star jump or jumping jack (as shown in figure 10*a*(i)). Furthermore, there is effectively no variation of pose in these sequences. This raises the question whether it would be more desirable to develop a more direct approach to motion classification. If one could classify the class of motion using the raw image data it would be no longer necessary to rely on a contour tracker. Such an approach might also solve the initialization problem for contour tracking. The development of such a method will be discussed in the following section.

4.3 Classifying motions directly from spatio-temporal features

As just mentioned, the aim is now to recognize biological motion directly from the spatio-temporal features of the image sequence. Black and Jepson (1998) use the optical flow field of the entire image to recognize gestures and expressions. One drawback of this method is that the flow field is not very well localized and can easily be corrupted by background motion. It turns out that representing the entire image sequence as a space-time cube or *XYT* cube, as opposed to analysing adjacent frames, is more appropriate for motion analysis. Niyogi and Adelson (1994*a,b*), for example, fit a spatio-temporal surface rather similar to the one shown in Fig. 4.6 to estimate the parameters of a stick-figure model. They use these parameters to recognize people by their gait. But as motivated in the introduction, our thesis is that motion recognition should not require any articulated model.

Without making any use of the underlying structure of the motion pattern Zelnik-Manor and Irani (2001) present a non-parametric approach. The imagery

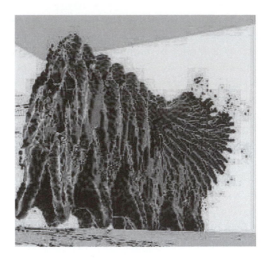

Fig. 4.6 Spatio-temporal surface. A sequence of mixed aerobics exercises (as shown in figure 10) is used to compute a space-time surface. The surface is extracted from the reprocessed sequence using an implementation of the 'marching cubes algorithm' (Schroeder *et al.* 1992). Note that in the latter part of the sequence the arm motion is clearly visible.

is analysed at three or four temporal scales and normalized spatial-temporal gradients at each scale are computed as

$$\frac{\nabla I(x, y, t)}{\nabla I(x, y, t)},$$
(3.1)

where image sequence is denoted by I. Hence at each of the L scales one gets a 3D feature vector on each voxel location. To reduce the computational complexity, they avoid estimating the joint density and treat each feature component and scale independently. The comparison of these feature histograms is very difficult because these histograms are typically dominated by feature points for which $|\nabla I|$ is almost zero. This is why they formulate a distance metric that uses a weighting factor for each histogram bin, i.e.

$$D(h, h') = \sum_i w_i (h(i) - h'(i))^2, \quad \text{where}$$
$$w_i = (h(i) - h'(i))^{-1}.$$
(3.2)

In the case that a number of sequences for each event type are available, they refine this distance measure by computing the mean and variance in each histogram bin and essentially computing cluster centres, each representing a class of motion. As mentioned before, points for which $|\nabla S|$ is almost zero swamp the statistic. This effectively causes a large amount of observation

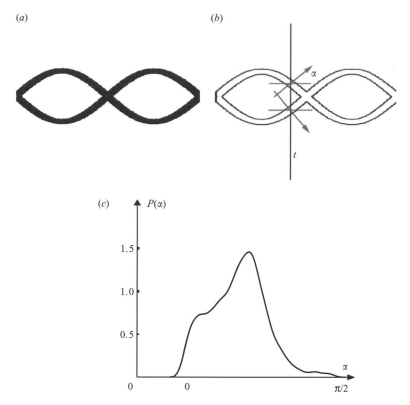

Fig. 4.7 Idealized braided pattern. (*a*) An idealized braided pattern of a person walking under a front-to-parallel view. (*b*) The angle of the outer normal to one curve, α, measures the velocity of the leg at time t. The other curve is a mirror image of the first hence the angles of both other normals are related. This is because the tan function is antisymmetric, i.e. $-\tan^{-1}(-x) = \tan^{-1}(x)$. It is also clear that the angles of the inner normals correspond to those of the outer normals. The distribution of $|\alpha|$ hence characterizes the braided pattern. (*c*) A typical learnt distribution of $|\alpha|$ from an epipolar slice taken from the experimental data.

noise. As can be observed in Fig. 4.8, the salient information is contained in the motion boundaries. This is why a conservatively set threshold can be applied to eliminate such data points from the statistic.

Motions like running, walking and skipping can be characterized by the different intrinsic velocities of leg movement. The slices of the XYT cube exhibit a braided pattern which characterizes each type of motion. Cipolla and Yamamoto (1990) use these slides for the stereoscopic tracking of bodies in motion and introduce the term epipolar slices. Because the epipolar slice is an entity in space time, the braided pattern is directly related to the velocity profile of the motion. The braided pattern of leg motion, for example, consists of two self-intersecting curves, one for each leg. Hence, the velocity of the leg can be computed by estimating the outer normal to the curve. This is also illustrated in Fig. 4.7. The angle α of the outer normal can be computed as

$$\tan(\alpha) = \frac{\delta_t I}{\delta_x I}.$$

For practical purposes $\delta_x I$ and $\delta_t I$ are computed from the bandpass-filtered data. And in order to suppress feature points that are not associated with the motion boundary α is only calculated where $|\nabla I|$ exceeds a threshold, i.e. $|\nabla I(x, t)| > C$, as

$$\tan(\alpha(x,t)) = \frac{(I * \delta_t \varphi)(x, t)}{(I * \delta_x \varphi)(x, t)}. \tag{3.3}$$

The threshold C can be set conservatively. Its only purpose is to prevent the distribution $p(|\alpha|)$ from being swamped by α-values that correspond to locations (x, t) at which the modulus of the gradient $|\nabla I(x, t)|$ is near zero. Because the tan function is antisymmetric, i.e. $-\tan^{-1}(-x) = \tan^{-1}(x)$, for every time t the modulus of α, $|\alpha|$, estimated from either curve, is identical. Hence the distribution of $|\alpha|$ will describe the velocity distribution of the motion pattern.

The distribution $p(|\alpha|)$ clearly depends on the position of the epipolar slice. Therefore a collection of slices will be used to characterize the motion pattern. The resulting feature vector consists of a set of skew factors $\gamma 1(I, y)$ computed from a slice at height y, i.e.

$$\gamma_1(I) := \{\gamma_1(I, y_1), \ldots, \gamma_1(I, y_N)\}, \tag{3.4}$$

where N is the number of epipolar slices taken from the space-time cube. Hence we compress the image sequence I to a feature vector of length N. The estimate of the third moment or skewness, γ_1 (see, for example, Scheffe 1959), of the distributions is defined as

$$\gamma_1(\{\alpha_1, \ldots, \alpha_N\}) = \frac{1}{N} \sum_{j=1}^{N} \left(\frac{\alpha_j - \overline{\alpha}}{\alpha}\right)^3. \tag{3.5}$$

The skewness of a distribution measures the degree of asymmetry. The measure does not depend on the location or scale (measured respectively by the mean $\overline{\alpha}$ and the variance σ). Hence a linear transformation of the distribution will not affect the skew factor γ_1. For a symmetrical distribution the skewness, γ_1, is evidently zero. A positive value of skewness signifies a distribution with an asymmetric tail extending to the right of the mean and vice versa. Three typical epipolar slices, ranging from fast to slow motions, are displayed in figure 8. Both the learnt distributions and the skewness, γ_1, allow us to discriminate between the three different velocity profiles. We therefore conclude that it is sufficient to compute the skewness of the learnt distribution of a collection of epipolar slices and treat the vector of the skew factors as a feature vector. Results of this method are shown in Figs 4.9 and 4.10. It should be

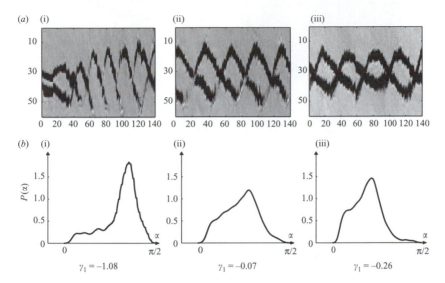

Fig. 4.8 Skewness of the $|\alpha|$ distributions. This figure illustrates the effect of estimating the skewness $\gamma_1(6)$ of the learnt distributions for $|\alpha|$. (*a*) Examples of typical epipolar slices for (i) running, (ii) skipping and (iii) walking. The corresponding distributions of $|\alpha|$ are shown in (*b*). The reader should note that all three representations of the data—the raw data, the learnt distribution of $|\alpha|$ and the skewness of the distribution—allow us to discriminate the three different motion patterns. In these examples the foreground pattern (in black) is clearly visible. But as this method is based on the estimation of normals the representation does not depend on the intensity difference between foreground and background as long as it exceeds the threshold C (see equation (3.3)).

noted that the vectors of skew factors shown in Fig. 4.9 give rise to a very natural interpretation of the characteristics of the three different motion types. This method orders these different walking styles in some kind of continuum where the two extremes are defined by running and walking. Here, we make use of the fact that the walking motions are periodic. In the next section we will demonstrate that the same method can be used to recognize non-repetitive motions when very short time intervals are used.

Many applications require the instantaneous classification of the type of motion. The skew vectors $\gamma_1(I)$ are computed for a set of consecutive frames or, in other words, of a spatio-temporal cube of a certain temporal length T. Apart from the noise of the measurement model itself, the distribution of the skew vectors $\gamma_1(I)$ for each class of motion will now depend on the length of the temporal window. This is due to the phase dependency of the motion itself. In a first experiment we attempt to classify each temporal window using a very basic model for the class densities. Like in the computation of the linear discriminant analysis in the previous section, the distributions of the skew

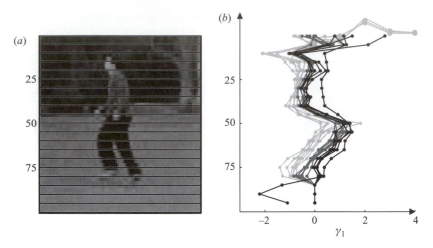

Fig. 4.9 Skew vectors $\gamma_1(I)$ for different walking styles. The skew vectors $\gamma_1(I)$ (3.5) are computed for a set of 20 epipolar slices. The exact position of the slices are indicated as light grey lines in (a). The skew vectors, $\gamma_1(I)$, for each of the sequences are presented in (b). The skew vectors are colour coded. Light grey corresponds to running, dark grey to skipping, and black to walking. It can be observed that the skew factors of top and bottom slices are implausible. This is a consequence of the naive threshold set in (see equation (3.3)). The amount of variation in the upper half of the body can be explained by the body motion with respect to the centroid of the body. As a result of computing the skew factors of the different epipolar slices, the different walking styles are ordered according to their average speed. In an experiment a linear discrimination analysis of the skew vectors $\gamma_1(I)$ for a set of four different people performing running, skipping and walking was used to demonstrate that the three different motion classes can be separated.

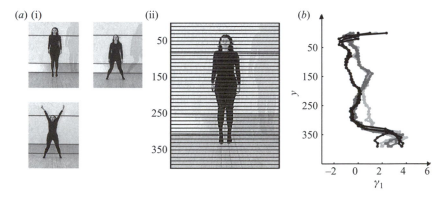

Fig. 4.10 Skew vectors $\gamma_1(I)$ for the aerobics motions. In these experiments the skew factors $\gamma_1(I)$ (see equation (3.4)) are computed for a set of 40 epipolar slices. The exact position of the slices is again indicated as light grey lines in (i). The skew vectors $\gamma_1(I)$ for each of the test sequences are presented in (b). The skew vectors are colour coded. Light grey corresponds to jumping, dark grey to a half-star jump and black to the full star-jump. It should be noted that although this method is more suitable for analysing leg motion (see text) the presence of arm motion is detected correctly. Moreover the fact that the skew factors are a relatively smooth function with respect to y indicates that the estimates are not particularly noisy.

vectors $\gamma_1(I)$ for each motion class are modelled as multivariate Gaussians with mean μ and diagonal covariance Σ. The Mahalanobis distance between the skew vectors $\gamma_1(I)$, computed for each interval of length T, and the learnt centres μ_i is used to classify the observed motion.

We believe that it is important to test the use of the skew vectors $\gamma_1(I)$ using a very basic classification technique. Unlike HMMs, such an approach discards, of course, the temporal information about the mean duration of each motion. But parameters for models with hidden parameters are usually learnt using some form of expectation maximization learning rule. These algorithms do not guarantee to find a local minimum and depend heavily on an initialization step. If the results obtained by a basic classifier are promising it will be possible to refine them using a more elaborate model.

We now benefit from the fact that it is no longer necessary to track the outline of the person in order to classify the type of motion. This allows us to test the newly developed method on examples that are considerably more complex than those used in Section 4.2. The first dataset contains sequences of four different people running, skipping and walking. Owing to the low contrast between foreground and background it would be difficult to track the outline of the people using an edge-based contour tracker. The second set of test sequences consists of a set of aerobics exercises similar to those used previously. But here we included the star jump as the third motion class.

All sequences of people walking were recorded at the same time and place. The group of people contained three males and one female all between 20 and 30 years old. In all, the dataset includes 77 sequences whose lengths vary between 2 s and 5 s. A simple blob tracker based on motion detectors was applied to locate the foreground window in every frame.

The second set of test sequences contains three different gymnastic exercises: jump, half-star jump and star-jump (or jumping jack) (see Fig. 4.10). These sequences do not require any preprocessing as the exercise is performed on the spot. Two sets of image sequences were analysed. The first set contains three sequences of a mixture of aerobics exercises shown in Fig. 4.10. The temporal length of the spatio-temporal cube T was chosen to be 25 fields or half a second. Like in the experiment shown in Fig. 4.10, a number of 40 epipolar slices were used to compute $\gamma_1(I)$. The distributions of the skew vector for each class, jumping, half-star and star-jump were learnt from a separate set of training sequences, each of which contained only one type of motion. In total, 114 half-second intervals were analysed. Out of these, eight were classified wrongly, which corresponds to an error rate of 7%.

These classification errors are due to measurement noise. To reduce this measurement noise we convolved each feature vector with a smoothing filter. This is justified by the following observations. First, we expect the true skew factors $\gamma_1(I, y)$, as mentioned before, to be continuous with respect to y. Second, the noise of the skew estimate on two adjacent slices $\gamma_1(I, y_i)$ and $\gamma_1(I, y_j)$ is assumed to be independent. One justification for this is that the support of the filters, $\delta_t\varphi$ and $\delta_x\varphi$, needed to compute α (see equation (3.3)), on the two adjacent slices are disjoint. As a result the number of misclassifications is reduced to three out of 114 samples. This corresponds to an error rate of 2.6%.

Finally we analysed sequences of a person playing basketball. Two sequences, each of which is 50 s long, were used. Like in the previous example the length of the spatio-temporal cube T was set to be 25 fields or half a second. The skew vectors $\gamma_1(I)$ were again convolved with a smoothing kernel. The foreground region was tracked using a simple blob tracker. The training data were obtained by labelling each half-second interval in one of the sequences as belonging to one of the following motion classes: walking, running, turning and throwing. As before, each of these motion classes was modelled by a multivariate Gaussian with diagonal covariance matrix. The resulting means for each of the motion classes are shown in Fig. 4.11. As can be seen in the figure, the distributions of

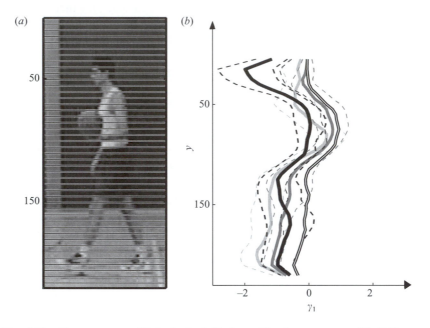

Fig. 4.11 Skew vectors $\gamma_1(I)$ for basketball player. The skew vectors $\gamma_1(I)$ (3.5) are computed for a set of 44 epipolar slices. The feature vectors are convolved with a smoothing filter to reduce the measurement noise (see text). As before, (*a*) shows the location of the epipolar slices. The distributions of the skew vectors of each motion class are modelled by a multivariate Gaussian with a diagonal covariance matrix. (*b*) The mean and standard deviation of each motion class. Four motion classes are used in this experiment: running (in light grey), walking (in dark grey), turning (in white or black) and throwing (in black). It can be easily observed that the throw is the only motion that involves a considerable amount of arm motion. The turning motion involves very little arm and leg motion. The motion classes running and walking, however, show some overlap.

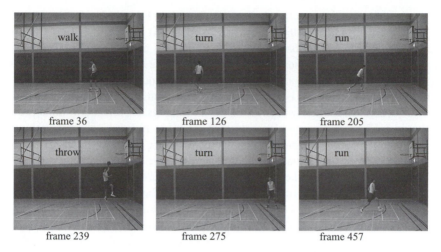

Fig. 4.12 An automatically annotated basketball sequence. Shown are single frames out of the automatically annotated sequence. The person runs towards the basket dribbling the ball. The ball is then thrown into the basket. After the ball is caught the person walks back. All of these stages are identified correctly. Only the decision between running and walking is sometimes ambiguous.

walking and running have some overlap. As a result, walking is occasionally misclassified as running. In total, 10 out of 99 samples are misclassified, which corresponds to a misclassification rate of 10%. All remaining classes of motion are identified correctly. Single frames of the sequence are shown in Fig. 4.12. Taking the difficulty of the sequence into account this is a very promising result. Potentially, this error rate results from the fact that during training some intervals that contain a transition from standing still to running were labelled as running. Assuming that the camera is stationary, this error rate can easily be reduced by taking prior information, such as the output from the blob tracker, into account. In comparison with the examples shown in the previous section, the task of visual tracking is a lot simpler. Here, a blob tracker like the one presented in Comaniciu *et al.* (2000) can be used to extract the motion trajectory of the foreground object.

4.4 Semantic information and context

The objective is now to give a higher-level interpretation of the imagery. As discussed in Section 4.1, this is required to establish the context of the scene. We now present an approach that uses the information contained in a semantic database to establish this context information. The overall approach consists of three main components: visual analysis, the mapping from vision to language and the search in the semantic database. Before details of these components can be given, the nature of the semantic database used here needs to be described. The current capability of the system will be discussed in Section 4.4d.

Here, WordNet (Fellbaum 1998) is employed as a semantic database. WordNet is an online lexical reference system whose design is inspired by current psycholinguistic theories of human lexical memory. As opposed to a normal dictionary, WordNet is a lexical ontology that attempts to organize lexical information hierarchically in terms of word meanings. Developed by hand over the past 17 years, it is a massive compilation of hierarchical relationships between each sense of every noun, verb, adjective and adverb in standard English. The 80 000 noun senses, for example, are organized into 11 hierarchies rooted by general concepts such as *entity, abstraction, human activity, event* and *group*. A word sense *C* may have any number of *subordinates*, which are specific types of *C*. For example, *object* is a subordinate of *entity*, and *natural-object, artefact* and *living-thing* are subordinates of *object*. Verbs have a similar set of hierarchies organized on the same principle of subordination, for example, *walking* is one way to *travel*. Each word also has a free-form, textual definition similar to a dictionary entry. These definitions are stored as strings without any indexing or structured content. The hierarchical structure of WordNet allows the formulation of efficient search algorithms. Starting at a very general root node, as for example, *artefact*, the visual information found in the entire scene is used to find a specific subordinate concept to describe a particular region.

One shortcoming of WordNet with respect to this particular application is that the definitions and glosses generally do not contain any descriptions of the objects' appearance. A chair, for example, is defined to be *a seat for one person, with a support of the back*. In order to address this problem we have tagged the concepts in WordNet with attribute values indicating whether they are visible, capable of motion and usually located indoors or outdoors. Topic attributes also indicate relevance to specific topics. The attribute information that describes the type of motion is more detailed. We differentiate between *no motion, continuous motion* and *random motion*. In the case of continuous motion we also specify the dominant direction of the motion. So, for example, the dominate direction of climbing is upward or vertical. Currently these attributes are added by hand to the database. The hierarchical structure of WordNet enables very efficient attribution, as the subordinates inherit attribute values. For our experiments, around 195 000 attribute values are assigned.

(a) Visual analysis

To initiate and conduct the semantic search, visual observables were extracted from the video. The challenge here is to find a set of visual observables. These were then mapped into language terms that aid the semantic search of WordNet. Visual analysis can produce information at a large range of semantic levels. The sole fact that the scene contains a set of parallel lines by itself is not very helpful for the visual search. The set of parallel lines, however, could indicate the presence of a man-made object. It is tempting to assume that image analysis can produce high-level semantic content, and map this information directly into WordNet. However, this is not feasible. For narrow, restricted problem domains, computer vision can indeed produce semantic content at the level of language. When the scope is a bit wider, as for example, in the broadcast video domain, the variety of objects and events present requires the development of tens of thousands of specialized object detectors.

Instead, our guiding principle was to use a small number of high-level object detectors, coupled with mid-level visual observables, to interpret the scene. We demonstrate later that by making extensive use of the semantic knowledge base and contextual information, a high-level scene description can be inferred from this combination of visual features. To formalize the semantic content of visual information, the extraction of visual descriptors was organized hierarchically (see Fig. 4.13). Edges, interest points, responses to filter banks, and segmented regions were considered to be *direct observables* and therefore form the basis of the visual information hierarchy (level 0). At level 1, information derived directly from image observables was computed and characterized. Level 2 consists of objects and events, which are recognized using data from the previous levels. Level 0 information is 2D, but carries little semantic information on its own. Level 1 information is more salient, but generally requires additional context to be meaningful. For the semantic search, level 2 information corresponds directly to semantic concepts in WordNet, while level 1 data are used to refine the search. We use three types of visual information across levels 1 and 2: people and their movements, other moving objects (e.g. vehicles) and stationary scene elements, such as

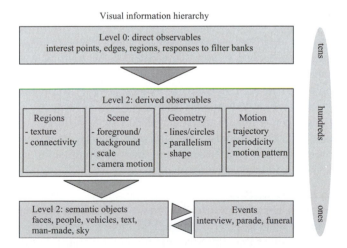

Fig. 4.13   The visual information hierarchy induced by semantic levels.

manmade objects and structures, and natural objects, such as sky, water and vegetation. People are detected using a face detector courtesy of Carnegie Mellon University (Rowley *et al.* 1998), although we also plan to integrate human body detectors in future work. Our scene and motion descriptors are now described in more detail.

(i) Scene characterization

The goal of scene characterization is to semantically categorize every object and element in the scene. This provides a starting point for the semantic search to add further specialization or detail to the categorization, and provides scene context to constrain the search. This characterization is a very difficult problem, however, as semantic context may be required even at this stage. Our approach was to define a small set of categories, some of which were very broad, that could be distinguished primarily by 2D appearance information. The categories spanned virtually all objects of interest except for people, which were handled with specialized detectors. Currently, our categories are *man-made objects, vegetation, water/sea/ocean, rock* and *sky*. Although the man-made category is very large, it corresponds to the 'artefact' hierarchy in WordNet, which contains all man-made objects. The presence of certain categories in a scene, such as water and sky, also provided evidence of scene context such as *outdoors*, which was useful in the semantic search as described later. Algorithms specifically designed for overall scene classification (Szummer and Picard 1998; Vailaya *et al.* 1998) could be easily integrated into the system, as well as other categories such as animals.

The categorization was formulated as an integrated problem of perceptual grouping, texture recognition and segmentation. While filter banks are useful for distinguishing between similar textures, the salient features of these broad texture categories are often embedded in the relationships between large-scale features such as regions. In previous work we have examined this problem (Hoogs *et al.* 2003), and developed a region-based approach for texture characterization. The algorithm outperforms filter banks when the range of appearance within each texture is large compared to the training images, as is generally the case in broadcast video.

The approach has been extended to video, using a maximum-likelihood formulation to combine texture class estimates across subsequent video frames after inter-frame homographies are estimated. At this stage, the scene is assumed to be static, or to contain only slowly moving objects. Example results are shown in Figs 4.15 and 4.18. Motion analysis is then applied to segment and characterize independently moving objects.

(ii) Motion characterization

Our system currently uses an extended version of the blob tracking approach presented in Comaniciu *et al.* (2000). The motion trajectory is computed based on the motion of the centroid of the foreground object. In the context of gesture analysis, suitable state space representations (Bobick and Wilson

1997) have been used to recognize a limited vocabulary of hand gestures. Rather than extracting a mathematical description of the motion trajectory we are interested in its characteristic. Is it, for example, a smooth horizontal motion or an erratic motion, which could indicate some kind of jumping or bouncing motion? Depending on how much we know about the camera and the scene, the motion trajectory allows us to estimate the speed of the motion, which can be a very important clue.

The discussion of recognizing motion patterns presented in Section 4.3 is of course highly relevant to this work. As opposed to the motion trajectory it is a local characteristic of the observed motion. We described techniques to recognize biological motion based on the spatio-temporal features of the image sequence. The structure and type of motion pattern also reveal whether a rigid or non-rigid object is being tracked. Furthermore, the periodicity of the motion can be computed. Polana and Nelson (1997) used a set of basic descriptors to recognize certain motion patterns. An approach to detect the periodicity of the motion is given in Liu and Picard (1998). Modal analysis (see Fig 4.2) provides another possibility to analyse the observed motion. The presence of harmonic modes and their time constants β indicates periodic motion. Currently the system uses only the dominant direction of the motion.

(b) Mapping from vision to language

To relate the disparate representations of visual observables and WordNet, we have defined the visual information hierarchy described in Section 4.4a, and established the relationship of each level to WordNet concepts. This formalism provides a grounded framework to contain visual information, linguistic information and their respective uncertainties and ambiguities. Specifically, level 2 observables corresponding to objects of interest are mapped directly to general concepts in WordNet, and become *elemental terms* (see Fig. 4.14). This is possible because the semantic meaning of each level 2 observable is clearly defined, and can be mapped directly to a word sense. Such observables of interest include human faces and manmade objects, which are mapped to nouns. Moving objects, including moving people, are mapped to verbs. The remaining level 2 observables are used as contextual search constraints as described below.

Elemental terms are very general, and provide entry points for searching WordNet. To find more specific concepts present in the video, level 1 observables are mapped to *pruning terms*, or words that are used to constrain the search as described below. Unlike level 2 observables, however, it is often impossible to map each level 1 observable to a single word sense because of the well-known difficulty of consistently mapping low-level, quantitative data onto symbolic terms. This problem is partially addressed by mapping some level 1 observables to multiple words that are synonyms.

Certain visual observables are mapped to attributes described earlier. Level 1 observables in this category include specific motion characteristics such as

visual observable	level	elemental	pruning	attribute
man-made	2	artefact, n, 1		
face	2	person, n, 1	person, human	
sky	2		sky, air	outdoors
motion	2	travel, v, 1	motion	
motion speed	1			fast, slow
motion direction	1			horizontal, up, down
motion type	1			smooth, erratic

Fig. 4.14 Selected mappings from visual observables to semantic terms. Elemental terms have a part of speech (n, noun or v, verb), and a sense number in WordNet. Motion maps to the elemental term travel, and motion characteristics map to quantized attribute values.

direction and speed. Some level 2 observables also map to attributes; for example, *sky* and *vegetation* map to the outdoors attribute. These level 2 observables do not become elemental terms, as we are not interested in categorizing them further in this work. Instead they provide scene context to constrain the search. Topics are mapped to both pruning terms and attribute terms; only a limited number of general topics are also attributes, as these are determined manually.

(c) Semantic search

As mentioned earlier, the objective of the semantic search is to find the most specific description of the scene elements supported by the evidence and topic context. Even with all observables in a common representation, there are still significant issues in searching WordNet. For example, the only difference between subordinates of the same node are their definitions, which are unstructured text. Natural language processing is required to extract information from definitions, and this process can be error prone. The length of the present article does not allow a detailed desciption of the search algorithm, but the main idea is to use the pruning information to find the most relevant concepts in the database. As a result of the search we obtain a ranked list of concepts. As will be seen later, these lists can of course contain concepts that have little or no relevance. The aim of the current work is to ensure relevant words are contained in the lists and have a sufficiently high ranking.

(d) Video annotation results

The purpose of our video annotation system is to derive semantic content descriptions. A video is currently segmented into clips (by hand in these experiments), and these clips are passed into the system. The scene characterization algorithm classifies these clips into the various categories. The face detector is applied in parallel, and supersedes segmentation results when humans are found. Next, the tracking algorithm, which is manually initialized in the current system, is applied to man-made regions and faces, to determine their motion. This visual information is translated into elemental, pruning and attribute terms as described in Section 4.4*b*. Simultaneously, topic terms are extracted from the transcript (this step is currently manual). Finally, semantic search is performed to determine the annotations. Once the search terminates, the 10 highest ranked concepts are output so that we can report performance measures as described below.

The first example, shown in Fig. 4.15, illustrates how the system makes use of the scene context. Three regions are segmented and classified. Region 1 (blue) is classified as 'water', region 3 erroneously as 'sky', and region 2 (light brown) as 'man-made'. Region 2 is contained within region 1. The topic information is 'crude oil', which is mentioned repeatedly in the commentary; this becomes a pruning term, but not a topic attribute because it is too specific. The man-made region maps directly to the elemental term 'artefact' and initiates a search through the 14 000 subnodes of artefact. The pruning terms 'sea' and 'water' are added because the man-made region is contained in the water region. As demonstrated by the output noun list, using relatively simple visual observables and basic topic information, the correct object label of {oil tanker, oiler,

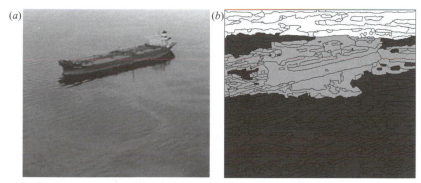

(a)   (b)

region 2, nouns:
water, crude oil: {oil tanker, oiler, tank ship, tanker}
sea, water: {milldam}, {Suez canal}, {abandoned ship, derelict}, {wreck}, {lifeboat}, {whaleboat}
water: {launch}, {frigate}, {bottom, freighter, merchant ship, merchant-man}

Fig. 4.15 The original image (a) is segmented into regions (b) classified as 'water' (dark grey), 'sky' (white) and 'man-made' (light grey). The man-made region (region 2) is contained within the water region. The top 10 concepts returned by the manmade search are shown in rank order, grouped by matched constraint terms shown in bold. The words listed within each set of brackets are synonyms and represent a single concept.
See Plate 2 of the Plate Section, at the centre of this book.

tank ship, tanker} is at the top of the ranked list. Without the 'crude oil' topic, the various types of boats are still detected as the most likely concepts, but with approximately equal likelihood.

Before discussing specific examples containing biological motion we present results of an initial study examining the system's ability to annotate a wide range of scenes. All clips in a contiguous news story about the *Exxon Valdez* oil spill were analysed. Typically, a 2–3 min story contains dozens of clips showing a wide range of subjects. Key frames from the clips of the story are shown in Fig. 4.16. Note the variety of scales, object types and scene content despite the common topic. No topic information was used in the search, however, as we were interested in the generic performance of the system.

Performance evaluation of this system has two levels. First, we assess the accuracy of the computed visual information. Then, we assess whether the semantic search found annotations that correctly improve upon the visual information. To measure the second stage, we manually examine the generated word lists to determine which words are appropriate descriptions of their corresponding scene elements. Currently we do not evaluate how specific the detected labels are. The system should be rewarded for finding more specific terms, and punished for finding overly specific terms. This will be addressed in future experiments.

The percentage of correct labels in the top 10 words is shown in Fig. 4.17. The extracted visual information is listed below each image above the line; the correct annotations found by the search are listed below the line. On approximately half of the clips, the semantic search found relevant annotations among the top 10 words. On the other half, one of two conditions applies. In some cases, such as the first clip, no objects corresponding to elemental terms were detected. Hence no search was performed, and the system output only visual analysis. In other cases, elemental terms were detected, but the additional visual evidence was insufficient to specialize the objects further. This occurred on clips 2, 3, 4, 6, 9 and 12. Another problem was of course errors caused by the segmentation. The detection of water in clips 10 and 11 was erroneous. In these particular examples, however, the system still produced the appropriate labels.

Finally, we discuss two examples that contain biological motion. In the example shown in Fig. 4.18 a man climbs a rock. A visual tracker is used to track the motion of the person (initialized manually in this example). The scene is segmented and classified into two regions, 'rock' and 'sky'. The person is misclassified as 'rock', but this error can be corrected when motion is present or the person is detected. The semantic search is conducted starting at the noun 'person', using the attribute term 'outdoors' derived from 'sky' and the pruning term 'rock'. This yields a list of nouns that contains the correct object label {rock climber}. The false positive 'punk rocker' is due to the ambiguity of the meaning of the word 'rock' in WordNet definitions (which are untagged strings). The verb search is conducted from the verb concept 'human motion', and constrained by the extracted motion attributes 'up' and

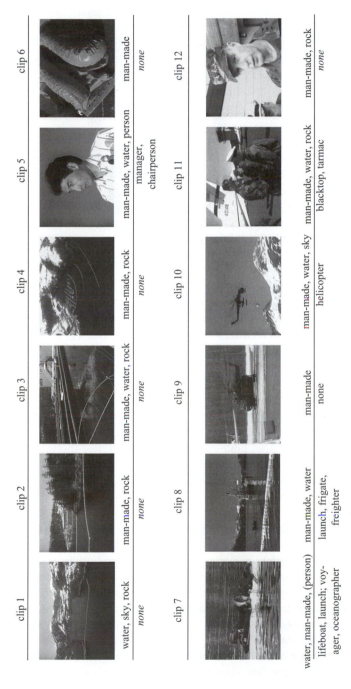

Fig. 4.16 A complete story containing 12 clips was analysed. One keyframe for each of the clips is shown with the extracted scene characteristics (above the line) and any correct semantic annotations in the top 10 found by the search.

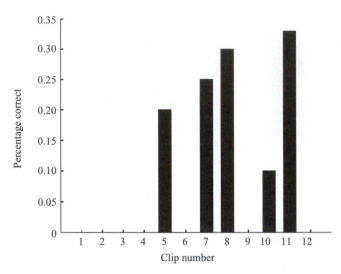

Fig. 4.17   Percentage of the top 10 concepts returned by the semantic search that are relevant to each clip.

'slow'. This yields a verb list including {ascend, come up, rise, uprise}, {scale} and {escalate}. The verb {climb} was also found, but was ranked just below the top 10 verbs. This illustrates the potential benefits of considering noun and verb searches jointly, which is a topic for future research. But in principle this example shows that the use of a semantic database can be useful, and frees us from learning very specific scenarios.

In Section 4.3 we detected the running motion (see Fig. 4.9) using the spatio-temporal pattern of the image sequence. Based on the motion of the centroid of the foreground blob we know that it is a fast motion in the horizontal direction. The semantic verb search using the pruning information *horizontal, articulated* and *fast* returns the words: march, pace, outride, romp, run, outrun, sprint and rush. Most of these words are an adequate description of the observed motion.

Our experiments show that with the existing set of visual analysis algorithms— face detector, scene characterization, motion tracking and semantic search— we can produce meaningful, non-trivial annotations on a wide variety of scenes. The results shown here are representative of our other experiments, and give an indication of the potential of the approach. Obviously, more experimentation needs to be performed, particularly to examine the trade-offs between topic context, the amount and levels of visual information and the specificity of the search. Currently, the system is limited by the visual algorithms, notably the lack of a person detector, motion track initialization and the segmentation algorithm. As stated earlier, information of the motion pattern is currently not used.

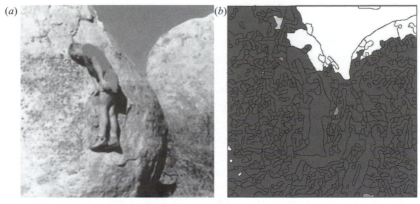

region 3, nouns:
rock: {rock 'n' roll musician, rocker}, {punk, punk rocker}, {groupie}, {cragsman, rock climber}, {pueblo}
region 3, verbs:
up: {emerge}, {ascend, come up, rise, uprise}, {bounce, jounce}, {swell, well}, {rocket, skyrocket}, {uplift}, {scale}, {escalade}, {ramp}, {ride}

Fig. 4.18   The original image (*a*) is segmented into regions (*b*) classified as 'rock' (red) and 'sky' (white), providing the attribute term 'outdoors'. The motion of the person is tracked and characterized as motion attribute terms 'upward' and 'slow'. Both a noun and a verb search are conducted using *person* and *human motion* as elemental terms. The most likely concepts returned by each search are shown in rank order, grouped by matched constraint terms shown in bold. See Plate 3 of the Plate Section, at the centre of this book.

Although WordNet was chosen because of its hierarchical structure we also need to consider other semantic databases. FrameNet (Baker *et al.* 1998), invented by C. Fillmore, for example, is based on the idea of semantic frames. Having more information of the possible or most probable noun–verb combinations will improve the analysis of events. Another idea is also to make extensive use of the audio information. Background noises, as for example, engine noise, could be processed in a similar fashion to the way that the visual information is used now. A number of researches have also collected co-occurrence information of words. This information would be useful to improve our current ranking. It would, for example, help to disambiguate the sense of rock in Fig. 4.18.

4.5 Conclusion

The aim of the work presented in this article is to explore mathematically rigorous approaches to recognize and classify biological motion. Guided by the principle that perception and classification should not be dealt with as two separate processes, the contour tracking framework was used to simultaneously track and classify the motion. We demonstrated how effectively ARPs can mimic certain biological motions (see Fig. 4.3). These learnt motion models could then be used as observation densities in an HMM. Other than in Bregler (1997), the discrete state variable of the HMM is not used for modelling the motion and can be used for classification. An automatic segmentation of a sequence containing more than one type of motion is demonstrated in Fig. 4.4. It is demonstrated that the Markov chain can be applied more effectively by using partial importance sampling.

Although the fusion of classification and perception itself is successful we concluded that the contour tracking framework is not a very robust method for tracking human beings. Apart from the problem of initialization, finely tuned motion models are needed for the classification of the type of motion. It would be advantageous to recognize a particular motion pattern directly from the spatiotemporal features in the image sequence, and not use any form of intermediate representation such as a spline contour or an articulated model. The method of extracting skew vectors from a set of epipolar slices turns out to be a very effective feature extraction method. The experiments demonstrate that the automatic segmentation of sequences containing more than one type of motion was successful. Now we are able to analyse more complex sequences, as for example, the basketball sequence shown in Fig. 4.12. One shortcoming of the new method is also that the skew vectors are not a viewpoint-invariant motion descriptor. This and a more systematic approach to the low-level feature extraction itself are the main topics for future research.

Finally the approach presented in Section 4.2 illustrates that it is possible to generate a higher-level description of the scene automatically. The examples in Fig. 4.18 show that a small number of low-level visual descriptors is sufficient to label the type of motion. This approach does not rely on objectspecific or event-specific learning and has the potential to scale up to a large problem domain. The objective of our current research is to extend the system's capability to recognize certain biological motions using the context information of the scene.

The work presented in Sections 4.2 and 4.3 was carried out by J. R. and A. B. at the University of Oxford. J.R. was supported by a Marie-Curie fellowship awarded by the European Union. The work presented in Section 4.4 was carried out by J. R., A. H. and G. S. at GE Global Research. This work was supported in full by the Advanced Research and Development Activity (ARDA). Any opinions, findings and conclusions or recommendations expressed in this material are those of the authors and do not necessarily reflect the views of the US Government. Furthermore we thank Steve Roberts (University of Oxford), Joseph Mundy (Brown University), George A. Miller, and Christiane D. Fellbaum (Princeton University) for fruitful discussions and guidance and John Schmiederer for implementation and experimental support.

References

Baker, C. F., Fillmore, C. J. and Lowe, J. B. (1998). The Berkeley FrameNet project. In *Proc. 36th A. Mtng of the Assoc. for Comput. Linguistics* and 17th Int. Conf. on Comput. Linguistics (ed. C. Boitet and P. Whitelock), pp. 86–90. San Francisco, CA: Morgan Kaufmann Publishers.

Baumberg, A. and Hogg, D. (1994). Learning flexible models from image sequences. In *Proc. 3rd European Conf. Computer Vision, Stockholm, Sweden*, pp. 299–308. Stockholm, Sweden: Springer.

Black, M. J. and Jepson, A. D. (1998). A probabilistic framework for matching temporal trajectories: condensation-based recognition of gestures and expressions. In *Proc. 5th European Conf. Computer Vision, Freiburg, Germany*, pp. 909–24.

Blake, A. and Isard, M. (1998). *Active contours*. Berlin: Springer.

Bloom, P. (2000). *How children learn the meaning of words*. Cambridge, MA: MIT Press.

Bobick, A. F. and Wilson, A. D. (1997). A state-based approach to the representation and recognition of gesture. *IEEE Trans. Pattern Analysis Machine Intell.* **19**, 1325–37.

Borgefors, G. (1988). Hierarchical chamfer matching: a parametric edge detection algorithm. *IEEE Trans. Pattern Analysis Machine Intell.* **10**, 849–65.

Bregler, C. (1997). Learning and recognizing human dynamics in video sequences. In *Proc. 11th IEEE Computer Vision and Pattern Recognition, San Taun, PR*, pp. 568–74.

Bülthoff, I. and Bülthoff, H. (2003). *Analytic and holistic processes in the perception of faces, objects, and scenes, chapter image-based recognition of biological motion, scenes and objects*. Norwood, NJ: Ablex Publishing Corporation.

Cipolla, R. and Yamamoto, M. (1990). Stereoscopic tracking of bodies in motion. *Image Vision Computing* **8**, 85–90.

Comaniciu, D., Ramesh, V. and Meer, P. (2000). Real-time tracking of non-rigid objects using mean shift. In *IEEE Computer Vision and Pattern Recognition, Hilton Head, SC*, vol. 2, pp. 142–9.

Deutscher, J., Blake, A. and Reid, I. (2000). Articulated body motion capture by annealed particle filtering. In *IEEE Computer Vision and Pattern Recognition, Hilton Head, SC*, pp. 126–33.

Fellbaum, C. (ed.) (1998). *WordNet*. Cambridge, MA: MIT Press.

Gavrila, D. (2000). Pedestrian detection from a moving vehicle. In *Proc. 6th European Conf Computer Vision, Dublin, Ireland*, pp. 37–49.

Gavrila, D. and Philomin, V. (1999). Real-time object detection for smart vehicles. In *Proc. 7th Int. Conf. on Computer Vision, Corfu, Greece*, pp. 87–93.

Gelb, A. (ed.) (1979). *Applied optimal estimation*. Cambridge, MA: MIT Press.

Gordon, N., Salmond, D. and Smith, A. (1993). Novel approach to nonlinear/non-Gaussian Bayesian state estimation. *IEEE Proc.* **140**, 107–13.

Grenander, U. (1976–1981). *Lectures in pattern theory I, II and III*. Berlin: Springer.

Hammersley, J. and Handscomb, D. (1964). *Monte Carlo methods*. London: Methuen.

Hoogs, A., Collings, R., Kaucic, R. and Mundy, J. (2003). A common set of perceptual observables for grouping, figureground discrimination and texture classification. *IEEE Trans. Pattern Analysis Machine Intell.* **25**(4).

Isard, M. and Blake, A. (1996). Contour tracking by stochastic propagation of conditional density. In *Proc. 4th European Conf. Computer Vision, Cambridge, UK*, vol. 1, pp. 343–56.

Johansson, G. (1976). Visual motion perception. *Sci. Am.* **232**, 76–89.

Karatzas, I. and Shreve, S. E. (1991). *Brownian motion and stochastic calculus*. Berlin: Springer.

Kass, M., Witkin, A. and Terzopoulos, D. (1987). Snakes: active contour models. In *Proc. 1st Int. Conf. on Computer Vision, London, UK*, pp. 259–68.

Kitagawa, G. (1996). Monte Carlo filter and smoother for non-Gaussian nonlinear state space models. *J. Comput. Graphical Statist.* **5**, 1–25.

Liu, F. and Picard, R. W. (1998). Finding periodicity in space and time. In *Proc. 6th Int. Conf. on Computer Vision, Bombay, India*, pp. 376–83.

Lütkepohl, H. (1993). *Introduction to multiple time series analysis*, 2nd edn. Berlin: Springer.

Niyogi, S. A. and Adelson, E. H. (1994*a*). Analyzing and recognizing walking figures in xyt. In *Proc 9th IEEE Computer Vision and Pattern Recognition, Seattle, WA*, pp. 469–74.

Niyogi, S. A. and Adelson, E. H. (1994*b*). Analyzing gait with spatiotemporal surfaces. In *Workshop on Non-Rigit Motion and Articulated Objects, Austin, TX*.

North, B., Blake, A., Isard, M. and Rittscher, J. (2000). Learning and classification of complex dynamics. *IEEE Trans. Pattern Analysis Machine Intell.* **22**, 1016–34.

Pearl, J. (1988). *Probabilistic reasoning in intelligent sytems*. San Fancisco, CA: Morgan Kaufmann Publishers.

Polana, R. and Nelson, R. (1997). Detection and recognition of peridic, non-rigit motion. *Int. J. Computer Vision* **23**, 261–82.

Rabiner, L. and Bing-Hwang, J. (1993). *Fundamentals of speech recognition*. Englewood Cliffs, NJ: Prentice-Hall.

Rittscher, J. and Blake, A. (1999). Classification of human body motion. In *Proc. 7th Int. Conf on Computer Vision, Corfu, Greece*, vol. 2, pp. 634–9.

Rowley, H. A., Baluja, S. and Kanade, T. (1998). Neural networkbased face detection. *IEEE Trans. Pattern Analysis Machine Intell.* **20**, 23–38.

Scheffe, H. (1959). *The analysis of variance*. New York: Wiley.

Schroeder, W. J., Zarge, J. A. and Lorensen, W. E. (1992). Decimation of triangle meshes. *Computer Graphics* **26**, 65–70.

Sidenbladh, H., Black, M. J. and Fleet, D. J. (2000). Stochastic tracking of 3D human figures using 2D image motion. In *Proc. 6th European Conf. Computer Vision, Dublin, Ireland*, vol. 2, pp. 702–18.

Szummer, M. and Picard, R. W. (1998). Indoor-outdoor image classification. In *IEEE International Workshop on Content Based Access of Image and Video Databases, in conjunction with ICCV'98*, pp. 42–51.

Toyama, K. and Blake, A. (2001). Probabilistic tracking in metric space. In *Proc. 8th Int. Conf. on Computer Vision, Vancouver, BC*, vol. 1, pp. 50–7.

Vailaya, A., Jain, A. and Zhang, H. (1998). On image classification: city vs. landscape. In *IEEE International Workshop on Content-based Access of Image and Video Databases, in conjunction with ICCV'98*, pp. 3–8.

Zelnik-Manor, L. and Irani, M. (2001). Event-based analysis of video. In *IEEE Computer Vision and Pattern Recognition, Hawaii.*

Glossary

ARP: autoregressive process
HMM: hidden Markov model

5

What imitation tells us about social cognition: a rapprochement between developmental psychology and cognitive neuroscience

Andrew N. Meltzoff and Jean Decety

Both developmental and neurophysiological research suggest a common coding between perceived and generated actions. This shared representational network is innately wired in humans. We review psychological evidence concerning the imitative behaviour of newborn human infants. We suggest that the mechanisms involved in infant imitation provide the foundation for understanding that others are 'like me' and underlie the development of theory of mind and empathy for others. We also analyse functional neuroimaging studies that explore the neurophysiological substrate of imitation in adults. We marshal evidence that imitation recruits not only shared neural representations between the self and the other but also cortical regions in the parietal cortex that are crucial for distinguishing between the perspective of self and other. Imitation is doubly revealing: it is used by infants to learn about adults, and by scientists to understand the organization and functioning of the brain.

Keywords: imitation; theory of mind; empathy; parietal cortex; mirror neurons; shared neural representations

5.1. Introduction

Our ability to imitate others' actions holds the key to our understanding what it is for others to be like us and for us to be like them. The past two decades of research have significantly expanded our knowledge about imitation at the cognitive and neurological levels. One goal of this article is to discuss striking convergences between the cognitive and neuroscientific findings. A second goal is to make a theoretical proposal. We wish to make a three-step argument:

 (i) imitation is innate in humans;
 (ii) imitation precedes mentalizing and theory of mind (in development and evolution); and
 (iii) behavioural imitation and its neural substrate provide the mechanism by which theory of mind and empathy develop in humans.

Metaphorically, we can say that nature endows humans with the tools to solve the 'other minds' problem by providing newborns with an imitative brain. In ontogeny, infant imitation is the seed and the adult theory of mind is the fruit.[1]

We are thus proposing a 'linking argument'. We think there is a large gap between mirror neurons and theory of mind. Monkeys have mirror neurons, but they lack a theory of mind, and they do not imitate. The missing link, we shall argue, is motor imitation. Through imitating others, the human young come to understand that others not only share behavioural states, but are 'like me' in deeper ways as well. This propels the human young on the developmental trajectory of developing an understanding of other minds.

This linking argument is missing from the literature. One can find excellent reviews about mirror neurons and common perception–action coding from both neuroscientific (Rizzolatti et al. 2002; Chapter 7 this volume) and cognitive (Prinz and Hommel 2002) perspectives. One can find theory of mind reviewed from both neuroscientific (Frith and Frith 1999) and cognitive (Astington and Gopnik 1991; Taylor 1996; Wellman and Gelman 1998; Flavell 1999) perspectives. What is missing is a proposal for how a neural mirror system begets theory of mind. In this paper we focus on a missing link—imitation.

5.2. Simple imitation and its neural substrate

(a) Evidence from developmental science: innate imitation

At what age can infants imitate facial acts, and how can they do so? Infants can see the adult's face but can not see their own faces. They can feel their own faces move, but have no access to the feelings of movement in the other. If they are young enough they will have never seen their own face. There are no mirrors in the womb. The holy grail for cognitive- and neuro-science theories of imitation is to elucidate the mechanism by which infants connect the felt but unseen movements of the self with the seen but unfelt movements of the other.

Classical theories such as that of Piaget (1962) considered facial imitation a cognitive milestone first passed at about 1 year. Piaget argued that infants learned to associate self and other through mirror play and tactile exploration of their own and others' faces. Mirrors made the unseen visible, rendering one's own body and that of the other in visual terms. Tactile exploration of faces rendered both self and other in tangible terms.

Over the past 25 years, empirical work from developmental science has forced a revision of the conventional view of imitation and challenged the theory that perceptual and motor systems are initially independent and uncoordinated in the human newborn (see Fig. 5.1).

To eliminate associative learning experiences, Meltzoff and Moore (1983, 1989) tested facial imitation using newborns in a hospital nursery. A large sample of newborns was tested ($n = 80$). The oldest infant in these studies was 72 hours old. The youngest was 42 minutes old. The results demonstrated

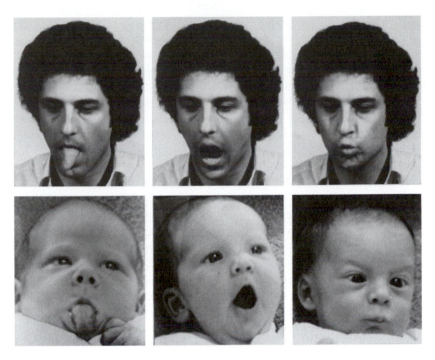

Fig. 5.1 Photographs of 12–21-day-old infants imitating facial expressions demonstrated by an adult. Imitation is innate in human beings, which allows them to share behavioural states with other 'like me' agents. (From Meltzoff and Moore (1977).)

successful facial imitation. This finding of early imitation came as a surprise to developmental psychology, which had long held the idea of independent visual and action spaces. It has now been replicated and extended in more than two dozen studies from 13 independent laboratories (see Meltzoff and Moore (1997) for a review). Evidently, the capacity for facial imitation is part of the innate endowment of human beings.

Several studies further illuminate the imitative capacity. One study showed that 12–21-day-old infants could imitate four different adult gestures: lip protrusion, mouth opening, tongue protrusion and finger movement (Meltzoff and Moore 1977). These results revealed that infants confused neither actions nor body parts. They accurately responded to tongue protrusion with tongue protrusion not lip protrusion (and vice versa) demonstrating that the specific *body part* could be identified. They also accurately responded to lip protrusion versus lip opening, showing that two different *action patterns* could be duplicated using the same body part.

Interestingly, the newborns' first response to seeing a facial gesture is activation of the corresponding body part (Meltzoff and Moore 1997). For example, when they see tongue protrusion, there is often a quieting of other body parts and an activation of the tongue. They do not necessarily protrude the tongue at first, but may elevate it or move it slightly in the oral cavity. The important point is that the tongue, rather than the lips or fingers, is energized before the movement is isolated. It is as if young infants isolate *what* part of their body to move before *how* to move it. Meltzoff and Moore (1997) call this 'organ identification'. Neurophysiological data show that visual displays of parts of the face and hands in monkeys activate specific brain sites (Perrett *et al.* 1987, 1992; Desimone 1991; Gross 1992; Gross and Sergent 1992; Rolls 1992). Thus, specific body parts could be neurally represented at birth and serve as a foundation for infant imitation.

Meltzoff and Moore (1997) describe a model of infant facial imitation. According to the model, there is a very primitive and foundational 'body scheme' that allows the infant to unify the seen acts of others and their own felt acts into one common framework. The infant's own facial movements are invisible to them, but they are not unperceived by them. Infants monitor their unseen facial acts through proprioception. Infants can link self and other through what Meltzoff and Moore (1977, 1983, 1997) termed a 'supramodal' representation of the observed body act. This representation allows them to imitate from memory: infants store a representation of the adult's act and subsequently compare their own acts to this internal model (Meltzoff and Moore 1992, 1994). This representation also allows them to correct their imitative movements to more faithfully match the target they see, which infants do when the adult model demonstrates novel actions such as tongue protrusion-to-the-side (Meltzoff and Moore 1994). A fuller exposition of the crossmodal equivalence metric used to establish self–other correspondences is provided elsewhere (Meltzoff and Moore 1997). The important point for the purposes of this paper is that infant imitation provides clear behavioural evidence for an innate link between the perception and production of human acts, which suggests shared neural representations.

(b) Evidence from neuroscience: mirror neurons and the neural bases for common coding

Compatible with the findings of newborn imitation, there is a large body of data from adult experimental psychology suggesting a common coding between perception and action (Prinz 1997, 2002; Viviani 2002). However, it is only in the past 15 years that neurophysiological evidence started to accumulate (Decety and Grézes 1999). The most dramatic discovery was that 'mirror neurons' in the monkey ventral premotor cortex discharge during the execution of goal-directed hand movements and also when the monkey observes similar hand actions (Rizzolatti *et al.* 1996a). Another region in the monkey brain containing neurons specifically responsive to the sight of actions performed by others is in the STS (Perrett *et al.* 1989; Jellema *et al.* 2002). These discoveries and others have boosted the search for a comparable mechanism in humans.

In humans, Fadiga *et al.* (1995) asked subjects to observe grasping movements performed by an experimenter. At the end of the observation period, TMS was applied to the subject's motor cortex and motor evoked potentials were recorded from their hand muscles. The pattern of muscular response to this stimulus was found to be selectively increased in comparison to control conditions, demonstrating increased activity in the motor system during the observation of actions. This finding was confirmed by neuromagnetic measures made with MEG over the premotor cortex while subjects observed another person manipulating an object (Hari *et al.* 1998). Using electroencephalography, similarities in signal desynchronization were found over the motor cortex during execution and observation of finger movements (Cochin *et al.* 1999). There are also PET studies in humans showing recruitment of premotor, parietal and temporal activation during action observation. In an experiment by Rizzolatti *et al.* (1996*b*), subjects observed the grasping of objects by an experimenter. In another condition, the subjects reached and grasped the same object themselves. Significant activation was detected in the left middle temporal gyrus and in the left inferior frontal gyrus in both conditions. Recently, a functional magnetic resonance imaging study also reported that observing actions activates the premotor cortex in a somatotopic manner, similarly to that of the classical motor cortex homunculus (Buccino *et al.* 2001). In summary, these studies all demonstrate activation of the motor/ premotor cortex during observation of actions. In humans, there is a kind of direct resonance between the observation and execution of actions, and the possible relation to monkey mirror neurons has been discussed (e.g. Iacobani *et al.* 1999; Rizzolatti *et al.* 2002; Chapter 7 this volume).

Humans do not simply directly resonate, however. Our goals affect how we process stimuli in the world. A series of studies performed by Decety's group show a top–down effect on the brain regions involved during the observation of the actions. More specifically, subjects were instructed to remember an action either for later imitation or for later recognition (Decety *et al.* 1997; Grézes *et al.* 1998, 1999). In the condition of encoding-with-the-intention-to-imitate, specific haemodynamic increase was detected in the SMA, the middle frontal gyrus, the premotor cortex and the superior and inferior parietal cortices in both hemispheres. A different pattern of brain activation was found when subjects were simply observing the actions for later recognition. Here the parahippocampal gyrus in the temporal lobe was activated. There is thus a top–down effect of intention upon the processing of observed action. Intending to imitate already tunes regions beyond simple motor resonance. Altogether, these studies strongly support the view that action observation involves neural regions similar to those engaged during actual action production. However, it is equally important that the pattern of cortical activation during encoding-with-the-intention-to-imitate is more similar to that of action production than the mere observation of actions. It is also noteworthy, as will be seen in Sections 5.4 and 5.5, that the right inferior parietal cortex is activated in conditions involving imitation.

Interestingly Perani *et al.* (2001) presented subjects with object-grasping actions performed by either a real hand or by means of 3D virtual reality or 2D TV screen. Results showed common activation foci in the left posterior parietal cortex and in the premotor cortex for observing both real-hand and artificial ones, with greater signal increase for the real-hand condition. A striking finding was the selective involvement of the right inferior parietal cortex and the right STG only in the real condition. We suggest that these regions play a part in the recognition of another's action and may be specific to registering human actions rather than the motions of mechanical devices.

Humans often imagine actions in the absence of motor execution. What are the neural correlates for imagined actions (Decety 2002)? Does it matter whether you imagine an action performed by the self or that same action performed by another person? Ruby and Decety (2001) asked subjects to imagine an action being performed by themselves (first-person perspective) or by another individual (third-person perspective). Both perspectives were associated with common activated clusters in the SMA, the precentral gyrus and the precuneus. However, there were differences depending on whether subjects were imagining their own versus another person's actions. First-person perspective taking was specifically associated with increased activity in the left inferior parietal lobule and the left somatosensory cortex, whereas the third-person perspective recruited the right inferior parietal lobule, the posterior cingulate and the frontopolar cortex. A similar pattern of activation was confirmed in a follow-up functional neuroimaging study involving more conceptual perspective-taking tasks (Ruby and Decety 2003). These results support the notion of shared representations of self and other, even in the case of imagined actions of self and other. The results also suggest a crucial role of the inferior parietal cortex in distinguishing the perspective of self and other.

(i) Going beyond mirror neurons

Human newborn imitation demonstrates an innate connection between the observation and execution of human acts. One assumption often made is that the mirror neurons discussed by Rizzolatti *et al.* (2002) are also innate. This assumption deserves scrutiny, however. Based on the evidence to date, it is possible that the mirror neurons found in adult monkeys are the result of learned associations. Consider the case of a mirror neuron that discharges to 'grasping-with-the-hand'. This same cell fires regardless of whether that act is performed by the monkey or is observed in another actor. A cell that discharges in both cases could mean that 'grasping' is an innate act; perhaps a cell is pre-tuned to this evolutionarily significant act whether performed by the self or the other. Alternatively, it could be based on the fact that the monkey has repeatedly observed itself perform this action. Observation and execution occur in perfect temporal synchrony whenever the monkey watches itself grasp an object. After such experience, the visual perception of grasping by another animal could activate neurons based on a visual equivalence class between the sight of one's own and another's hand. Monkeys are known to be capable of such visual generalizations and categorization. Thus, mirror neurons could result from learning by association and visual generalization.

It is crucial to investigate the ontogeny of mirror neurons. One needs to determine whether monkeys are born with functioning mirror neurons that activate the first time the animal sees an act, which would be equivalent to the newborn work done by Meltzoff and Moore (1983, 1989) with 42-minute-old human infants. To the best of our knowledge this work has not been done with newborn monkeys. Thus, we are left with unfinished empirical work. There is behavioural evidence of an innate observation–execution system in humans (imitation) but work is lacking on the neural basis in this newborn population; and there is research addressing the neural bases for an observation–execution system in monkeys (mirror neurons), but work is lacking on the innateness question.

A further interesting question for the future is whether innate human imitation relies chiefly on neural machinery in the premotor cortex (akin to monkey mirror neurons), or, alternatively, on neural systems involving the inferior parietal lobule (which have been shown to be crucial in human studies involving the processing of similarities and differences between the actions of self and other). The infancy work shows that young babies *correct* their imitative behaviour, which suggests an active comparison and lack of confusion between self and other (Meltzoff and Moore 1997). It also shows that infants can store a model and imitate *from memory* after delays as long as 24 hours (Meltzoff and Moore 1994; Meltzoff 1999), which requires more than simple visual-motor resonance. These features of human imitation may go beyond the workings of the mirror neurons *per se*. Furthermore, monkeys do not imitate (Tomasello and Call 1997; Byrne 2002; Whiten 2002), although they certainly have the basic mirror neuron machinery. Something more is needed to prompt and support behavioural imitation, especially the imitation of novel actions and imitation from memory without the stimulus perceptually present. This may involve the inferior parietal lobe, which is implicated in registering both the similarity and the distinction between actions of the self and other.

5.3 Knowing you are being imitated by the other: self–other relations

Human beings do not only imitate. They also recognize when they are being imitated by others. Such reciprocal imitation is an essential part of communicative exchanges. A listener often shows interpersonal connectedness with a speaker by adopting the postural configuration of the speaker. If the speaker furrows his or her brow, the listener does the same; if the speaker rubs his chin, the listener follows. Parents use this same technique, however unconsciously, in establishing intersubjectivity with their preverbal infants. Imitation seems to be intrinsically coupled with empathy for others, broadly construed.

(a) Evidence from developmental science: emotional reactions to being imitated

Adults across cultures play reciprocal imitative games with their children. Some developmentalists have focused exclusively on the temporal turn-taking embodied in these games (Trevarthen 1979; Brazelton and Tronick 1980). Timing is important, but we think these games are uniquely valuable owing to the structural congruence between self and other. Physical objects may come under temporal control. Only people who are paying attention to you and acting intentionally can match the form of your acts in a generative fashion. Only people can act 'like me'.

Meltzoff (1990) tested whether infants recognize when another acts 'like me' and the emotional value of this experience. One experiment involved 14-month-old infants and two adults. One of the adults imitated everything the baby did; the other adult imitated what the previous baby had done. Each adult copied one of the infants, so each acted like a perfect baby. Could the infants distinguish which adult was acting just like the self?

The results showed that they could. They looked longer at the adult who was imitating them; smiled more at this adult; and most significantly, directed testing behaviour at that adult (for similar results, see also Asendorph (2002) and Nadel (2002)). By testing we mean that infants often modulated their acts by performing sudden and unexpected movements to check if the adult was following what they did. The Marx brothers are famous for substituting a person who imitates in place of a true reflection in a mirror. The actor in such a situation systematically varies his acts to see if the other is still in congruence. Infants acted in this same way, testing in a concerted fashion whether the other person would follow everything they did.

Further research revealed that even very young infants are attentive to being imitated. However, we found an important difference between the younger and the older infants. Although younger infants increase the particular gesture being imitated, they do not switch to mismatching gestures to see if they will be copied. For example, if an adult systematically matches a young infant's tongue protrusion, her attention is attracted and she generates more of this behaviour, but does not switch to gestures to test this relationship. The older infants go beyond this interpretation and treat the interaction as a matching game that is being shared.

By saying that the older infant appreciates the shared matching game, we mean that the relationship is being abstractly considered and the particular behaviours are substitutable. It is not the notion that tongue protrusion leads to tongue protrusion (a mapping at the level of a particular behaviour), but the abstract notion that the other is doing 'the same as' me. By 14 months, infants undoubtedly know that adults are not under their total control, and part of the joy of this exchange is the realization that although the infant does not actually control the other, nonetheless the other is choosing to do just what I do.

Together these two factors may help to explain why older infants will joyfully engage in mutual imitation games for 20 minutes or more—much longer and with greater glee than watching themselves in a mirror. The infants recognize the difference between self and other and seem to be exploring the sense of agency involved—exploring who is controlling whom in this situation.

(b) Evidence from neuroscience: imitation and the neural basis of differentiating actions of self and other

The developmental work shows that infants not only imitate but also know when they are being imitated by others. This is interesting because the situation in the physical world is the same—there are two bodies in correspondence with one another—whether one is the imitator or the imitatee. An external observer might not know who imitated whom. How does the brain keep track of this? What is the neural basis for distinguishing the self's imitation of the other from the other's imitation of the self?

Decety *et al.* (2002) designed a PET study focusing on this question. In the two imitation conditions, the subjects either imitated the experimenter's actions on objects or saw their own actions imitated by him. Three control conditions were used: (i) action-generation control: subjects allowed to freely manipulate the objects any way they wanted to; (ii) observing action control: subjects simply watching the demonstrator's actions; or (iii) visual-motor mismatch control: subjects performed actions while watching the other person simultaneously performing mismatched movements.

Several regions were involved in the two imitation conditions compared to the control conditions, namely the STG, the inferior parietal lobule, and the medial prefrontal cortex. Interestingly for our view linking imitation and mentalizing, the medial prefrontal cortex is known to be activated in tasks involving mentalizing (Frith and Frith 1999; Blakemore and Decety 2001). The inferior parietal lobule also proved to be a key region (see Fig. 5.2). When the two imitation conditions were contrasted to the control condition in which subjects acted differently from the experimenter, a lateralization of the activity was found in this region. The left inferior parietal lobule was activated when subjects imitated the other, while the right homologous region was associated with being imitated by the other. In comparing the imitation and control conditions, activation was also detected in the posterior part of the STG, known to be involved in the visual perception of socially meaningful hand gestures (Allison *et al.* 2000). This cluster was found in both hemispheres when contrasting the imitation conditions to the action-generation control condition. However, it was only present in the left hemisphere when the condition of being imitated was subtracted from the condition of imitating the other. This lateralization in the STG is an intriguing finding. We suggest that the right STG is involved in visual analysis of the other's actions, while its

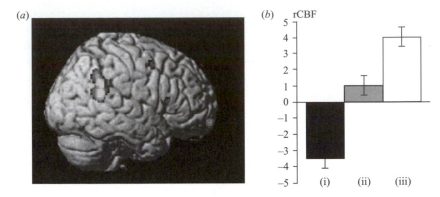

Fig. 5.2 (*a*) Right inferior parietal lobule activation when subjects saw their actions being imitated superimposed on an average MRI. (*b*) The relative haemodynamic variation during self action, when subjects acted at will (i), when they imitated the actions demonstrated by the experimenter (ii), and when they saw their actions being imitated by the experimenter (iii). Note the dramatic increase in right inferior parietal lobe activation in this last condition. rCBF indicates regional cerebral blood flow. (Adapted from Decety *et al.* (2002).) See Plate 4 of the Plate Section, at the centre of this book.

homologous region in the left region is concerned with analysis of the other's actions in relation to actions performed by the self.

The activation of the inferior parietal cortex in imitation is at least partially attributable to the sense of agency involved. That the inferior parietal cortex is involved in the feeling of agency is supported by converging evidence from neuropsychology (Kinsbourne 2002), and other neuroimaging studies (e.g. Ruby and Decety 2001; Chaminade and Decety 2002; Farrer and Frith 2002; Farrer *et al.* 2003), as well as from abnormalities in self–other distinctions found in schizophrenic patients (e.g. Spence *et al.* 1997). All these studies have pointed out the specific involvement of this region in tasks that require subjects to distinguish actions produced by the self from those produced by another agent. This, of course, is the essential ingredient in knowing 'who is imitating whom'—and is a common situation in parent–child games and empathic resonance.

There is also much evidence that the prefrontal cortex plays a key role in self-consciousness, including self-agency (i.e., I am the initiator of the action, thought, or desire) and self-ownership (i.e., it is my body that is moving). These high-level functions tap executive-function resources, including inhibition, which are necessary for the initiation and the maintenance of nonautomatic cognitive processes (Ferstl and von Cramon 2002). Lesions of the prefrontal cortex may cause dysfunction in self-monitoring and lead to what Lhermitte *et al.* (1986) termed the 'environmental dependency syndrome.' We suggest that the prefrontal cortex, via its reciprocal connections with the parietal lobe, plays a central role in coordinating self and other representations by monitoring signals from executive and sensory regions and identifying the source of perceptions (internal or external).

5.4 Reading others' goals and intentions

Persons are more than dynamic bags of skin that I can imitate and which imitate me. In the mature adult notion, persons have internal mental states—such as beliefs, goals and intentions—that predict and explain human actions. Recently, attention has turned to the earliest developmental roots and neural substrate of decoding the goals and intentions of others.

(a) Evidence from developmental science: infants' understanding of others' goals and intentions

Developmental psychologists have attempted to use preferential-looking procedures to explore infants' understanding of goals (see Gergely *et al.* 1995; Woodward *et al.* 2001; Chapter 2 this volume). These visual tests assess infants' ability to recognize discrepancies from visible goal states, such as grasping one object versus another, or moving towards/away from a visible location in space. These studies do not involve adopting the goals of others and using them as the basis for self action. Nor do they involve inferring unseen goals and intentions, such as drawing a distinction between what a person means to do versus what they actually do (a crucial distinction in the law and morality).

Meltzoff (1995) introduced a more active procedure to address these issues. The procedure capitalizes on imitation, but it uses this proclivity in a new, more abstract way. It investigates infants' ability to read below the visible surface behaviour to the underlying goals and intentions of the actor. It also assesses infants' capacity to act on the goals that they inferred.

One study involved showing 18-month-old infants an unsuccessful act, a failed effort (Meltzoff 1995). For example, the adult 'accidentally' under- or overshot his target, or he tried to perform a behaviour but his hand slipped several times; thus the goal state was not achieved. To an adult, it was easy to read the actor's intentions although he did not fulfil them. The experimental question was whether infants also read through the literal body movements to the underlying goal of the act. The measure of how they interpreted the event was what they chose to re-enact. In this case the correct answer was not to copy the literal movement that was actually seen, but to copy the actor's goal, which remained unfulfilled.

The study compared infants' tendency to perform the target act in several situations: (i) after they saw the full target act demonstrated, (ii) after they saw the unsuccessful attempt to perform the act, and (iii) after it was neither shown nor attempted. The results showed that 18-month-old infants can infer the unseen goals implied by unsuccessful attempts. Infants who saw the unsuccessful attempt and infants who saw the full target act both produced target acts at a significantly higher rate than controls. Evidently, young toddlers can understand our goals even if we fail to fulfil them. They choose to imitate what we meant to do, rather than what we mistakenly did do.

In further work, 18-month-old infants were shown an adult trying and failing to pull apart a dumbbell-shaped object, but they were handed a trick toy. The toy had been surreptitiously glued shut before the study began. When infants picked it up and attempted to pull it apart, their hands slipped off the ends of the cubes. This, of course, matched the surface behaviour of the adult. However, this imitative match at the behavioural level did not satisfy them. They sought to fulfil the adult's intention. The infants repeatedly grabbed the toy, yanked on it in different ways, and appealed to their mothers and the adult. Fully 90% of the infants immediately ($M < 2$ s) looked up at an adult after failing to pull apart the trick toy, and they vocalized while staring directly at the adult.

If infants are picking up the underlying goal or intention of the human act, they should be able to achieve the act using a variety of means. Meltzoff tested this with a dumbbell-shaped object that was too big for the infants' hands. The infants did not attempt to imitate the surface behaviour of the adult. Instead they used novel ways to struggle to get the gigantic toy apart. They put one end of the dumbbell between their knees and used both hands to pull upwards, or put their hands on the inside faces of the cubes and pushed outwards, and so on. They used different means than the experimenter, but their actions were directed towards the same end. This fits with the hypothesis that infants had inferred the goal of the act, differentiating it from the literal surface behaviour that was observed.[2]

In the adult psychological framework, people and other animate beings have goals and intentions, but inanimate devices do not. Do infants carve the world in this way? To assess this, Meltzoff designed an inanimate device made of plastic and wood (Meltzoff (1995), experiment 2). The device had poles for arms and mechanical pincers for hands. It did not look human, but it traced the same spatiotemporal path that the human actor traced and manipulated the object much as the human actor did (see Fig. 5.3). The results showed that infants did not attribute a goal or intention to the movements of the inanimate device when its pincers slipped off the ends of the dumbbell. Infants were no more (or less) likely to pull the toy apart after seeing the failed attempt of the

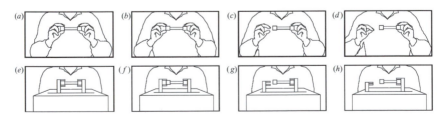

Fig. 5.3   Human demonstrator (*a–d*) and inanimate device performing the same movements (*e–h*). Infants attribute goals and intentions to the person but not the inanimate device. (From Meltzoff (1995).)

inanimate device than they were in baseline levels when they saw nothing. This was the case despite the fact that infants pulled the dumbbell apart if the inanimate device successfully completed this act. Evidently, infants can pick up certain information from the inanimate device, but not other information: they can understand successes, but not failures. (This makes sense because successes lead to a change in the object, whereas failures leave the object intact and therefore must be interpreted at a deeper level.)

This developmental research shows that infants distinguished between what the adult meant to do and what he actually did. They ascribed goals to human acts; indeed, they inferred the goal even when it was not attained. This differentiation between behaviour versus goals and intentions lies at the core of our mentalizing, and it underlies our moral judgements. The infants in these experiments were already exhibiting a fundamental aspect of our adult framework: the acts of persons (but not the motions of inanimates) are construed in terms of goals and intentions.[3]

(b) Evidence from neuroscience: means and goals

This research shows that even infants draw a distinction between observed behaviour and the goals towards which it is heading. We designed a functional neuroimaging experiment to differentiate the neural correlates of two key components of human actions, the goals and the means to achieve it (Chaminade *et al.* 2002). The 'goal' in this experiment was operationalized as the end state of the object manipulation and the 'means' as the motor programme used to achieve this end. Actions consisted of sequentially moving Lego blocks from a start position to a specific place in a Lego construction. Depending on the experimental conditions, subjects were asked to imitate a human model who presented either: (i) the goal only, (ii) the means only, or (iii) the whole action. The control condition involved free action, during which the subject could manipulate the Lego blocks at will, and thus did not involve imitation.

The results revealed partially overlapping clusters of increased regional cerebral blood flow in the right dorsolateral prefrontal area and in the cerebellum when subjects imitated either the goal or the means. Moreover, specific activity was detected in the medial prefrontal cortex when only the means were presented (and the *goal* had to be inferred); whereas there was increased activity in the left premotor cortex when only the goal was presented (and the *means* had to be inferred). The finding of the involvement of the right dorsolateral prefrontal cortex in our imitation tasks is consistent with its role in the preparation of forthcoming action based on stored information (Pochon *et al.* 2001). Interestingly, the medial prefrontal region was primarily activated in the experimental condition involving inferences about goals. The medial prefrontal region is known to play a critical role in inferring others' intentions and is consistently involved in mentalizing tasks (Blakemore and Decety 2001). Its activation during our imitation task suggests that observing the means used by an actor prompts the observer to construct/infer the goals towards which this human agent is aiming. The fact that the same neural regions are activated in imitation and mentalizing tasks fits with the ideas we advanced earlier in this paper (see Section 5.1).

5.5 Theoretical speculations

The conundrum of social cognition stems from the simple truth that persons are more than physical objects. Giving a person's height and the shape of his fingerprint does not exhaust our description of that person. We have skipped their psychological makeup. A longstanding question is how we come to know others as persons like ourselves.

We suggest that infant imitation provides an innate foundation for social cognition. Imitation indicates that newborns, at some level of processing no matter how primitive, can map actions of other people onto actions of their own body. Human acts are especially relevant to infants because they look like the infant feels himself to be and because they are events infants can intend. When a human act is shown to a newborn, it may provide the first recognition experience, 'something familiar! That seen event is like this felt event'.

(a) Developmental science: innate imitation and 'like me' processing as the root of mentalizing

We are now in a position to see how the imitative mind and brain may contribute to the development of mentalizing. We offer a three-step developmental sequence as follows.

(i) *Innate equipment*. Newborns can recognize equivalences between perceived and executed acts. This is that starting state, as documented by newborn imitation (Meltzoff and Moore 1997).

(ii) *First-person experience*. Through everyday experience infants map the relation between their own bodily acts and their mental experiences. For example, there is an intimate relation between 'striving to achieve a goal' and the concomitant facial expression and effortful bodily acts. Infants experience their own unfulfilled desires and their own concomitant facial/postural/vocal reactions. They experience their own inner feelings and outward facial expressions and construct a detailed bidirectional map linking mental experiences and behaviour.

(iii) *Inferences about the experiences of others*. When infants see others acting 'like me', they project that others have the same mental experience that is mapped to those behavioural states in the self.

In sum, given the innate state (step no. (i)) and the knowledge that behaviour X maps to mental state X' in their own experience (step no. (ii)), infants have relevant data to make inferences about relations between the visible behaviour of others and the underlying mental state (step no. (iii)).

Infants would not need the adult theory of mind innately specified. Infants could infer the internal states of others through an analogy to the self. Infants imbue the acts of others with 'felt meaning', because others are intrinsically recognized as 'like me'.

(b) Neuroscience: the importance of the human inferior parietal cortex in representing self–other relations

Imitation indicates a common coding between the observation and execution of acts. However, that is not the end of the story. Infants also correct their imitative behaviour, which indicates that their representation of the target is kept distinct from the representation of their own movements. Similarly, infants recognize being imitated by others, and they 'test' whether the other will follow what they do. Here, again, there is a recognition of self–other equivalence, but not a total confusion between the two. Thus, one highly relevant issue concerns how the self-versus-other distinction operates within these shared representations and which neural mechanisms are engaged in integrating and discriminating the representations activated from within and those activated by external agents.

Our functional neuroimaging studies on imitation were designed to explore both what is common as well as distinct between self and other. The results highlight the role of the posterior part of the STG and the inferior parietal cortex, in conjunction with medial prefrontal and premotor areas. Indeed, all of our imitation tasks across several studies activate the posterior part of the temporal cortex and the medial prefrontal cortex. It is noteworthy that the former region is activated by tasks that require detection of biological agents (Griffiths et al. 1998; Grossman et al. 2000; Grézes et al. 2001). The latter region is consistently activated in mentalizing tasks involving the attribution of intentions to oneself and to others (Frith and Frith 1999; Blakemore and Decety 2001), as well as in executive functioning (a cluster of high-order capacities, including selective attention, behavioural planning and response inhibition; e.g. Siegal and Varley 2002).[4]

In our studies, there was more increase in the left inferior parietal lobule when subjects imitated the other, and more increase in the right homologous region when they saw that their actions were imitated by the other. We suggest that the left inferior parietal lobule computes the sensory-motor associations necessary to imitate, which is compatible with the literature on apraxia (Halsband 1998), whereas the right inferior parietal lobule is involved in recognizing or detecting that actions performed by others are similar to those initiated by the self and determining the locus of agency for matching bodily acts.

This proposal about the importance of the right inferior parietal lobule fits with the clinical neuropsychological evidence that it is important for body knowledge and self-awareness and that its lesion produces disorders of body representation such as anosognosia, asomatognosia or somatoparaphrenia (Berlucchi and Aglioti 1997). Ramachandran and Rogers-Ramachandran (1996) reported cases of patients with right parietal lesions in whom the denial of hemiplegia applies both to their own condition and to the motor deficits of other patients. This indicates that availability of an efficient body schema is necessary not only for recognizing one's own behavioural states but also for understanding those states in others.

It is interesting to note that the ability to represent one's own thoughts and to represent another's thoughts are intimately tied together, and they may have similar origins within the brain (Keenan *et al.* 2000). Thus it makes sense that self-awareness, empathy, identification with others, and more generally inter-subjective processes, are largely dependent upon right hemisphere resources, which are the first to develop Measurements of cerebral metabolism in children (aged between 18 days to 12 years) indicate a right hemispheric predominance, mainly due to neural activity in the posterior associative areas, suggesting that the right hemisphere's functions develop earlier than the left hemisphere (Chiron *et al.* 1997).

Finally, in light of our neuroimaging experiments, we suggest that the right inferior parietal lobule plays a key role in the uniquely human capacity to identify with others and appreciate the subjective states of conspecifics as both similar to and differentiated from one's own (Decety and Chaminade 2003; Ruby and Decety 2003). This may well be a qualitative difference between human and non-human primates, not just a quantitative one (Povinelli and Prince 1998; Tomasello 1999). In other words, the adult human framework is not simply one of resonance. We are able to recognize that everyone does not share our own desires, emotions, intentions and beliefs. To become a sophisticated mentalizer one needs to analyse both the similarities and differences between one's own states and those of others. That is what makes us human.

Acknowledgements

The authors thank T. Chaminade and C. Harris for help on the work presented here, and B. Repacholi for valuable comments. They gratefully acknowledge support from NIH (HD-22514) and from the Talaris Research Institute and the Apex Foundation, the family foundation of B. and J. McCaw.

Endnotes

1. We use the terms 'theory of mind' and 'mentalizing' interchangeably in this paper.
2. Work with older children, in the 3–6 year age range, also underscores the importance of goals in children's imitation (Bekkering *et al.* 2000; Gleissner *et al.* 2000), and the present work shows that goal detection is connected to imitation right from infancy.

3. None the less, both infants and adults sometimes make confusions. People some-times attribute goals to their computer (because it exhibits certain functionality), and one could build a robot that fooled children and even adults; consider Star Trek androids. However, in the present case an inanimate device was used that only mimicked the spatiotemporal movements of a hand, and did not look or otherwise act human. The results of Meltzoff (1995) dovetail with the finding that there are certain neural systems activated by human actions and not similar movements produced by a mechanical device (Decety *et al.* 1994; Perani *et al.* 2001; Castiello *et al.* 2002), and the demonstration that infants process animate body parts differently from inanimate objects (e.g. Brooks and Meltzoff 2002).

4. Prefrontal, inferior parietal and temporoparietal areas have evolved tremendously in humans compared to non-human primates (Passingham 1998). The parietal cortex is roughly 'after' vision and 'before' motor control in the cortical information-processing hierarchy (Milner 1998). The inferior parietal lobule is a heteromodal association cortex which receives input from the lateral and posterior thalamus, as well as visual, auditory, somaesthic and limbic input. It has reciprocal connections to the prefrontal and temporal lobes (Eidelberg and Galaburda 1984). It is claimed by some scholars (e.g. Milner 1997), following Brodmann (1907), that the human superior parietal lobe, taken alone, is equivalent to the whole of the monkey poste-rior parietal cortex. If so, the monkey and human inferior parietal lobes may not be fully equivalent. This is a highly speculative position, but it is interesting in light of the role we have found for the inferior parietal lobe in representing the relationship between self and other. Further information on the evolution and development of this brain region is needed.

References

Allison, T., Puce, A. and McCarthy, G. (2000). Social perception from visual cues: role of the STS region. *Trends Cogn. Sci.* **4**, 267–78.

Asendorph, J. B. (2002). Self-awareness, other-awareness, and secondary representa-tion. In *The imitative mind: development, evolution, and brain bases* (ed. A. N. Meltzoff and W. Prinz), pp. 63–73. New York: Cambridge University Press.

Astington, J. W. and Gopnik, A. (1991). Theoretical explanations of children's under-standing of the mind. *Brit. J. Devl. Psych.* **9**, 7–31.

Bekkering, H., Wohlschlandauml;ger, A. and Gattis, M. (2000). Imitation of gestures in children is goal-directed. *Q. J. Exp. Psychol.* **53A**, 153–64.

Berlucchi, G. and Aglioti, S. (1997). The body in the brain: neural bases of corporeal awareness. *Trends Neurosci.* **20**, 560–4.

Blakemore, S.-J. and Decety, J. (2001). From the perception of action to the under-standing of intention. *Nature Rev. Neurosci.* **2**, 561–7.

Brazelton, T. B. and Tronick, E. (1980). Preverbal communication between mothers and infants. In *The social foundations of language and thought* (ed. D. R. Olson), pp. 299–315. New York: Norton.

Brodmann, K. (1907). Beitrandauml;ge zur histologischen Lokalisation der Grosshirnrinde. Sechste Mitteilung: die cortoxygliederung der Menschen. *J. Psychol. Neurol. Lpz* **10**, 231–6.

Brooks, R. and Meltzoff, A. N. (2002). The importance of eyes: how infants interpret adult looking behavior. *Dev. Psychol.* **38**, 958–66.

Buccino, G., Binkofski, F., Fink, G. R., Fadiga, L., Fogassi, L., Gallese, V., *et al.* (2001). Action observation activates premotor and parietal areas in a somatotopic manner: an fMRI study. *Eur. J. Neurosci.* **13**, 400–04.

Byrne, R. W. (2002). Seeing actions as hierarchically organized structures: great ape manual skills. In *The imitative mind: development, evolution, and brain bases* (ed. A. N. Meltzoff and W. Prinz), pp. 122–40. New York: Cambridge University Press.

Castiello, U., Lusher, D., Mari, M., Edwards, M. and Humphreys, G. W. (2002). Observing a human or a robotic hand grasping an object: differential motor priming effects. In *Common mechanisms in perception and action: attention and performance* XIX (ed. W. Prinz and B. Hommel), pp. 315–33. New York: Oxford University Press.

Chaminade, T. and Decety, J. (2002). Leader or follower? Involvement of the inferior parietal lobule in agency. *NeuroReport* **13**, 1975–78.

Chaminade, T., Meltzoff, A. N. and Decety, J. (2002). Does the end justify the means? A PET exploration of the mechanisms involved in human imitation. *NeuroImage* **15**, 318–28.

Chiron, C., Jambaque, J., Nabbout, R., Lounes, R., Syrota, A. and Dulac, O. (1997). The right brain hemisphere is dominant in human infants. *Brain* **120**, 1057–65.

Cochin, S., Barthelemy, C., Roux, S. and Martineau, J. (1999). Observation and execution of movement: similarities demonstrated by quantified electroencephalography. *Eur. J. Neurosci.* **11**, 1839–42.

Decety, J. (2002). Is there such thing as a functional equivalence between imagined, observed, and executed action? In *The imitative mind: development, evolution, and brain bases* (ed. A. N. Meltzoff and W. Prinz), pp. 291–310. New York: Cambridge University Press.

Decety, J. and Grandézes, J. (1999). Neural mechanisms subserving the perception of human actions. *Trends Cogn. Sci.* **3**, 172–8.

Decety, J. and Chaminade, T. (2003). Neural correlates of feeling sympathy. *Neuropsychologia* **41**, 127–38.

Decety, J., Chaminade, T., Grandézes, J. and Meltzoff, A. N. (2002). A PET exploration of the neural mechanisms involved in reciprocal imitation. *NeuroImage* **15**, 265–72.

Decety, J., Perani, D., Jeannerod, M., Bettinardi, V., Tadary, B., Woods, R., *et al.* (1994). Mapping motor representations with positron emission tomography. *Nature* **371**, 600–2.

Decety, J., Grandézes, J., Costes, N., Perani, D., Jeannerod, M., Procyk, E., *et al.* (1997). Brain activity during observation of actions: influence of action content and subject's strategy. *Brain* **120**, 1763–77.

Desimone, R. (1991). Face-selective cells in the temporal cortex of monkeys. *J. Cogn. Neurosci.* **3**, 1–8.

Eidelberg, D. and Galaburda, A. M. (1984). Inferior parietal lobule. *Arch. Neurol.* **41**, 843–52.

Fadiga, L., Fogassi, L., Pavesi, G. and Rizzolatti, G. (1995). Motor facilitation during action observation: a magnetic stimulation study. *J. Neurophysiol.* **73**, 2608–11.

Farrer, C. and Frith, C. D. (2002). Experiencing oneself vs another person as being the cause of an action: the neural correlates of the experience of agency. *NeuroImage* **15**, 596–603.

Farrer, C., Franck, N., Georgieff, N., Frith, C. D., Decety, J. and Jeannerod, M. (2003). Modulating the experience of agency: a PET study. *NeuroImage* **18**, 324–33.

Ferstl, E.C. and von Cramon, D.Y. (2002). What does the frontomedian cortex contribute to language processing: coherence or theory of mind? *Neuroimage* **17**, 1599–612.

Flavell, J. H. (1999). Cognitive development: children's knowledge about the mind. *A. Rev. Psychol.* **50**, 21–45.

Frith, C. D. and Frith, U. (1999). Interacting minds: a biological basis. *Science* **286**, 1692–95.

Gergely, G., Nandádasdy, Z., Csibra, G. and Bandírandá, S. (1995). Taking the intentional stance at 12 months of age. *Cognition* **56**, 165–93.

Gleissner, B., Meltzoff, A. N. and Bekkering, H. (2000). Children's coding of human action: cognitive factors influencing imitation in 3-year-olds. *Dev. Sci.* **3**, 405–14.

Grézes, J., Costes, N. and Decety, J. (1998). Top-down effect of strategy on the perception of human biological motion: a PET investigation. *Cogn. Neuropsychol.* **15**, 553–82.

Grézes, J., Costes, N. and Decety, J. (1999). The effects of learning and intention on the neural network involved in the perception of meaningless actions. *Brain* **122**, 1875–87.

Grézes, J., Fonlupt, P., Bertenthal, B., Delon-Martin, C., Segebarth, C. and Decety, J. (2001). Does perception of biological motion rely on specific brain regions? *NeuroImage* **13**, 775–85.

Griffiths, T. D., Rees, G., Green, G. R. G., Witton, C., Rowe, D., Büchel, C., *et al.* (1998). Right parietal cortex is involved in the perception of sound movement in humans. *Nature Neurosci.* **1**, 74–9.

Gross, C. G. (1992). Representation of visual stimuli in inferior temporal cortex. In *Processing the facial image* (ed. V. Bruce, A. Cowey and A. W. Ellis), pp. 3–10. New York: Oxford University Press.

Gross, C. G. and Sergent, J. (1992). Face recognition. *Curr. Opin. Neurobiol.* **2**, 156–61.

Grossman, E., Donnelly, M., Price, R., Pickens, D., Morgan, V., Neighbor, G., *et al.* (2000). Brain areas involved in perception of biological motion. *J. Cogn. Neurosci.* **12**, 711–20.

Halsband, U. (1998). Brain mechanisms of apraxia. In *Comparative neuropsychology* (ed. A. D. Milner), pp. 184–212. Oxford: Oxford University Press.

Hari, R., Forss, N., Avikainen, S., Kirveskari, E., Salenius, S. and Rizzolatti, G. (1998). Activation of human primary motor cortex during action observation: a neuromagnetic study. *Proc. Natl Acad. Sci. USA* **95**, 15061–65.

Iacobani, M., Woods, R. P., Brass, M., Bekkering, H., Mazziotta, J. C. and Rizzolatti, G. (1999). Cortical mechanisms of human imitation. *Science* **286**, 2526–28.

Jellema, T., Baker, C. I., Oram, M. W. and Perrett, D. I. (2002). Cell populations in the banks of the superior temporal sulcus of the macaque and imitation. In *The imitative mind: development, evolution, and brain bases* (ed. A. N. Meltzoff and W. Prinz), pp. 267–90. New York: Cambridge University Press.

Keenan, J.P., Wheeler M.A., Gallup, G.G. and Pascual-Leone, A. (2000). Self-recognition and the right prefrontal cortex. *Trends in Cognitive Science* **4**, 338–44.

Kinsbourne, M. (2002). The role of imitation in body ownership and mental growth. In *The imitative mind: development, evolution, and brain bases* (ed. A. N. Meltzoff and W. Prinz), pp. 311–30. New York: Cambridge University Press.

Lhermitte, F., Pillon, B. and Serdaru, M.D. (1986). Human autonomy and the frontal lobes: Part 1: Imitation and utilization behavior; a neurophysychological study of 75 patients *Annals of Neurology* **19**, 326–34.

Meltzoff, A. N. (1990). Foundations for developing a concept of self: the role of imitation in relating self to other and the value of social mirroring, social modeling, and self practice in infancy. In *The self in transition: infancy to childhood* (ed. D. Cicchetti and M. Beeghly), pp. 139–64. Chicago, IL: University of Chicago Press.

Meltzoff, A. N. (1995). Understanding the intentions of others: re-enactment of intended acts by 18-month-old children. *Dev. Psychol.* **31**, 838–50.

Meltzoff, A. N. (1999). Origins of theory of mind, cognition, and communication. *J. Commun. Disord.* **32**, 251–69.

Meltzoff, A. N. and Moore, M. K. (1977). Imitation of facial and manual gestures by human neonates. *Science* **198**, 75–8.

Meltzoff, A. N. and Moore, M. K. (1983). Newborn infants imitate adult facial gestures. *Child Dev.* **54**, 702–09.

Meltzoff, A. N. and Moore, M. K. (1989). Imitation in newborn infants: exploring the range of gestures imitated and the underlying mechanisms. *Dev. Psychol.* **25**, 954–62.

Meltzoff, A. N. and Moore, M. K. (1992). Early imitation within a functional framework: the importance of person identity, movement, and development. *Infant Behav. Dev.* **15**, 479–505.

Meltzoff, A. N. and Moore, M. K. (1994). Imitation, memory, and the representation of persons. *Infant Behav. Dev.* **17**, 83–99.

Meltzoff, A. N. and Moore, M. K. (1997). Explaining facial imitation: a theoretical model. *Early Dev. Parenting* **6**, 179–92.

Milner, A. D. (1997). Neglect, extinction, and the cortical streams of visual processing. In *Parietal lobe contributions to orientation in 3D space* (ed. P. Thier and H. O. Karnath), pp. 3–22. Heidelberg: Springer.

Milner, A. D. (1998). Streams and consciousness: visual awareness and the brain. *Trends Cogn. Neurosci.* **2**, 25–30.

Nadel, J. (2002). Imitation and imitation recognition: functional use in preverbal infants and nonverbal children with autism. In *The imitative mind: development, evolution, and brain bases* (ed. A. N. Meltzoff and W. Prinz), pp. 42–62. New York: Cambridge University Press.

Passingham, R. E. (1998). The specializations of the human neocortex. In *Comparative neuropsychology* (ed. A. D. Milner), pp. 271–98. Oxford: Oxford University Press.

Perani, D., Fazio, F., Borghese, N. A., Tettamanti, M., Ferrari, S., Decety, J., *et al.* (2001). Different brain correlates for watching real and virtual hand actions. *Neuro-Image* **14**, 749–58.

Perrett, D. I., Mistlin, A. J. and Chitty, A. J. (1987). Visual neurons responsive to faces. *Trends Neurosci.* **10**, 358–64.

Perrett, D. I., Harries, M. H., Bevan, R., Thomas, S., Benson, P. J., Mistlin, A. J., *et al.* (1989). Frameworks of analysis for the neural representation of animate objects and actions. *J. Exp. Biol.* **146**, 87–113.

Perrett, D. I., Hietanen, J. K., Oram, M. W. and Benson, P. J. (1992). Organization and functions of cells responsive to faces in the temporal cortex. In *Processing the facial image* (ed. V. Bruce, A. Cowey and A. W. Ellis), pp. 23–30. New York: Oxford University Press.

Piaget, J. (1962). *Play, dreams and imitation in childhood.* New York: Norton.

Pochon, J.-B., Levy, R., Poline, J.-B., Crozier, S., Lehéricy, S., Pillon, B., *et al.* (2001). The role of dorsolateral prefrontal cortex in the preparation of forthcoming actions: an fMRI study. *Cerebral Cortex* **11**, 260–6.

Povinelli, D. J. and Prince, C. G. (1998). When self met other. In *Self-awareness* (ed. M. Ferrari and R. Sternberg), pp. 37–107. New York: Guilford Press.

Prinz, W. (1997). Perception and action planning. *Eur. J. Cogn. Psychol.* **9**, 129–54.

Prinz, W. (2002). Experimental approaches to imitation. In *The imitative mind: development, evolution, and brain bases* (ed. A. N. Meltzoff and W. Prinz), pp. 143–62. New York: Cambridge University Press.

Prinz, W. and Hommel, B. (eds) (2002). *Common mechanisms in perception and action: attention and performance* XIX. New York: Oxford University Press.

Ramachandran, V. S. and Rogers-Ramachandran, D. (1996). Denial of disabilities in anosognosia. *Nature* **382**, 501.

Rizzolatti, G., Fadiga, L., Gallese, V. and Fogassi, L. (1996*a*). Premotor cortex and the recognition of motor actions. *Cogn. Brain Opin.* **3**, 131–41.

Rizzolatti, G., Fadiga, L., Matelli, M., Bettinardi, V., Paulesu, E., Perani, D., *et al.* (1996*b*). Localization of grasp representations in humans by PET. 1. Observation versus execution. *Exp. Brain Opin.* **111**, 246–52.

Rizzolatti, G., Fadiga, L., Fogassi, L. and Gallese, V. (2002). From mirror neurons to imitation, facts, and speculations. In *The imitative mind: development, evolution, and brain bases* (ed. A. N. Meltzoff and W. Prinz), pp. 247–66. New York: Cambridge University Press.

Rolls, E. T. (1992). Neurophysiological mechanisms underlying face processing within and beyond the temporal cortical visual areas. In *Processing the facial image* (ed. V. Bruce, A. Cowey and A. W. Ellis), pp. 11–21. New York: Oxford University Press.

Ruby, P. and Decety, J. (2001). Effect of subjective perspective taking during simulation of action: a PET investigation of agency. *Nature Neurosci.* **4**, 546–50.

Ruby, P. and Decety, J. (2003). What you believe versus what you think they believe: A neuroimaging study of conceptual perspective-taking. *Eur. J. of Neurosci.* **17**, 2475–80.

Siegal, M. and Varley, R. (2002). Neural systems involved in theory of mind. *Nature Rev. Neurosci.* **3**, 463–71.

Spence, S. A., Brooks, D. J., Hirsch, S. R., Liddle, P. F., Meehan, J. and Grasby, P. M. (1997). A PET study of voluntary movement in schizophrenic patients experiencing passivity phenomena (delusions of alien control). *Brain* **120**, 1997–2011.

Taylor, M. (1996). A theory of mind perspective on social cognitive development. In *Handbook of perception and cognition:*, vol. 13. Perceptual and cognitive development (ed. R. Gelman and T. Au), pp. 283–329. New York: Academic.

Tomasello, M. (1999). *The cultural origins of human cognition*. Cambridge, MA: Harvard University Press.

Tomasello, M. and Call, J. (1997). *Primate cognition*. New York: Oxford University Press.

Trevarthen, C. (1979). Communication and cooperation in early infancy: a description of primary intersubjectivity. In *Before speech: the beginning of interpersonal communication* (ed. M. Bullowa), pp. 321–47. New York: Cambridge University Press.

Viviani, P. (2002). Motor competence in the perception of dynamic events: a tutorial. In *Common mechanisms in perception and action: attention and performance* XIX (ed. W. Prinz and B. Hommel), pp. 406–42. New York: Oxford University Press.

Wellman, H. M. and Gelman, S. A. (1998). Knowledge acquisition in foundational
    domains. In *Handbook of child psychology:*, vol. 2. Cognition, perception, and
language (ed. D. Kuhn and R. Siegler), pp. 523–73. New York: Wiley.
Whiten, A. (2002). The imitator's representation of the imitated: ape and child. In *The
    imitative mind: development, evolution, and brain bases* (ed. A. N. Meltzoff and
W. Prinz), pp. 98–121. New York: Cambridge University Press.
Woodward, A. L., Sommerville, J. A. and Guajardo, J. J. (2001). How infants make
    sense of intentional action. In *Intentions and intentionality: foundations of social
    cognition* (ed. B. F. Malle, L. J. Moses and D. A. Baldwin), pp. 149–69. Cambridge,
    MA: MIT Press.

Glossary

MEG: magnetoencephalography
PET: positron emission tomography
SMA: supplementary motor area
STG: superior temporal gyrus
STS: superior temporal sulcus
TMS: transcranial magnetic stimulation

6

Action generation and action perception in imitation: an instance of the ideomotor principle

Andreas Wohlschläger, Merideth Gattis, and Harold Bekkering

We review a series of behavioural experiments on imitation in children and adults that test the predictions of a new theory of imitation. Most of the recent theories of imitation assume a direct visual-to-motor mapping between perceived and imitated movements. Based on our findings of systematic errors in imitation, the new theory of goal-directed imitation (GOADI) instead assumes that imitation is guided by cognitively specified goals. According to GOADI, the imitator does not imitate the observed movement as a whole, but rather decomposes it into its separate aspects. These aspects are hierarchically ordered, and the highest aspect becomes the imitator's main goal. Other aspects become sub-goals. In accordance with the ideomotor principle, the main goal activates the motor programme that is most strongly associated with the achievement of that goal. When executed, this motor programme sometimes matches, and sometimes does not, the model's movement. However, the main goal extracted from the model movement is almost always imitated correctly.

Keywords: imitation; ideomotor principle; action perception; action generation

6.1. Introduction

Imitation (when actors match their own movements to those of others) plays an important part in skill acquisition, and not merely because it avoids time-consuming trial-and-error learning. Observing and imitating is also a special case of the translation of sensory information into action. The actor must translate a complex dynamic visual input pattern into motor commands in such a way that the resulting movement visually matches the model movement, even when the motor output is only partly, or not at all, visible to the actor. For that reason, imitation is one of the most interesting instances of perceptual-motor coordination.

Although humans are very successful in imitating many complex skills, the mechanisms that underlie successful imitation are poorly understood. The translation problem is particularly interesting in children, because they must perform the translation despite the obviously great differences in orientation, body size, limb lengths and available motor skills. Additionally, these differences result in very different dynamic properties (e.g. Meltzoff 1993). Nevertheless, children spontaneously and continuously try to imitate the customs and skills manifested by the adults and peers in their environment.

The debate about whether the ability to imitate is learned (see Miller and Dollard 1941; Skinner 1953; Piaget 1962) or innate has a long history. Meltzoff and Moore (1977) concluded that the matching of others' visible movements with one's own movements is an inborn ability because it can be observed in neonates. Although some could replicate the finding of imitation in neonates (see Field *et al.* 1982; Vinter 1986; Reissland 1988; Heimann 1989; Meltzoff and Moore 1989), many others failed (Hayes and Watson 1981; McKenzie and Over 1983; Koepke *et al.* 1983; Neuberger *et al.* 1983; Lewis and Sullivan 1985) or showed that it is restricted to tongue protrusion (Kaitz *et al.* 1988; Heimann *et al.* 1989; Abravanel and DeYong 1991).[1]

Based on earlier findings, Meltzoff and Moore (1994) developed an influential theory—the theory of AIM—that assumes a supra-modal representational system, which merges the perceptual and the action systems. This supra-modal representational system is thought to match visual information with proprioceptive information. The AIM theory is in line with the recently common view that, in imitation, perception and action are coupled by a direct perceptual-motor mapping (see, for example, Butterworth 1990; Gray *et al.* 1991). In addition, AIM is the only theory, so far, that addresses the processes that allow the transfer of perceived actions into motor programmes.

A direct perceptual-motor mapping is also supported by neurophysiological findings. The so-called mirror neurons (di Pellegrino *et al.* 1992) in the monkey's pre-motor area F5 are potential candidates for a neural implementation of an observation–execution matching system, because they fire both during the observation and during the execution of particular actions. Support for a similar system in humans comes from the finding of a motor facilitation during action observation (Fadiga *et al.* 1995) and from increased brain activity in Broca's area during imitation (Iacoboni *et al.* 1999), an area that is thought to be the human homologue of monkey's pre-motor area F5.

Unfortunately, direct-mapping theories, including AIM, cannot account for certain findings in human imitation behaviour. For example, 18-month-old children not only re-enact an adult's action, but are also able to infer what the adult intended to do when the model fails to perform a target act (Meltzoff 1995). These findings suggest that young children comprehend the equivalence between acts seen and acts done not only on an inter-modal sensorial level, but also on a higher cognitive, intentional level. Although direct mapping can cope with *that* finding by making a few additional assumptions, *other* robust findings are harder to explain using direct-mapping approaches. Imitation, especially in children, sometimes consistently and systematically deviates from the model movements. First, it is well documented that although young children spontaneously imitate adults in a mirror-like fashion, older children tend to transpose left and right (Swanson and Benton 1955; Wapner and Cirillo 1968). Hence, if direct mapping is the basic process for imitation, it is either less 'direct' in younger children than in older ones (and that is not only counterintuitive but also contradicts the developmental function of direct mapping in theories such as AIM), or it should more appropriately be called 'direct mirroring' in younger children rather than 'direct mapping.' Second, a hand-to-ear test (originally developed for aphasics by Head (1920)) repeatedly showed that young children prefer to imitate both ipsi-lateral movements (e.g. left hand touching left ear) and contra-lateral (e.g. left hand to right ear) movements with an ipsi-lateral response (Schofield 1976). Clearly, it is not the movement (ipsi lateral versus contra lateral) that is mapped. But if body parts instead of movements were to be mapped onto each other, then in the case of contra-lateral movements imitated ipsi laterally (the so-called CI-error; see Bekkering *et al.* 2000) one of the two body parts involved would be mapped incorrectly—either hand or ear.

The reason for the avoidance of cross-lateral movements in children is not due to an immature bifurcation, as Kephart (1971) suggested. Recently, we showed that bimanual contra-lateral movements (i.e. left hand to right ear and, at the same time, right hand to left ear) are imitated contra laterally quite often and more frequently than unimanual contra-lateral movements are, even though the bimanual movements require a double crossing of the body midline and hence should be avoided even more, not less, often (experiment 1 in Bekkering *et al.* (2000)).

A replication of this standard experiment in which our imitation procedure was embedded in a song-and-dance game (see Appendix A for song text) allowed us to get more data per child, because we could repeat the original imitation procedure (consisting of the six hand movements three times each in random order) three times without losing the children's attention. As Table 6.1 and Fig. 6.1 show, neither the relative amount of CI-errors, nor the relative

Table 6.1 Average error rates for different error types and for each of three successive blocks. Friedman tests showed no difference in the error rates between blocks (overall: $\chi_r^2 = 1.21$, d.f. = 2, $p = 0.294$, bimanual: $\chi_r^2 = 0.32$, d.f. = 2, $p = 0.854$, and unimanual: $\chi_r^2 = 0.03$, d.f. = 2, $p = 0.987$).

error type	block 1 (%)	block 2 (%)	block 3 (%)
overall rate	21.6	17.3	15.5
CI bimanual	14.5	14.0	12.3
CI unimanual	31.5	30.3	30.1

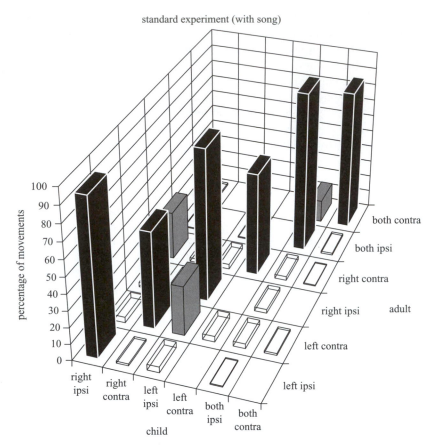

Fig. 6.1 The movements made by an adult model on the right axis and the movements imitated by the child on the left axis. The black boxes on the diagonal represent the percentages of mirror-matching movements, the most frequent type of imitation for each model movement. The grey boxes represent the percentages of other types of imitation movement that deviated significantly from 0. Transparent boxes represent the percentages of types of imitation movement, which appear with statistically insignificant frequency (according to the Kolmogoroff test, setting $\alpha = 0.1$). Note that 'left' and 'right' are defined with respect to bodies. Thus, when a child 'correctly' mirrors a left-hand movement, he or she uses his or her right hand.

lower amount of CI-errors with bimanual than with unimanual movements decreases with extensive practice ($T_0' = 19$, $N_0 = 15$, $u = -2.86$, $p < 0.01$, Cureton test; see Lienert 1973).

In a further experiment, we were able to show that unimanual contra-lateral movements are perfectly imitated contra laterally, if throughout the session only one ear is touched (experiment 2 in Bekkering *et al.* (2000)). Based on these findings, and supported by the observation that children almost always touched the correct ear (correct was defined in the mirror sense, because children spontaneously imitate ipsi-lateral movements in a mirror fashion), we speculated that children primarily imitate the goal of the model's action while paying less attention to, or not caring about, the course of the movement. However, if the goal is non-ambiguous (both ears are touched simultaneously) or if there is only one goal (only one ear is touched), then aspects of the movement come into play. In other words: in imitation it is primarily the goal of an act that is imitated; how that goal is achieved is only of secondary interest. Of course, perceiving the goal of an action would be a prerequisite for such a GOADI. Indeed, recent research showed that six-month-old infants already selectively encode the goal object of an observed reaching movement (Woodward 1998; Woodward and Sommerville 2000). Hence, these results demonstrate that in action observation children perceive the goals from a very early age.

We tested our proposal of GOADI by a variation of the hand-to-ear task that allowed the removal of the goal objects of the model's movement. Instead of touching the ears, the model now covered one of two adjacent dots stuck to the surface of a table with either the ipsi- or the contra-lateral hand (experiment 3 in Bekkering *et al.* (2000)). Results were similar to those of the hand-to-ear task. Children always covered the correct dot; but they quite often used the ipsi-lateral hand when the model covered the dot contra laterally. However, when the same hand movements were performed with the dots removed, children imitated almost perfectly ipsi-lateral with ipsi-lateral movements and contra-lateral with contra-lateral movements.

Thus, it seems that in imitation the presence or absence of goal objects for the model's movement has a decisive influence on imitation behaviour. Goal-oriented movements seem to be imitated correctly with respect to the goal; but the movement itself is frequently ignored. Movements without goal objects or with a single, non-ambiguous goal object are imitated more precisely. It seems that if the goal is clear (or absent), then the course of the movement plays a more central role in imitation. One might also say therefore, that the movement itself becomes the goal.

6.2 The theory of goal-directed imitation

Our theory of GOADI does not make a principled differentiation between object-oriented movements and movements lacking a goal object. It rather suggests:

(i) *Decomposition*. The perceived act is cognitively decomposed into separate aspects.
(ii) *Selection of goal aspects*. Owing to capacity limitations, only a few goal aspects are selected.

(iii) *Hierarchical organization*. The selected goal aspects are hierarchically ordered. The hierarchy of goals follows the functionality of actions. Ends, if present (e.g. objects and treatments of the latter) are more important than means (e.g. effectors and movement paths).

(iv) *Ideomotor principle*. The selected goals elicit the motor programme with which they are most strongly associated. These motor programmes do not necessarily lead to matching movements, although they might do so in many everyday cases.

(v) *General validity*. There is no essential difference in imitation behaviour between children, adults and animals. Differences in accuracy are due to differences in working memory capacity.

GOADI not only explains the imitation data, but also gives imitation a more functional nature. Direct mapping, however, has a rather automatic taste. GOADI allows imitators to learn from models even if the differences in motor skills or in body proportions are so great that the imitator is physically unable to make the same movement as the model. Whatever movement the imitator uses, the purpose of learning by imitation can be regarded as being fulfilled as soon as he reaches the same goal as the model.

GOADI is, however, primarily based upon very recent findings; and most of its assumptions still need to be tested. It is the aim of this paper to review the evidence for the theory in general and to provide further evidence by proving some of its specific assumptions.

6.3 Goal selection or perceptual deficit?

In particular, we first have to examine whether the observed deviations in imitation behaviour might not be specific to imitation, but instead simply due to a perceptual discrimination deficit.

According to GOADI, in imitation the model's action is cognitively decomposed into sub-goals and goals, in the sense that the imitator can infer the intentions of the model (Meltzoff 1995; Woodward 1998).[2] Because the children we investigated almost always reached the correct ear or dot, one can be sure that they have perceived and represented the ultimate goal of the movement. However, one-third of the children showed no contra-lateral movements while imitating. Therefore, it remained unclear whether they had perceived and represented the course of the movement and simply did not consider imitating it because of its sub-goal status or, alternatively, whether they had not built up any representation of the movement's course.

If the error pattern we observed in imitation is due to a perceptual deficit, then children should experience difficulties in matching photographs depicting the end state of the movement. In particular, children should make more errors with photographs showing unimanual contra-lateral movements than with photographs depicting ipsi-lateral ones. Therefore, we showed photographs of an adult woman and a 3-year-old boy depicting the end states of the six movements used in the standard experiment. The experimenter randomly chose one photograph of the woman and asked the child to point to the photograph in which the boy showed the same movement by saying 'Wo macht der Bub das gleiche wie die Frau?' ('In which one is the boy doing the same thing as the woman?').

Fig. 6.2 shows the frequency at which each of the six photographs of the boy was chosen for each photograph of the adult. We found that children produced an average error rate of 34.5%. When presented with unimanual photographs, children chose the matching photograph 51.7% of the time, which is well above chance level (25%, because there are four unimanual photographs and children virtually never matched bimanual photographs with unimanual ones) and more frequent than choosing nonmatching ones (Friedman test, $\chi_r^2 = 37.84$, d.f. = 15, $p < 0.001$). More important, the several types of error did not differ in their frequency of appearance, neither in general nor in particular for any of the four unimanual photographs of the adult (general: $\chi_r^2 = 16.48$, d.f. = 11, $p < 0.124$, right ipsi and right contra: $\chi_r^2 = 0.55$, $p < 0.761$, left ipsi: $\chi_r^2 = 2.36$, $p < 0.307$, left contra: $\chi_r^2 = 0.59$, $p < 0.744$, d.f. = 2 for all of the latter tests). Because the CI-errors (32.9%) were as frequent as IC-errors (34.5%), we conclude that there is no specific perceptual deficit for unimanual contra-lateral movements and that the particularly high error-rate for CI-errors (none the less leading to matching ears) specifically occurs under imitation and not in a more perceptually oriented task.

This interpretation must, however, be qualified. In the imitation task, the children saw the whole movement and not just the end state as in the photograph-matching task. It is probable that the error pattern in imitation also changes when children have to imitate static instead of dynamic models. Perhaps the dynamic part of the gesture is distracting; in this case, the children could even improve when imitating static models. Although Head (1920) has already demonstrated, at least for aphasics, that there is no fundamental difference between the imitation of real models and the imitation of their photographs, he did not analyse imitation behaviour using our methods. In addition, one cannot use photographs when investigating the role of the dynamic part of the model's act. Instead, one should use static real models, because otherwise the size and dimensionality (two-dimensional versus three-dimensional) would be confounded with the factor of interest: static versus dynamic model gesture. Thus, we decided to use an adult model instead of photographs to test the relevance of dynamic information in imitation tasks.

We used two variations of the standard experiment. In the first variant—the static or closed-eyes condition—children had to close their eyes during the movement phase of the model's gesture until the adult had reached the end position of the movement. When the model had reached the end position, she asked the child to open his or her eyes, and the child imitated the movement.

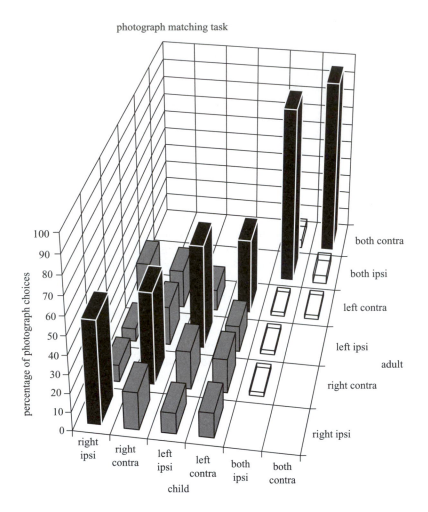

Fig. 6.2 Results of a photograph-matching task. The adult's photograph presented by the experimenter is shown on the right axis and the boy's photographs chosen by the child on the left axis. The black boxes on the diagonal represent the percentages of matching choices, the most frequent choice for each of the adult's photographs. The grey boxes represent the percentages of other choices that deviated significantly from 0. Transparent boxes represent percentages of choices made with statistically insignificant frequency. Note that 'left' and 'right' are defined with respect to bodies. Thus, when the adult photograph depicts a right-handed movement, a correct choice would be the boy's photograph depicting the corresponding right-handed movement.

If this condition—when compared with the data of the standard experiment—did not yield any difference in the error pattern, then the question would be if the dynamic phase of the model's gesture plays any role. Therefore, we introduced a second condition—the cueing condition. This was the opposite of the closed-eyes condition; more attention was drawn to the movement phase by first stretching the hand(s) used out towards the child, rather than moving it (them) directly to the ear(s): the model first stretched out the appropriate hand(s) straight (i.e. ipsi laterally) towards the child and waited until the child imitated that movement. Next, the experimenter moved the stretched-out hand(s) to the ear(s); and the child continued the imitation.

Thus, together with the standard experiment, we have three different levels of information about the movement phase: (i) no information in the closed-eyes condition; (ii) medium or normal information in the standard experiment; and (iii) salient information in the cueing condition. In addition, the cueing condition tests assumption (i) of GOADI, according to which the model movement is decomposed into several goal aspects. A fragmentation of the model movement should assist the decomposition of the model's act and, thus, reduce potential neglect of the movement aspect.

Fig. 6.3 shows the frequency of each of the six imitated movements for each model movement in both conditions. In the closed-eyes condition, children generated 100.0%, 61.5%, 89.3%, 53.6%, 100.0% and 100.0% mirror-matching movements when presented with the left-ipsi, left-contra, right-ipsi, right-contra, both-ipsi and both-contra model movements, respectively. Again, we considered mirror-matching movements to be correct imitations. The children thus produced an average error rate of 16.0%. Only two types of error, both CI-errors, occurred with significant frequency: the left-handed ipsi-lateral imitation of the left-handed contra-lateral movement (38.5%) and the right-handed ipsi-lateral imitation of the right-handed contra-lateral movement (39.3%). Note that with these errors the ears touched by the child are still mirror matching the ears touched by the adult model. Unimanual CI-errors (average 38.9%) were as frequent for left-handed as for right-handed model movements ($T_0' = 8$, $N_0 = 3$, $p = 0.375$, Pratt's exact test).

In the cueing condition, children always imitated the stretching of the hand(s) correctly. For the left-ipsi, left-contra, right-ipsi, right-contra, both-ipsi and both-contra model movements, they showed 96.3%, 92.6%, 82.1%, 74.1%, 92.3 and 92.6% mirror-matching movements. As in the previous experiments, we considered mirror-matching movements to be correct imitations. Children thus produced an average error rate of 11.7%. However, here only one type of error, again a CI-error occurred with significant frequency: the right-handed ipsi-lateral imitation of the right-handed contra-lateral movement (22.2%). It is important to note that in this error the ear touched by the child is still the 'mirror match' of the ear touched by the adult model.

When compared with the cueing condition, the overall error rate of the closed-eyes condition was slightly, but not significantly higher ($T_0' = 16.5$, $N_0 = 6$, $p = 0.375$, Pratt's exact test). However, an individual comparison of the two types of CI-error between conditions shows that the error rates were clearly higher in the closed-eyes condition (left CI-error: $T_0' = 0$, $N_0 = 6$, $p = 0.001$, right CI-error: $T_0' = 4$, $N_0 = 6$, $p = 0.05$). This can be seen in

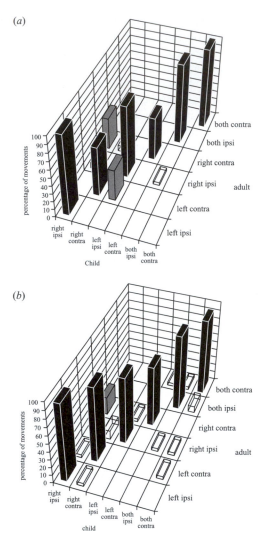

Fig. 6.3 The movements made by the adult model on the right axes and the movements made by the child on the left axes. (*a*) The results of the closed-eyes condition, in which the children had to keep their eyes closed until the adult had reached the end positions. (*b*) The results of the cueing condition, in which the adult stretched out her hand(s) towards the child before moving it (them) to the ear(s). In this condition, the children also had to imitate the stretching of the hand. The black boxes on the diagonal represent the percentages of mirror-matching movements, the most frequent type of imitation for each model movement in both conditions. The grey boxes represent the percentages of other types of imitation movement whose frequency of appearance deviated significantly from 0. Transparent boxes represent percentages of types of imitation movement appearing with statistically insignificant frequency. It is important to note that 'left' and 'right' are defined with respect to bodies. Thus, when a child correctly mirrors a left hand movement, he or she uses his or her right hand.

the complete absence of left-ipsi-lateral imitations of left-contra-lateral movements in the cueing condition.

The closed-eyes condition replicated the error pattern of the standard experiment: the main and only error types that occurred with significant frequency were CI-errors leading to mirror-matching ear contact. Thus, the movement phase of the gestures is neither necessary to cause the standard error pattern, nor distracting, because children did not improve in the closed-eyes condition.

In the cueing condition, the children imitated the stretching of the hand perfectly. This is what we expected, because hands were always stretched ipsi laterally. Moreover, cueing led to a reduction of the CI-errors. In fact, only one type of CI-error was left: the right-handed ipsi-lateral imitation of the right-handed contra-lateral movement. When this type of error occurred, children held the left hand stretched out in front of them (the mirror-matching imitation of the stretched right model hand) while touching the right ear with the right hand.

This (unexpected) type of error lends very strong support to GOADI. With this error type, children simultaneously imitated the sub-goal with the left hand and the main goal with the right hand. This not only shows that they decomposed the movement into goal and sub-goal, it also shows that both the goal and the sub-goal elicit their own, separate motor programme. The reason for the asymmetry of that error (it only occurred for right-handed contra-lateral model movements) is, however, unclear. It may have something to do with the fact that in that case the ear is touched with the dominant hand, a point we will return to later.

The above experiment shows that the imitator decomposes the model movement into several goal aspects. However, because sub-goal and goal were sequenced in time (a point we already commented on in Gattis *et al.* (1998)), it is unclear whether goals become goals because of their recency or because of their saliency. If goals were goals only because of their recency, then GOADI's assumption (iii) of a hierarchy of goals could simply be replaced by a recency effect.

To test assumption (iii) of GOADI, we used a new type of gesture (Gattis *et al.* 2002). Instead of touching her ears, the model now moved one hand either ipsi laterally or contra laterally to the left or to the right side of her head, just next to her ears (Gleissner (1998) and Gleissner *et al.* (2000) showed that, although the overall error rate decreases, the error pattern stays unchanged when moving the hands next to the ears instead of touching them). Just as her hand reached this position, she either clenched her hand into a fist or extended her fingers to open her palm. Thus, we introduced a new goal—open versus closed hand—that was reached at the same time as (not sequential to!) another goal, the position of the hand relative to the head. Because it is more salient, we expected the opening of the hand to become the main goal and the position of the hand relative to the head to become the sub-goal. If this were the case, then the children should make no (or hardly any) errors in the opening of the hand. By contrast, they should more or less ignore the position of the hand relative to the head, because the position of the hand relative to the head now should be a sub-goal.

Apart from testing whether in imitation children really extract the goals of the model's movement or whether they just imitate the most recent aspect of the movement, this experiment also tests whether the selection of a goal at the expense of a sub-goal only occurs for goals in space (left versus right). At present, the goals that the children pursued are always defined by a position in space, such as in the hand-to-ear task or in the experiment with the dots on the table (see Bekkering *et al.* 2000). If we are to develop a more general theory of imitation, it is necessary to show that its validity goes beyond spatially defined goals.

Fig. 6.4 shows the frequency of each of the eight imitated movements for each model movement. We arranged the diagram in such a way that the mirror-matching movements are on the diagonal, because for each model movement the mirror-matching movements were the most frequently imitated movements (100.0%, 72.7%, 84.4% and 63.3% versus 93.9%, 78.8%, 84.8% and 72.7% for the left-ipsi, left-contra, right-ipsi and right-contra model movement with open versus closed hand, respectively). Based on our assumption that the mirror-matching movements are the correct imitations, we calculated that the children thus produced an average rate of error of 18.6%. For our further analyses of each model movement, we only considered erroneous movements of the child appearing with a frequency that significantly deviated from zero. No errors remained for the opening/closing of the hand. The overall error level was identical for both the open-handed and the closed-handed model movements (15.2%). Within each group of movements (open-handed versus closed-handed), the same five error types were left. These were the left-ipsi and left-contra imitations of left-contra movements, the right-ipsi imitations of right-ipsi movements, and the right-ipsi and right-contra imitations of right-contra movements (note that a 'correct' imitation would have required mirroring). None of these five types of error differed significantly between open-handed and closed-handed model movement conditions ($T_0' = 0$, $N_0 = 1$, $p = 0.5$, $T_0' = 10$ $N_0 = 2$, $p = 0.25$, $T_0' = 10$, $N_0 = 2$, $p = 0.25$, $T_0' = 11$, $N_0 = 4$, $p = 0.188$, $T_0' = 0$, $N_0 = 4$, $p = 0.063$, for the respective types of error). Thus, we collapsed errors across open-handed and closed-handed movements for further analyses. Statistically, the five types of error occurred with equal frequency (10.6%, 9.1%, 10.6%, 18.2% and 12.1%, $\chi_r^2 = 0.42$, d.f. = 4, $p = 0.981$). We further collapsed errors according to the categories: 'movement errors' (preserving the position of the hand relative to the head) and 'position errors' (preserving the type of movement, i.e. ipsi lateral versus contra lateral).[3] These two categories also did not differ in frequency (movement errors: 14.4%, position errors: 10.6%, $T_0' = 29$, $N_0 = 9$, $p = 0.436$).

This experiment showed that the primary imitation of goals at the expense of sub-goals is not restricted to left–right tasks. When introducing a new, salient feature (an open hand with extended fingers versus a hand closed into a fist)

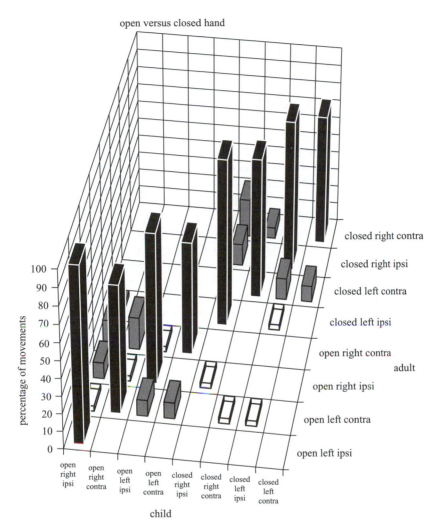

Fig. 6.4 The movements made by the adult model on the right axis and the movements made by the child on the left axis. The black boxes on the diagonal represent the percentages of mirror-matching movements, the most frequent type of imitation for each model movement. The grey boxes represent the percentages of other types of imitation movement whose frequency of appearance deviated significantly from 0. The transparent boxes represent percentages of types of imitation movement appearing with statistically insignificant frequency.

in our standard paradigm, it is this feature that is now imitated without error. More importantly, the main goal of our earlier experiments, the position of the hand relative to the head, has now obviously become a sub-goal because it was erroneously imitated just as often as the former sub-goal 'type of movement'.

In addition, we demonstrated that it is not the recency of a movement that makes it the main goal in imitation. The final spatial position of the hand was reached at the same time as the final configuration (open versus closed hand).

6.4 The ideomotor principle in imitation

Whereas the above experiments were primarily concerned with the perceptual component of imitation, the following experiment tries to investigate the motor component of imitation. According to GOADI, the model movement is decomposed into its different aspects. If this has taken place and if the imitator has (subjectively) decided on the main goal, our question here is how this goal is translated into the motor programme that (more or less erroneously) mimics the model's movement. In assumption (iv), GOADI states that the goal directly elicits the motor programme with which it is most strongly associated. This idea goes back to William James's analysis of voluntary actions (see Prinz 1990). If we want to elicit a voluntary action, we only need to think of the action's effects (e.g. pushing a button, grasping a cup, etc.), and the rest is accomplished by the motor system. The motor system, in turn, then uses the motor programme that has the strongest relation to the intended effect (this is the ideomotor principle). The strength of the association with the intended effect can be either innate or acquired through learning, in the sense that the particular motor programme is most frequently used to elicit the intended outcome.

Assumption (iv) of GOADI, however, still needed to be tested. We therefore varied the dot experiment (experiment 3 in Bekkering *et al.* (2000)) by replacing the dots with movable objects (see Wohlschläger and Bekkering 2002*b*). In the dot experiment, children had to imitate ipsi- and contra-lateral movements towards two adjacent dots stuck to the surface of a table. In addition to having replaced the dots with movable objects, we varied the character of the movement the model made towards these objects. In the experimental condition, the model grasped and lifted the objects. In the control condition, which was similar to the dot experiment (see experiment 3 in Bekkering *et al.* (2000)), the model almost touched the objects by pointing to them with her index finger. If the assumption regarding the elicitation of the motor programme most strongly associated with the main goal is correct, then we would expect the same error pattern as in the dot experiment (or as in the standard experiment). This should be true for both the control and the experimental condition. Conversely, we would expect that with grasping, children would use their dominant hand more frequently, because that is the hand most frequently used for grasping. In the control condition we would not expect such a tendency for the dominant hand, because we did not observe it in the dot experiment (experiment 3 in Bekkering *et al.* (2000)). We thus predict that in the grasping condition (not in the pointing condition), errors would increase in the cases in which the tendency to use the dominant hand for grasping coincides with the tendency to reach for objects with the ipsi-lateral hand. For right-handed subjects, this condition is met when the model grasps an object on its left side contra laterally with its right hand. In that case, the object is located to the right of the child, and he or she should almost inevitably be driven to use his or her right hand to grasp the object ipsi laterally.

Fig. 6.5 shows the frequency of each of the six imitated movements for each model movement in both conditions. We arranged both diagrams in such a way that the mirror-matching movements are on the diagonal, although now it was only in the pointing condition that for each model movement mirror-matching movements were the most frequent movements imitated. In the grasping condition, children generated 100.0%, 50.0%, 66.7%, 25.0%, 100.0% and 79.2% mirror-matching movements when presented with the left-ipsi, left-contra, right-ipsi, right-contra, both-ipsi and both-contra model movements, respectively.

Children produced an average error rate of 30.6%. Four types of error occurred with significant frequency: left-handed ipsi-lateral imitation of the left-handed contra-lateral movement (50.0%), right-handed contra-lateral imitation of the right-handed ipsi-lateral movement (33.3%), right-handed ipsi-lateral imitation of the right-handed contra-lateral movement (75.0%), and bimanual ipsi-lateral imitation of the bimanual contra-lateral model movement (20.8%). With bimanual contra-lateral model movements, we made an unexpected observation. Children sometimes grasped the objects ipsi laterally and then, after lifting, crossed their arms while still holding the objects. This type of imitation was treated as 'correct' imitation. One-third of the correct imitations of bimanual contra-lateral model movements were imitated in this unexpected way. Despite these errors, children always grasped the correct object. Three of these error types were CI-errors and the fourth was an IC-error. Unimanual CI-errors (average 62.5%) were more frequent than bimanual CI-errors ($T_0' = 0$, $N_0 = 5$, $p = 0.05$). In addition, unimanual CI-errors were more frequent when the child used the right hand (75.0%) than when he or she used the left hand (50.0%) for imitation ($T_0' = 0$, $N_0 = 5$, $p = 0.05$).

In the pointing condition, children generated 100.0%, 75.0%, 100.0%, 66.7%, 100.0% and 95.8% mirror-matching movements when presented with the left-ipsi, left-contra, right-ipsi, right-contra, both-ipsi and both-contra model movements, respectively. Children produced an average error rate of 10.4%. Only two types of error occurred with significant frequency: left-handed ipsi-lateral imitation of the left-handed contra-lateral movement (20.8%) and right-handed ipsi-lateral imitation of the right-handed contra-lateral movement (29.2%). These two error types were the unimanual CI-errors. Hence, despite these errors, children always pointed to the correct object. The CI-errors (average 30.6%) were as frequent for the child's left-handed as for the child's right-handed movements ($T_0' = 8$, $N_0 = 7$, $p = 0.133$, Pratt's exact test).

When compared with the pointing condition, the overall error rate of the grasping condition was significantly higher ($u = 2.04$, $p = 0.05$). All four error

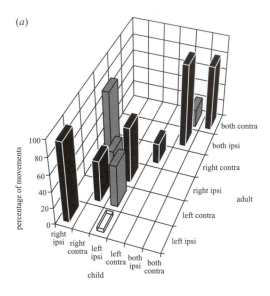

(a)

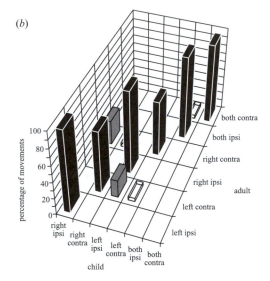

(b)

Fig. 6.5 The movements made by the adult model on the right axis and the movements made by the child on the left axis. (a) The results of the grasping condition, in which the model as well as the children grasped and lifted the objects on the table. (b) The results of the pointing condition, in which the model as well as the children only pointed towards the objects on the table. The black boxes on the diagonal represent the percentages of mirror-matching movements, generally the most frequent type of imitation, but not for every model movement in the grasping condition. The grey boxes represent the percentages of other types of imitation movement occurring with a frequency that deviated significantly from 0. The transparent boxes represent a type of imitation movement appearing with statistically insignificant frequency.

types of the grasping condition had a higher error rate when compared with the respective error types in the pointing condition. The rate of the bimanual CI-error in the pointing condition did not significantly deviate from zero. The IC-error in the grasping condition was not observed in the pointing condition. The right-handed CI-error rate was significantly higher in the grasping condition than in the pointing condition ($u = 1.86$, $p = 0.05$). Concerning the left-handed CI-error rate, there was no significant difference between the two conditions ($u = 1.48$, $p = 0.69$).

The experiment clearly confirmed another prediction of GOADI. Once the imitator has identified the goal of the model act, this goal elicits the motor programme most strongly associated with it. When imitating the grasping of objects (or the pointing towards objects), children always grasped (or pointed to) the correct object. Thus, as expected, the treatment of the object (grasping or pointing to) was the highest goal in the hierarchy. More important, however, is the fact that when we used grasping rather than pointing as the model act, the children showed a clear preference for using the dominant right hand. Such a preference was neither observed in any of the previous experiments, nor in the pointing condition. The preference for the right hand led to a strong increase (of around 45% when compared with the standard experiment or to the pointing condition) in the error rate for the condition in which the preference for the right hand met the preference for ipsi-lateral movements: the imitation of a right-handed, contra-lateral model movement.

This preference for the dominant right hand in the grasping condition received very strong corroboration by an unexpected finding. The preference was so strong that the children even produced a significant portion of errors in a condition in which they had shown no (or almost no) errors, either in the previous experiments or in the pointing condition. When the adult ipsi laterally grasped the object to her right, children quite frequently (in one-third of the cases) contra laterally grasped the corresponding object (which was located to their left) with their right hand. In this case, the preference for the dominant hand was obviously sometimes even stronger than the preference for ipsi-lateral movements. No such tendency was observed in the pointing condition.

Another unexpected finding also confirms GOADI and is a nice illustration of our theory of GOADI. When the model grasped both objects with crossed arms, children ended up in 80% of the cases by holding the two objects with crossed arms. This is not a surprise, because it is in line with our previous findings. However, in one-third of these cases, the children first grasped the objects ipsi laterally and only afterwards crossed their arms. This unexpected finding shows that the model's act was decomposed into a main goal (grasping both objects) and a sub-goal (crossing the arms). The main goal then was pursued first, followed by the pursuit of the sub-goal. In that sequence, which was, however, reversed with respect to the model's act, both the main goal and the sub-goal elicited the motor programme most strongly associated with their achievement.

6.5 Imitation in adults

The theory of GOADI is thought to be valid for all individuals, irrespective of age and developmental state. Hence, one should be able to show the same pattern of imitation 'errors' in adults. Of course, in such simple tasks as touching the contra-lateral ear, we do not expect adults to show the same overall level of errors that we found in children. Nevertheless, if the goal-directed theory of imitation is generally valid, some (probably weaker) effects in adult's imitation behaviour should be detectable. This was indeed the case in a speeded response version of the hand-to-ear task in adults: adults also showed significantly ($T_0' = 7$, $N_0 = 10$, $p < 0.05$) more CI-errors than IC-errors (see Fig. 6.6).

We also replicated another one of our core experiments—covering dots on a table—in adults (see Wohlschläger and Bekkering 2002*a*), expecting to find a reflection of the children's error pattern at a lower level in adults and in their RTs. To be able to measure RTs precisely, we slightly modified the task. First, we used finger movements instead of whole hand movements. Second, the model movements were not presented by the experimenter but on a computer screen. Subjects were instructed to put their hands next to each other on the table and to imitate the depicted downward finger movement as quickly as possible after the presentation of one of the stimuli. As in the experiment with children, there were two conditions. In one condition, the stimuli contained two dots, one of which was covered by one of the fingers at the end of an either ipsi-lateral or contra-lateral downward movement. In the other condition, the stimuli depicted the same movements, but no dots were present.

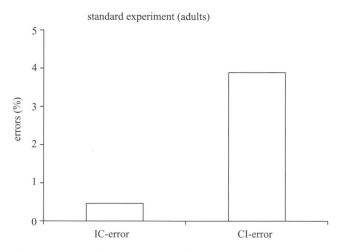

Fig. 6.6 The amounts of IC-errors and CI-errors adults made in a unimanual speeded response version of the standard hand-to-ear task. Stimuli were presented on a computer monitor and the hand movements were recorded using a magnetic positioning system (POLHEMUS FASTRAK).

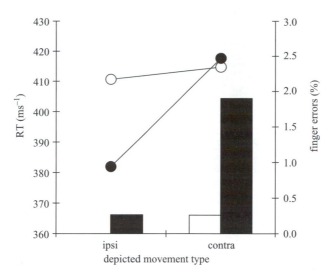

Fig. 6.7 Results of the covering-dots experiment in adults. Imitating contra lateral was slower (lines) and more finger errors (columns) were made, but only if dots were present. Black circles represent with-object results; open circles represent without-object results.

Results showed that, although adults make almost no errors (0.6%), these few errors mainly (77.8%) occur with stimuli depicting contra-lateral movements towards dots (CI-error). Second, RTs were faster for ipsi-lateral movements, but only if dots were present (see Fig. 6.7). These and the above results from the hand-to-ear task, which basically replicate the findings in children, show that in adults dots also as action goals are activating the direct, ipsi-lateral motor programme, which leads to faster responses and sometimes even to errors.

Although adults show the same pattern of errors as children in simple actions, more complex actions are needed to investigate the *general validity* and the *hierarchical organization* of our goal-directed theory of imitation. In the experiments reported above, the actions comprised only two variable aspects: the goal object and the effector. It transpired that an increase to three variable and independent aspects (goal *object*, *effector* and *movement path*) is sufficient to cause considerable amounts of errors also in adults.

The action we used was more complex but nevertheless quite simple. It consisted of moving a pen upside down into one of two cups (*object*). In either case, the pen was rotated by 180°. The experimenter served as the model and he either used his right or his left hand (*effector*). In addition, he either turned the pen clockwise or counter-clockwise (*movement path*) to bring it into an upside-down position at the end of the movement (see Fig. 6.8).

In a pilot study, we did not tell the subjects about the three different aspects of the movement, because we wanted to find out which hierarchical order the

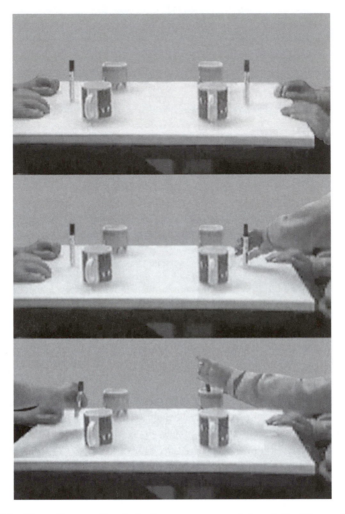

Fig. 6.8 Three frames of an imitation sequence used for adults. The model on the right uses the left hand to put the pen upside down into the right cup by turning it counter-clockwise. The imitator uses the right hand and turns the pen clockwise to put it into the left cup (not shown). In this example, the imitator perfectly mirrored the model movement. However, most subjects failed to do so. For details see text.

subjects apply spontaneously. However, an analysis of the errors revealed that although subjects start with the expected hierarchy (least errors with object followed by effector followed by movement path), after some tens of trials, they reordered their hierarchy individually, always in favour of one aspect at the cost of the others. Hence we decided to fully explain the experiment to the subjects, except for the very first trial. In the first trial, the experimenter made

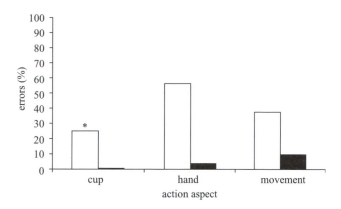

Fig. 6.9 Spontaneous (open bars) and repeated (black bars) imitation of an action with three aspects in adults. The asterisk indicates spontaneous errors significantly below chance level (50%). For details see text.

one of the eight possible movements without instructing the subjects to imitate. Instead he asked, 'Kannst Du das auch?' ('Can you do that too?'). Only after the first trial were subjects fully instructed about the purpose of the experiment and about each individual aspect of the movement by stressing that it was important to imitate all aspects as precisely as possible. Thus, we could analyse and compare spontaneous imitation with repeated imitation.

Results (see Fig. 6.9) showed that in spontaneous imitation the only aspect that was imitated correctly above chance level was the object (binomial probability $p < 0.05$). Likewise, the object was imitated most correctly, followed by the effector, followed by the movement path in repeated imitation (linear contrast: $t = 1.98$, d.f. $= 7$, $p < 0.05$). Obviously, the goal of an action is so strong that the other aspects of an action are more or less neglected, even if the subject knows explicitly about all aspects and tries his/her best to copy all of them as exactly as possible.

In a further series of experiments, we increased the number to four variable aspects: the goal *object*, the *treatment* of the object, the *effector* and the *movement path*. We added the fourth aspect—treatment—because the corresponding experiment in children (grasping versus pointing, see above) showed that apart from the object itself, its treatment plays a decisive part for imitation behaviour. Again, in repeated imitation, subjects showed the least errors with respect to the object, followed by treatment, followed by effector and followed by movement (linear contrast: $t = 4.16$, d.f. $= 15$, $p < 0.01$). As predicted, the only aspects that were imitated correctly in spontaneous imitation were the object and its treatment (binomial probability: $p < 0.001$; see Fig. 6.10 for the results). A control task showed that the differential effects in repeated imitation were not due to perceptual deficits. When we blocked the trials in such a way that in each block only one aspect varied while the others were

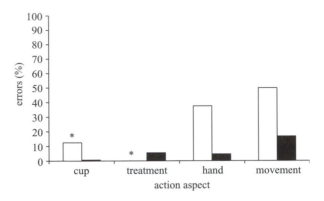

Fig. 6.10 Spontaneous (open bars) and repeated (black bars) imitation of an action with four aspects in adults. The asterisks indicate spontaneous errors significantly below chance level (50%). For details see text.

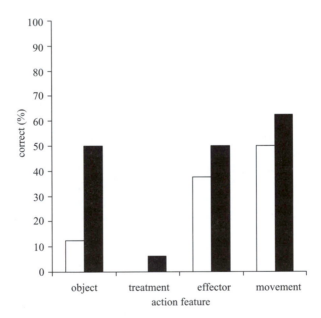

Fig. 6.11 Spontaneous imitation of an action with four aspects in adults. Open bars: objects differ in both colour and location; black bars, objects differ in location only. For details see text.

held constant (subjects were informed about the varying aspect at the beginning of each block), subjects showed approximately the same amount of errors for every aspect. In spontaneous imitation, however, we could show that the choice of the object is indeed a choice for object identity and not for object location. When using four cups of the same colour (*not* as in Fig. 6.8), so that the objects only differed by location, only treatment was left as the single aspect that was imitated correctly above chance level (Wohlschläger and Bekkering 2002*b*; Fig. 6.11).

6.6. Conclusions

The experiments we have reported demonstrate the importance of objects and their treatments in human imitation, both for children and adults. The experiments widely confirmed our theory of GOADI. They showed that it is primarily the treatment of an object that is imitated in object-oriented actions, whereas the choice of the effector and the movement path are following the so-called *ideomotor principle*: the motor programme most strongly associated with the achievement of the goal is executed during the execution of the imitative act and it is probably already activated during the observation of the action that is imitated later (Fadiga *et al*. 1995). The study of brain activity during the covering-dot task (Wohlschläger and Bekkering 2002*a*) in adults recently showed that the human homologue of the monkey's mirror-neuron area is more active during the imitation of object-oriented than non-object-oriented actions (Koski *et al*. 2002). Hence, one may conclude here that there is a mirror-neuronsystem in humans too, and that it is used for imitation. This does not mean that the mirror-neuron system is doing the imitation: despite the fact that it was discovered in monkeys, monkeys do not imitate. However, when conceiving imitation as an imitation of the goals of an action, then it makes sense that the mirror-neuron system is involved in imitation, because it is essentially a system for representing actions (irrespective of whether just observed or executed) in terms of action goals, i.e. object plus treatment.

According to GOADI and confirmed by the data presented above, actions involving objects are imitated in such a way that the same treatment is given to the same object, thereby ignoring the motor part of the action. Of course, in everyday life the model acts in an efficient and direct way on the object. If the imitator copies the action goal and if this action goal in turn activates the most direct motor programme in the imitator, then both actions resemble each other in all aspects, leading to an impressive, mirror-like behaviour. When there is no object, the movements themselves become the goal and they are also imitated in a mirror-like fashion. It is probably the frequently observed parallelism between the movements of the model and the imitator that led to direct-mapping theories. However, according to GOADI, this similarity between the movements of the model and the imitator is only superficial and incidental: the underlying similarity is a similarity of action goals.

Imitating goals and/or intentions of course requires that the imitator understands the action of the model. In our view, action understanding is a prerequisite for imitation. It is a necessary but not a sufficient condition for imitation to occur. Within a goal-directed theory (as opposed to direct-mapping explanations) it is possible to explain why imitation sometimes occurs and sometimes does not. *Because* action understanding precedes imitation the observer can decide whether or not he wants to imitate the goals of the model. In addition, a goal-directed theory of imitation also gives room for creativity in imitation, because the way the goal is achieved is left to the imitator, whereas direct-mapping approaches have a rather automatic taste. When the model observes the imitator achieving the same goal in a more efficient way it might, in turn, cause the model to imitate the new movement of the former imitator. This type of creativity, based on the decoupling of ends and means and on mutual imitation, probably plays a very important part in the evolution of culture and technique.

Although using action goals as the core concept, GOADI does not say anything about the representation of the intentions of the model in the imitator. In our view, the representation of intentionality or any theory of mind is not necessary to explain imitation (see Gattis *et al.* (2002) for a different interpretation). We have so far only investigated rather simple actions. However, GOADI could also be applied to more complex actions and action sequences. Byrne's concept of 'imitation as behaviour parsing' (see Chapter 8 of this volume) is very close to our theory of GOADI. Byrne also assumes that the elements of an action sequence that will be learned by imitation have to already be in the repertoire of the observer. This corresponds to GOADI's ideomotor principle. His studies of imitation in gorillas also show that the actual movement is less important than the action outcome (e.g. the hand the imitator uses does not depend on the hand the model uses; Byrne and Byrne 1991).

Although the experiments reported here widely confirm GOADI and, at the same time, illustrate the shortcomings of the AIM theory of Meltzoff and Moore (1994), some sort of mapping mechanism must still be involved in imitation. The ability to identify limbs and body parts and to map those to the parts of our own body is perhaps inborn. AIM is primarily based on imitation performances in neonates. Presumably, neonates need to develop successful GOADI behaviour by learning through experience. In fact, our theory may require the assumption of a coarse direct limb-to-limb mapping, But it is probably only a coarse mapping of visual input to motor output, because neither the side of the body, nor the number of effectors, nor even the type of movement is consistently mapped. In addition, and as already noted above, the direct-mapping approaches hold the notion of automaticity and mainly address the question of how the input is translated into a motor output matching the input. They do not address more complex questions such as when imitation occurs, or who imitates whom. GOADI does not (yet) address these questions either; but it is open to that meta-level of imitation, because it uses action goals as the central explanatory component. Thus, by using GOADI one can easily build a hypothesis about the meta-level of imitation. For instance, one might speculate that the minimum necessary condition for the occurrence of imitation is that the goal of the model's act is within the range of the imitator's desires.

The differentiation between goals and sub-goals (or ends and means) parallels the distinction made by Tomasello *et al.* (1993) between emulation and imitation. Whereas emulation refers to the reproduction of the goal, imitation also includes the reproduction of the model's strategies for achieving the goal. By contrast, Byrne and Russon (1998) argue that it is the complexity of the goal hierarchy that decides whether almost all aspects of an action (programme-level imitation) or only a few of them (action-level imitation) are imitated.

Let us now turn to some of GOADI's implications. First, GOADI has adaptive implications. In general, a model and its imitator have different body and limb sizes, which results in differences in their dynamic properties. In addition, they usually also differ in their available motor skills. Thus, for the imitator, it is more reasonable to concentrate on the goal of a movement and try to reach it somehow in his own manner (perhaps even with several trials), and it is less reasonable to focus on the course of the movement. A second and more practical implication concerns teaching. Teachers who want to teach by imitation should keep in mind that it is probably more useful to demand the achievement of the ends rather than the means from their pupils. When they serve as models, they should encourage pupils to focus on the goal, rather than on the movement. Recent research results recommend this method for the acquisition of motor skills (Wulf 1998).

In summary, the experiments reported here widely confirm the assumptions of GOADI. We assume that there is no principle difference in imitation behaviour between children and adults beyond the fact that children probably have a smaller working memory capacity and hence disregard more aspects of a model's movement than adults do.[4]

We thank Brigitte Gleißner and Monika Benstetter for the conduction of the experiments and Megan Otermat for proof-reading.

Endnotes

1. Anisfeld (1996) argues that if infants' imitative behaviour is restricted to a single gesture, it is perhaps more parsimonious to explain it as a specific, directly elicited response. The increase in tongue protrusion after modelling might also be explained by its inhibition during the attentive observation of the model (Anisfeld 1991).
2. By 'inferring the intention of the model', we do not want to imply that the imitator has an explicit representation of the model's intention as a mental state of the model. This question is mainly relevant for predicting the action outcome of one's conspecifics but it is irrelevant for imitating it.
3. Though theoretically possible, there were no double errors.
4. For example, when asked to imitate the cross-lateral, bimanual hand-to-ear movement, adults of course imitate correctly, but—unless this aspect is drawn to their attention—they do not care which arm is in front.

Appendix A: Song Text

Boys' version
Auf der Wiese, auf der Wiese
Läuft ein kleiner Mann.
Hat zwei Hände, hat zwei Füße,
Läuft so schnell er kann.

(Refrain):
Läuft ganz schnell im Kreis herum,
Fällt dabei auch gar nicht um.
Schau den kleinen Mann mal an,
Was der Mann noch alles kann:

(Imitation)
Auf der Straße, auf der Straße
Läuft der kleine Mann.
Hat zwei Augen, Mund und Nase,
Läuft so schnell er kann.
(Refrain, Imitation)
In die Pfütze, in die Pfütze
Läuft der kleine Mann.
Auf dem Kopf hat er 'ne Mütze,
Läuft so schnell er kann.

(Refrain, Imitation)

Girls' version
Auf der Wiese, auf der Wiese
Läuft 'ne kleine Frau.
Hat zwei Hände, hat zwei Füße,
Läuft so schnell sie kann.

(Refrain):
Läuft ganz schnell im Kreis herum,
Fällt dabei auch gar nicht um.
Schau die kleine Frau mal an,
Was die Frau noch alles kann:

(Imitation)
Auf der Straße, auf der Straße
Läuft die kleine Frau.
Hat zwei Augen, Mund und Nase,
Läuft so schnell sie kann.
(Refrain, Imitation)
In die Pfütze, in die Pfütze
Läuft die kleine Frau.
Auf dem Kopf hat sie 'ne Mütze,
Läuft so schnell sie kann.
(Refrain, Imitation)

Text: Andreas Wohlschläger
Tune: Brigitte Gleissner

References

Abravanel, E. and DeYong, N. G. (1991). Does object modeling elicit imitative-like gestures from young infants? *J. Exp. Child Psychol.* **52**, 22–40.

Anisfeld, M. (1991). Neonatal imitation. *Devl. Rev.* **11**, 60–97.

Anisfeld, M. (1996). Only tongue protrusion modeling is matched by neonates. *Devl. Rev.* **16**, 149–61.

Bekkering, H., Wohlschläger, A. and Gattis, M. (2000). Imitation of gestures in children is goal-directed. *Q. J. Exp. Psychol.* A **53**, 153–64.

Butterworth, G. (1990). On reconceptualizing sensorimotor development in dynamic system terms. In *Sensory motor organizations and development in infancy and early childhood* (ed. H. Bloch and B. I. Bertenthal), pp. 57–73. Dordrecht, The Netherlands: Kluwer.

Byrne, R. W. and Byrne, J. M. E. (1991). Hand preferences in the skilled gathering task of mountain gorillas (*Gorilla g. beringei*). *Cortex* **27**, 521–46.

Byrne, R. W. and Russon, A. E. (1998). Learning by imitation: a hierarchical approach. *Behav. Brain Sci.* **21**, 667.

di Pellegrino, G., Fadiga, L., Fogassi, L., Gallese, V. and Rizzolatti, G. (1992). Understanding motor events: a neurophysiological study. *Exp. Brain Res.* **91**, 176–80.

Fadiga, L., Fogassi, L., Pavesi, G. and Rizzolatti, G. (1995). Motor facilitation during action observation: a magnetic stimulation study. *J. Neurophysiol.* **73**, 2608–11.

Field, T. M., Woodson, R., Greenberg, R. and Cohen, D. (1982). Discrimination and imitation of facial expressions by neonates. *Science* **218**, 179–81.

Gattis, M., Bekkering, H. and Wohlschläger, A. (1998). When actions are carved at the joints. *Behav. Brain Sci.* **21**, 691–2.

Gattis, M., Bekkering, H. and Wohlschläger, A. (2002). Goal-directed imitation. In *The imitative mind: development, evolution and brain bases* (ed. A. N. Meltzoff and W. Prinz), pp. 183–205. New York: Cambridge University Press.

Gleissner, B. (1998). Imitation of hand gestures to body parts is guided by goals rather than perceptual-motor mapping. Unpublished diploma thesis. Ludwig-Maximilians-University, Munich.

Gleissner, B., Meltzoff, A. N. and Bekkering, H. (2000). Children's coding of human action: cognitive factors influencing imitation in 3-year-olds. *Devl Sci.* **3**, 405–14.

Gray, J. T., Neisser, U., Shapiro, B. A. and Kouns, S. (1991). Observational learning of ballet sequences: the role of kinematic information. *Ecol. Psychol.* **3**, 121–34.

Hayes, L. A. and Watson, J. S. (1981). Neonatal imitation: fact or artifact? *Devl Psychol.* **17**, 655–60.

Head, H. (1920). Aphasia and kindred disorders of speech. *Brain* **43**, 87–165.

Heimann, M. (1989). Neonatal imitation, gaze aversion, and mother–infant interaction. *Infant Behav. Dev.* **12**, 495–505.

Heimann, M., Nelson, K. E. and Schaller, J. (1989). Neonatal imitation of tongue protrusion and mouth opening: methodological aspects and evidence of early individual differences. *Scand. J. Psychol.* **30**, 90–101.

Iacoboni, M., Woods, R. P., Brass, M., Bekkering, H., Mazziotta, J. C. and Rizzolatti, G. (1999). Cortical mechanisms of human imitation. *Science* **286**, 2526–28.

Kaitz, M., Meschulach-Sarfaty, O., Auerbach, J. and Eidelman, A. (1988). A reexamination of newborns' ability to imitate facial expressions. *Devl Psychol.* **24**, 3–7.

Kephart, N. C. (1971). *The slow learner in the classroom*. Columbus, OH: Charles Merill.

Koepke, J. E., Hamm, M., Legerstee, M. and Russell, M. (1983). Neonatal imitation: two failures to replicate. *Infant Behav. Dev.* **6**, 97–102.

Koski, L., Wohlschläger, A., Bekkering, H., Woods, R. P., Dubeau, M.-C., Mazziotta, J. C., *et al.* (2002). Modulation of motor and premotor activity during imitation of target-directed actions. *Cerebr. Cortex* **12**, 847–55.

Lewis, M. and Sullivan, M. W. (1985). Imitation in the first six month of life. *Merrill-Palmer Q.* **31**, 315–33.

Lienert, G. A. (1973). *Verteilungsfreie Methoden in der Biostatistik*, vol. 1. Meisenheim am Glan: Anton Hain.

McKenzie, B. E. and Over, R. (1983). Young infants fail to imitate facial and manual gestures. *Infant Behav. Dev.* **6**, 85–95.

Meltzoff, A. N. (1993). The centrality of motor coordination and proprioception in social and cognitive development: from shared actions to shared minds. In *The development of coordination in infancy* (ed. G. J. P. Savelsbergh), pp. 463–96. The Netherlands: North-Holland.

Meltzoff, A. N. (1995). Understanding the intentions of others: re-enactment of intended acts by 18-month-old children. *Devl Psychol.* **31**, 838–50.

Meltzoff, A. N. and Moore, M. K. (1977). Imitation of facial and manual gestures by human neonates. *Science* **198**, 75–8.

Meltzoff, A. N. and Moore, M. K. (1989). Imitation in newborn infants: exploring the range of gestures imitated and the underlying mechanism. *Devl Psychol.* **25**, 954–62.

Meltzoff, A. N. and Moore, M. K. (1994). Imitation, memory and the representation of persons. *Infant Behav. Dev.* **17**, 83–99.

Miller, N. E. and Dollard, J. (1941). *Social learning and imitation.* New Haven, CT: Yale University Press.

Neuberger, H., Merz, J. and Selg, H. (1983). Imitation bei Neugeborenen: eine kontroverse Befundlage (Imitation in neonates: a controversial finding). *Z. Entwicklungspsychol. Pädagog. Psychol.* **15**, 267–76.

Piaget, J. (1962). *Play, dreams and imitation in childhood.* New York: Norton. [Translated by C. Gattegno and F.M. Hodgson. Original work published 1945.]

Prinz, W. (1990). A common coding approach to perception and action. In *Relationships between perception and action* (ed. O. Neumann and W. Prinz), pp. 167–201. Berlin: Springer.

Reissland, N. (1988). Neonatal imitation in the first hours of life: observations in rural Nepal. *Devl Psychol.* **24**, 464–9.

Schofield, W. N. (1976). Do children find movements which cross the body midline difficult? *Q. J. Exp. Psychol.* **28**, 571–82.

Skinner, B. F. (1953). *Science and human behavior.* New York: Macmillan.

Swanson, R. and Benton, A. L. (1955). Some aspects of the genetic development of right–left discrimination. *Child Dev.* **26**, 123–33.

Tomasello, M., Kruger, A. C. and Ratner, H. H. (1993). Cultural learning. *Behav. Brain Sci.* **16**, 495–552.

Vinter, A. (1986). The role of movement in eliciting early imitations. *Child Dev.* **57**, 66–77.

Wapner, S. and Cirillo, L. (1968). Imitation of a model's hand movements: age changes in transpositions of left–right relations. *Child Dev.* **39**, 887–95.

Woodward, A. L. (1998). Infants encode the goal object of an actor's reach. *Cognition* **69**, 1–34.

Woodward, A. L. and Sommerville, J. A. (2000). Twelve-month-old infants interpret action in context. *Psychol. Sci.* **11**, 73–7.

Wohlschläger, A. and Bekkering, H. (2002*a*). Is human imitation based on a miror-neurone system? Some behavioural evidence. *Exp. Brain Res.* **143**, 335–41.

Wohlschläger, A. and Bekkering, H. (2002*b*). The role of objects in imitation. In *Mirror neurons and the evolution of brain and language* (ed. M. Stamenor and V. Gallese), 5.101–14. Amsterdam: John Benjamins.

Wulf, G. (1998). Bewußte Kontrolle stört Bewegungslernen. *Spektrum der Wissenschaft* **4**, 16–22.

Glossary

AIM: active intermodal mapping
CI-errors: contra-ipsi-errors
GOADI: goal-directed imitation
IC-errors: ipsi-contra-errors
RT: response time

7

The manifold nature of interpersonal relations: the quest for a common mechanism

Vittorio Gallese

It has been proposed that the capacity to code the 'like me' analogy between self and others constitutes a basic prerequisite and a starting point for social cognition. It is by means of this self/other equivalence that meaningful social bonds can be established, that we can recognize others as similar to us, and that imitation can take place.

In this article I discuss recent neurophysiological and brain imaging data on monkeys and humans, showing that the 'like me' analogy may rest upon a series of 'mirror-matching' mechanisms. A new conceptual tool able to capture the richness of the experiences we share with others is introduced: the *shared manifold* of intersubjectivity. I propose that all kinds of interpersonal relations (imitation, empathy and the attribution of intentions) depend, at a basic level, on the constitution of a shared manifold space. This shared space is functionally characterized by automatic, unconscious embodied simulation routines.

Keywords: empathy; imitation; mirror neurons; mind reading; simulation

7.1 Introduction

Intersubjectivity is one of the most controversial topics within the ongoing debate in the cognitive sciences. Various modalities of normal and pathological interpersonal relations are the focus of many different disciplines such as neuroscience, cognitive and developmental psychology, philosophy of mind, and psychiatry. *Imitation*, *empathy* and *mind reading* denote, among others, different levels and modes of interaction by means of which individuals establish meaningful bonds with others; therefore, they have been variously used to characterize mechanisms and modes of intersubjective relation.

Why has intersubjectivity progressively gained the centre of the stage? Because more and more scholars are experiencing a growing sense of discomfort with respect to the heuristic value of accounts of human cognition exclusively focusing on a solipsistic, monadic dimension. Intersubjective relations are interesting not only because they capture an essential trait of the human mind—its social character—but also, and even more importantly, because they provide a greater opportunity to understand how the *individual* mind develops and works.

Imitation, empathy and mind reading are different in many respects. When we engage in re-enacting the observed behaviour of someone else, we translate the *observed* actions into executed ones. When we empathize with others, we understand what others are feeling, be it a particular *emotion* or *sensory state*. Finally, when we witness the actions of others, we supposedly understand their meaning and the reasons that possibly promoted them. In these three different types of interpersonal relation we are confronted with *apparently different* objects (actions, emotions and sensations, and thoughts, respectively), and we reply with different modalities (actions, feelings and thoughts, respectively). It therefore seems legitimate to assume that imitation, empathy and mind reading depend on totally different mechanisms.

I suggest a different perspective. I demonstrate that imitation, empathy and mind reading do share, *at a basic level*, a crucial common feature: they all depend on the constitution of a shared meaningful intersubjective space. I propose that the shared manifold space—orthogonal to imitation, empathy and to the attribution of intentions—relies on a specific functional mechanism, which is probably also a basic feature of how our brain/body system models its interactions with the world: embodied simulation.

Furthermore, I clarify how embodied simulation can be characterized from a neurobiological perspective, by proposing that the mirror-matching neural system, originally discovered in the premotor cortex of monkeys—but also present in the human brain—might be part of the neural correlate of simulation, and therefore provide an integrated neuroscientific account of the basic aspects of intersubjectivity.

7.2 Social identity: Why it matters

From the very beginning of our life, the social dimension seems to play a very powerful role within the network of interactions shaping our view of the world. Social behaviour is not peculiar to primates; it is diffuse across species very different from humans, such as bees and ants. Within different species, social interactions certainly play different roles, and are probably subsumed by different mechanisms. Nevertheless, central to all social species and, within more evolved species of primates, central to all social cultures of whatever complexity, is the notion of *identity* of the individuals within those species and cultures. It follows, that *all* levels of social interaction that can be employed to characterize cognition in single individuals must intersect or overlap, to enable the development of mutual recognition and intelligibility.

As humans, we implicitly 'know' that all human beings have four limbs, walk in a certain way, act and *think* in special ways. If we share the same culture, we will, for example, all tattoo our body in a special striped fashion, pierce different parts of our body, or wear the same striped scarf when attending the games of our favourite soccer team. If we share with other individuals a given perspective on how our society should be governed, together with other citizens sharing our views, we will vote for the same political party.

Social identity can therefore be articulated at many different levels of complexity: it can be analysed by means of increasingly complex tests in which different species might score differently. However, whatever their complexity might be, identity relations are necessary to allow the sense of belonging to a larger community of other organisms. Why is this so? Why in the course of evolution has this feature been preserved?

Identity is important within a group of social individuals because it provides them with the capacity to better *predict* the consequences of the ongoing and future behaviour of others. The attribution of identity status to other individuals automatically contextualizes their behaviour. This, in turn, reduces the variables to be computed, thus optimizing the employment of cognitive resources by reducing the 'meaning space' to be mapped. By contextualizing content, identity reduces the amount of information our brain has to process. In Section 7.3 I examine the issue of identity from a developmental perspective.

7.3 Investigating social cognition: The developmental cognitive revolution

One of the major contributions to our understanding of human social cognition has been provided during recent decades by research in developmental psychology. Developmental psychology has literally revolutionized our way of looking at newborns and infants as cognitive agents. These results have shown, among other things, that at the very beginning of our life we are capable of performances which, if and when instantiated by adult individuals, we would readily ascribe to the most abstract resources of our cognitive system.

One aspect of infants' proclivity to 'abstraction' is their astonishing capacity to operate cross-modal mapping of sensory information. Three-week-old infants are able to visually identify pacifiers that they previously felt having sucked on them when blindfolded (Meltzoff and Borton 1979). What was previously experienced as *haptically different* was later recognized as being *visually different*. Other studies have shown that infants can easily map the intensity and timing of sensory stimulation independently from the modality through which it is conveyed, be it somatosensory, visual or auditory (for a review of this literature, see Stern 1985). Cross-modal transfer seems, therefore, to be a basic capacity we are born with, or that, at the very least, we develop very early.

This capacity appears to be crucial for the development of social cognition, because it is exploited to constitute interpersonal bonds. As shown by Meltzoff and Moore, newborns as young as 18 hours old can reproduce mouth and face movements displayed by the adult they are facing (Meltzoff and Moore 1977; see also Meltzoff and Moore 1997; Meltzoff 2002). What is remarkable is that this behaviour is instantiated by body parts such as the mouth to which newborns have no visual access. Infants, nevertheless, can re-enact the observed behaviour as displayed by the adult demonstrator. The visual information about the observed behaviour is translated into motor commands for reproducing it.

Meltzoff and Moore (1997) have defined this apparently innate mechanism as AIM. According to Meltzoff (2002), intermodal mapping can be conceived of as a 'supramodal act space', unconstrained by any particular mode of inter-action, visual or motor. Modes of interaction as diverse as seeing or doing something *must* share some peculiar feature making the process of equival-ence carried out by AIM possible.

Early imitation appears to constitute a further example of infants' capacity to establish equivalence relations between different modalities of experience. The importance of early imitation for our understanding of social cognition is that it shows that interpersonal bonds are established at the very onset of our life, when no subjective representation can yet be entertained by the organism, because a *conscious subject* of experience is not yet constituted.

The absence of a self-conscious subject does not preclude, however, the constitution of a primitive '*self–other* space', a paradoxical form of intersub-jectivity without subjects. The infant shares this 'we-centric' space with the other individuals inhabiting his world.

The discoveries of developmental psychology are also of vital importance in our discussion of social cognition for another reason: these data show that our cognitive system is capable of conceiving an 'abstract' multimodal way to map apparently unrelated sensory sources of information, well before the development and mastery of language (the cognitive tool of abstraction *par excellence*) and of more sophisticated forms of social interaction.

7.4 Early and mature imitation

A striking feature of the early type of imitation discovered by Meltzoff and co-workers is that it cannot be elicited after the third month or so of life. Later on, however, a more mature form of imitation will develop, one implying the capacity to fully grasp the meaning and relevance of what is to be imitated (see Chapter 6, this volume).

It is this second type of imitation which stirs the debate among psycholo-gists and primatologists concerning whether such behaviour can also be ascribed to non-humans, or if it has to be considered a unique endowment of our species (for a discussion of imitation from an ethological point of view, see Whiten and Custance 1996; Tomasello and Call 1997; Byrne 1995; Visalberghi and Fragaszy 1990, 2001; see Chapter 8 this volume).

I will not delve into this controversial debate here. Rather, what I would like to emphasize is the following aspect: early and mature forms of imitation in humans share a basic feature, which is independent of the presence of highly developed cognitive faculties such as language, or from the capacity to identify the individual to be imitated as a *different self*.

What is common between a neonate who replies to his mother sticking out her tongue with an equivalent behaviour, and the skilled repetition by an adolescent of the piano chords as demonstrated by the piano teacher? Both instances of imitative behaviour are made possible only by the capacity to solve the computational difficulties inherent in any type of interpersonal mapping, due to the different perspectives of demonstrator and imitator (see Chapter 9 of this volume). If I want to reproduce the behaviour of someone else, no matter how complex it is, or whether I understand it or not, I always need to translate my external perspective of the demonstrator into my own personal body perspective. This problem can, however, be overcome if both the actions of the demonstrator and of the imitator share a basic neural format. Later on we will see that this is exactly the case. For the time being what we can say is that the basic feature shared by early and mature forms of imitative behaviours is the presence of a shared, multimodal, *we-centric*, blended space. In Section 7.5, this basic feature is also shown to lie at the core of a different mode of interpersonal relation: empathy.

7.5 Empathy

When we observe other acting individuals, we are exposed to a full range of *expressive* power, which is not confined to what their actions are, but it also encompasses the emotions and feelings they display. When this occurs, an affective meaningful interpersonal link is automatically established (see Chapter 11 of this volume). Empathy constitutes precisely the capacity to establish this link (for a recent discussion of the historical origin of the notion of empathy, see Prigman 1995; Gallese 2001, 2003*a,b*).

The empathic link is not confined to our capacity to understand when someone is angry, happy or sad. Empathy, if conceived, as I am doing, in a broader sense, also enables us to understand what is happening when someone else is experiencing sensations such as pain, touch or tickling.

Again, the results of developmental psychology research are highly relevant in showing that this particular type of interpersonal relationship is present at a very early age. Starting from the second month of age, the infant engages with the mother in what Stern (1985) has called 'affective attunement': a cross-modal matching of interpersonal affective expressions. More precisely, what is matched is not a particular aspect of the other person's behaviour—as typically occurs in imitation. What is matched is '. . . some aspect of the behaviour that reflects the person's feeling state' (Stern 1985). These expressions can be different in form and intensity (body movements, facial expressions, vocalizations), but they all share the same affective dimension of emotional resonance. Incidentally, it is worth noting that according to Lipps (1903), empathy (Einfühlung) can be conceived of as a sort of 'inner imitation'.

Since the very beginning of our life we therefore inhabit a *shared multi-dimensional interpersonal space*, which, I posit, also constitutes a substantial part of our social semantic space during adulthood. When we observe other acting individuals, and face their full range of *expressive* power (the way they act, the emotions and feelings they display), a meaningful embodied interpersonal link is automatically established.

The point is *how* to characterize this special form of *understanding*. Do we apply our capacity for mental logic? Do we apply *theories* to figure out what kind of emotion or sensation is expressed and felt by the individual we are facing? In principle, we can certainly achieve this goal in the aforementioned ways. However, we must note that in everyday life we are able to 'decode' the *quality* of the sensations or emotions embedded in the witnessed behaviour of others without the need to exert any conscious cognitive effort. The meaning of the expressions of affective behaviour seems to be automatically understood by the observer without the necessity of any intervening complex cognitive mediation. How is this possible? And what is the functional mechanism at the basis of our capacity for empathy, as I have defined it? In Section 7.7, I propose that this mechanism can also be envisaged as a kind of simulation.

7.6 Mind reading

Inter-individual relations have played a fundamental role in the evolution of primate cognition. Humphrey (1976) originally suggested that the intelligence of primates primarily evolved to solve social problems. This view is supported by empirical data. Several studies have revealed the unique capacity of non-human primates to understand the *quality* of the relationships within their social group, not only in terms of kin, but also in terms of coalitions, friendship and alliances. As pointed out by Tomasello and Call (1997), primates can categorize and understand third-party social relationships. The evolution of this cognitive trait seems to be related to the necessity to deal with the social complexities that arose when individuals living in groups had to compete for scarce and patchily distributed resources.

An ever-increasing literature has raised questions about the possibility that the social behaviour of non-human primates might be driven by intentions and that their understanding of others' behaviour might be intentional. There is general agreement that monkeys and apes behave *as if* possessing objectives and goals. However, unless human their awareness of purpose is not assumed.

(a)

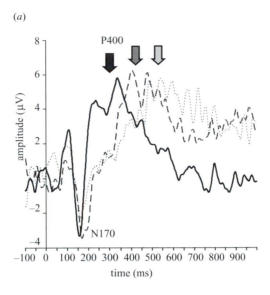

(b)

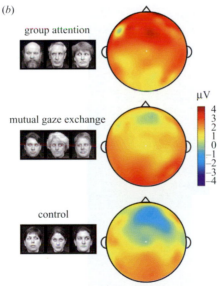

group attention

mutual gaze exchange

μV

control

Plate 1. ERPs elicited to a social attention task. (*a*) ERP waveforms elicited to three conditions: solid line, group attention; dashed line, mutual gaze exchange; dotted line, control. The arrows indicate a late peak of ERP activity that follows the N170 ERP (P400), which changes its latency as a function of viewing condition. (*b*) Voltage maps for the three viewing conditions generated at the peak of P400 activity for the group attention condition (black arrow in (*a*)). The group attention condition shows fronto-temporal positivity, whereas the other two conditions show small posterior positivities. (See Chapter 1, p. 13.)

(a)

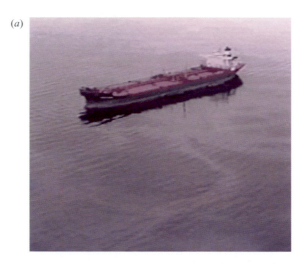

(b)

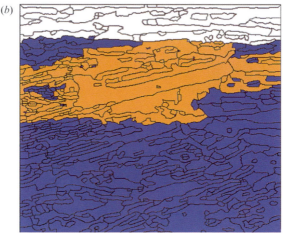

region 2, nouns:
water, crude oil: {oil tanker, oiler, tank ship, tanker}
sea, water: {milldam}, {Suez canal}, {abandoned ship, derelict}, {wreck}, {lifeboat}, {whaleboat}
water: {launch}, {frigate}, {bottom, freighter, merchant ship, merchant-man}

Plate 2. The original image (a) is segmented into regions (b) classified as 'water' (blue), 'sky' (white) and 'man-made' (light brown). The man-made region (region 2) is contained within the water region. The top 10 concepts returned by the manmade search are shown in rank order, grouped by matched constraint terms shown in bold. The words listed within each set of brackets are synonyms and represent a single concept.
(See Chapter 4, p. 99.)

(*a*)

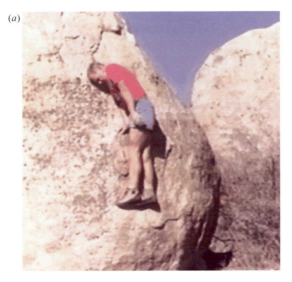

(*b*)

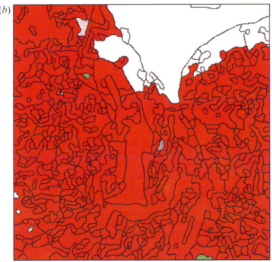

region 3, nouns:
rock: {rock 'n' roll musician, rocker}, {punk, punk rocker}, {groupie}, {cragsman, rock climber}, {pueblo}
region 3, verbs:
up: {emerge}, {ascend, come up, rise, uprise}, {bounce, jounce}, {swell, well}, {rocket, skyrocket}, {uplift}, {scale}, {escalade}, {ramp}, {ride}

Plate 3. The original image (*a*) is segmented into regions (*b*) classified as 'rock' (red) and 'sky' (white), providing the attribute term 'outdoors'. The motion of the person is tracked and characterized as motion attribute terms 'upward' and 'slow'. Both a noun and a verb search are conducted using *person* and *human motion* as elemental terms. The most likely concepts returned by each search are shown in rank order, grouped by matched constraint terms shown in bold. (See Chapter 4, p. 103.)

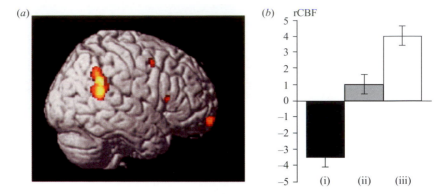

Plate 4. (*a*) Right inferior parietal lobule activation superimposed on an average MRI. (*b*) The relative haemodynamic variation during self action, when subjects acted at will (i), when they imitated the actions demonstrated by the experimenter (ii), and when they saw their actions being imitated by the experimenter (iii). Note the dramatic increase in right inferior parietal lobe activation in this last condition. rCBF indicates regional cerebral blood flow. (Adapted from Decety *et al.* (2002). See Chapter 5, p. 118.)

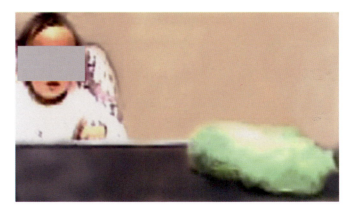

Plate 5. The green blob. This object could move around and make noise on its own. (From Johnson *et al.* 2003. See Chapter 10, p. 230.)

The capacity to understand conspecifics' behaviours as goal related provides considerable benefits to individuals, as they can predict others' actions. The advantage of such a cognitive skill would also allow individuals to influence and manipulate the behaviour of conspecifics (see the Machiavellian Intelligence hypothesis; Whiten and Byrne 1997).

The problem of intentionality in primates was almost simultaneously and independently raised by Humphrey (1978, 1980) and Premack and Woodruff (1978). The traditional view in the cognitive sciences holds that human beings are able to understand the behaviour of others in terms of their *mental states* by exploiting what is commonly designated as 'Folk Psychology'. The capacity for attributing mental states—intentions, beliefs and desires—to others has been defined as ToM (Premack and Woodruff 1978). The attributes of 'Folk Psychology' have been largely identified with the notion of ToM (see Carruthers and Smith 1996; Chapter 3 of this volume). A common trend on this topic has been to emphasize that non-human primates, apes included, do not rely on mentally based accounts for others' behaviour (Hayes 1998; Povinelli *et al.* 2000).

The notion of ToM has been addressed from many different perspectives. ToM has been characterized in terms of a domain-specific ability, supported by an innate, encapsulated and specific module, whose function is segregated from the other intellectual capacities of the individual (Leslie 1987; Baron-Cohen 1995; Fodor 1992, 1994; Chapter 3 of this volume).

A different view holds that ToM constitutes the final stage of a developmental process in which different scientific theories about the world and its inhabitants are tested and eventually discarded to adopt new ones (see the 'child-as-scientist' hypothesis by Gopnik and Meltzoff 1997). Both accounts of ToM are often collectively identified under the heading TT.

Finally, according to a radically different perspective, the capacity to interpret others' behaviour in a meaningful way is conceived as the result of a *simulation routine* by means of which we can *purposely pretend* to be in the other's 'mental shoes' and use our own mind as a model for the mind of others (Gordon 1986; Harris 1989; Goldman 1989, 1992, 1993*a,b*, 2000).

All of these different perspectives on mind reading make distinct assumptions about the brain mechanisms at the basis of this distinctive cognitive feature and, even more importantly from a neuroscientific perspective, about its phylogenetic aspects. The TT approach basically emphasizes the cognitive discontinuity between human beings and other non-human primates. ToM is considered to be a sort of 'mental Rubicon', sanctioning the uniqueness of human cognitive capacities.

The simulationist approach, however, seems to make greater allowance for a possible evolutionary continuity between behaviour reading and mind reading. This perhaps explains why Simulation Theory has progressively gained a larger consensus among neuroscientists and among those cognitive scientists—still not the majority!—fully aware of the intimate relationship between brain mechanisms and cognition.

It is nevertheless an oversimplification to address the issue of how individuals understand the behaviour of others only in terms of a confrontation between behaviour readers and mind readers. To say that human beings mind read, while other animals do not, simply denies the possibility that mind reading can be considered part of a more general model of cognition.

If a process such as ToM really underpins our understanding of others' behaviour, this cognitive feature must still have evolved from a non-human ancestor who shared with the present primates, humans included, several cognitive features. The behavioural study of social cognition of non-human primates and the enquiry of the neural mechanisms supporting it are therefore necessary for a thorough understanding of how the human mind evolved and how it works.

It is reasonable to suggest that this evolutionary process proceeded along a line of continuity (see Gallese and Goldman 1998; Gallese 2000*a,b*, 2001; Gallese *et al*. 2002*a*). This suggests that we should pursue a different heuristic: investigating whether apparently different cognitive strategies may be underpinned by similar functional mechanisms. This is the precise aim of this paper.

Whenever we are exposed to behaviours of others requiring our response, be it reactive or simply attentive, we seldom engage in *explicit and deliberate interpretative acts*. The majority of the time our understanding of the situation is immediate, automatic and almost reflex-like.

According to the TT approach, when faced with the problem of understanding the meaning of others' behaviour, adult human beings must *necessarily* translate the sensory information about the observed behaviour into a series of *mental representations* that share, with language, the propositional format. This enables one to ascribe to others' intentions, desires and beliefs, and therefore to understand the *mental antecedents* of their overt behaviour.

According to this view if, while sitting in a public house I see someone reaching for a pint of ale, I will immediately realize that my neighbour is going to sip some ale from it. The point is, how do I do it? In order to interpret the behaviour of the person sitting beside me in the public house, I must translate his biological motions into a series of mental representations regarding his *desire* to drink beer, his *belief* about the fact that the glass sitting on the table is indeed full of beer, and his *intention* to bring it to the mouth in order to sip beer from it.

Though perhaps a bit caricatured, this account essentially captures how TT characterizes interpersonal relations. I think that the view heralded by classic cognitivism, according to which our capacity of understanding the intentions determining others' behaviour is *solely determined* by metarepresentations created by ascribing propositional attitudes to others, is biologically implausible. The traditional TT perspective on mind reading exemplifies, or perhaps better, *modularizes* within this particular aspect of cognition, a more general view on the mind: a *disembodied* one. I think that there is now enough empirical evidence to reject a disembodied theory of the mind as biologically implausible.

We observe other people behaving and, most of the time, we understand what they are doing and what they are going to do. The crucial point is to clarify what the term 'understanding' means. The observed behaviour is obviously the starting point of any understanding. But the way we characterize *what* we are supposed to understand constrains the quality and structure of our understanding. Much depends on the nature of *what* we are supposed to understand.

The point is that the behaviour of others is not *objectively given* and expressed by *objectively given creatures*. If we accept this distinction between apparent/real aspects of reality, we must also accept that the brain, in order to *represent an external objective reality*, must operate according to the normative dictates of rationality. According to this disembodied view of the human mind, the invisible attitudes governing the ostensive behaviour of others *must be interpreted* by employing the cognitive tool-kit of the rational mind.

However, things look quite different. We now know that there is no such thing as an objective reality that our brain is supposed to represent. For example, there are no objective colours in the world, colour being the result of the wavelength reflectance of objects, the surrounding lighting conditions, the colour cones in our eyes, and the neural circuitry connected to those colour cones. *There is no colour out there independent of us.*

The same argument holds for interpersonal relations. *There can be no other persons out there independent of us.* When we try to understand the behaviour of others, our brain is not representing an *objective external personal reality*. Our brain *models the behaviour of others, much the same as it models our own behaviour*. The results of this modelling process enable us to understand and predict what the behaviour of others is. This point will become clearer later, when introducing neuroscientific data.

If Folk Psychology were the only game in town, a further difficulty we would have to overcome would be the problem of explaining the remarkable capacities of infants and children to 'tune in' in meaningful ways to their social environment, at an age at which the supposed capacity to ascribe propositional attitudes is not yet in place.

I am not, of course, maintaining that we *never* ascribe intentions, desires or beliefs in an *explicit* way. What I am saying is that these explicit forms of mind reading, whatever they might be, are at best only one part of our 'mental social space'. This space is multidimensional, with different dimensions individuating different types of *relational specification* defining the various kinds of interactions of the individual (a biological system) with 'the world outside'.

Relational specifications constitute the almost infinite number of ways that we can *act upon* the world, or *simulate* doing so. The same different types of interaction, when ascribed to others, pertain to different beings, which, nevertheless, we feel, recognize and 'represent' as *persons similar to us*. The point is that we do not *necessarily* need to apply theories of any kind to do this.

My proposal is that all these different levels of organism–organism interactions, whatever the complexity of the relational specifications defining them might be, rely first on the same basic functional mechanism: *embodied simulation*. Embodied simulation enables the constitution of a shared and common background of *implicit certitudes* about ourselves and, simultaneously, about others. In Section 7.7 I demonstrate that embodied simulation is a pervasive brain mechanism, intimately related to apparently 'abstract' aspects of human cognition.

7.7 The many sides of simulation

The *Oxford English Dictionary* provides three different definitions of 'simulation':

 (i) The action or practice of simulating, with intent to deceive; false pretence, deceitful profession.
 (ii) A false assumption or display, a surface resemblance or imitation, of something.
(iii) The technique of imitating the behaviour of some situation or process (whether economic, military, mechanical, etc.) by means of a suitably analogous situation or apparatus, esp. for the purpose of study or personnel training.

   The first two definitions convey the idea of simulation as of something fake, something supposedly aimed to deceive, by *pretending to be similar* to what really differs in many respects. The third definition conveys a totally different meaning: namely, it characterizes simulation as a process meant to produce a better understanding of a given situation or state of affairs, by means of modelling it.

   The third definition of simulation appears to be much closer than the previous ones to the etymology of the word. Indeed 'to simulate' comes from the Latin '*simulare*', which in turn derives from '*similis*', which means 'like', 'similar to'. The third definition of simulation, incidentally, also defines the prevalent epistemic approach of the classic Greek–Roman western world: knowledge is conceived as a process in which the knower *assimilates* what he is supposed to know (see the Latin expression *similia similibus, or* the Greek verb *homologhêin*). (For a discussion of the philosophical history of simulation, see Romano 2002.)

   I will use the term *simulation* in a way that is close to the third definition given above: *an implicit mechanism meant to model the objects and events that the mechanism itself is supposed to control while interacting with them*. The term interaction is considered here in its broadest sense. Simulation is a *control functional mechanism*, its function being the modelling of the objects to be controlled. Indeed, a current authoritative view on motor control envisages simulation as the mechanism employed by forward models to predict the sensory consequences of impending actions (see Chapter 14, this volume). According to this view, the predicted consequences are the simulated ones.

It should be clear that the way I characterize simulation is different from the notion of simulation discussed by the proponents of Simulation Theory. According to Simulation Theory, the pretend state used by the interpreter in order to understand the behaviour of the agent is the result of a deliberate and voluntary act on the side of the interpreter. The simulation process I am discussing is instead *automatic*, *unconscious* and *pre-reflexive*.

Furthermore, I argue that simulation is not a prerogative of the motor system. In other words, simulation is not just confined to the executive control strategies presiding over our functioning in the world, but is a basic functional mechanism, used by vast parts of the brain. I propose that simulation, that is, how we model reality, is the only epistemic strategy available to organisms such as ourselves deriving their knowledge of the world by means of interactions with the world. What we call the *representation of reality* is not a copy of what is objectively given, but an interactive model of what cannot be known in itself. Of course, this also holds for the social interpersonal reality in which we spend all our lives.

Perception requires the capacity to predict forthcoming sensory events. Similarly, action requires the capacity to predict the consequences of action. Both predictions are the result of unconscious and automatic simulation processes. The advantage of this theory is that it is extremely parsimonious: if my theory is correct, a single mechanism—embodied simulation—can provide a common functional framework for all the apparently different aspects of interpersonal relations.

In the next section I review the neuroscientific evidence showing that simulation is a pervasive functional characteristic of the monkey and human brain.

(a) Mental imagery

As human beings we have the capacity to imagine worlds that we have or have not seen before, to imagine doing things that we did or did not do before. The power of our imagination is seemingly infinite. Indeed, mental imagery has long been considered as one of the most characteristic aspects of the human mind, in that it was thought to best epitomize its disembodied nature.

However, in the light of neuroscientific research, things look quite different. We have learned from neuroscience that visual imagery shares, with visual perception, several features (for comprehensive reviews see Farah 2000; Kosslyn and Thompson 2000). For example, the time employed to scan a visual scene is matched by the time employed to mentally imagine the same scene (Kosslyn *et al.* 1978). Furthermore, and more importantly, brain imaging studies show that when we engage in imagining a visual scene, we activate regions in the brain that are normally active when we actually perceive the same visual scene (Farah 1989; Kosslyn *et al.* 1993; Kosslyn 1994), including areas supposedly involved in mapping low-level visual features, such as the primary visual cortex (Le Bihan *et al.* 1993).

As with visual imagery, motor imagery also shares many features with its actual counterpart (Jeannerod 1994). Mentally rehearsing a physical exercise induces an increase of muscle strength comparable to that attained by a real exercise (Decety et al. 1989; Yue and Cole 1992). When we engage in imagining performing a given action, several bodily parameters behave similarly to when we actually carry out the same action. Decety et al. (1991) have shown that heartbeat and breathing frequency increase during motor imagery of physical exercise. Furthermore, as with real physical exercise, they increase linearly with the increase of the imagined effort. Finally, brain imaging experiments have shown that motor imagery and real action both activate a common network of brain motor centres such as the primary motor cortex, premotor cortex, the SMA, the basal ganglia and the cerebellum (Roland et al. 1980; Fox et al. 1987; Decety et al. 1990; Parsons et al. 1995; Porro et al. 1996; Roth et al. 1996; Schnitzler et al. 1997).

All these data show that typical human cognitive activities, such as visual and motor imagery, far from being of exclusive symbolic and propositional nature, rely on and depend upon the activation of sensorimotor brain regions. Visual imagery is equivalent to simulating an actual visual experience and motor imagery is equivalent to simulating an actual motor experience. There is, however, an important point to bear in mind: in mental imagery the simulation process is not automatic and implicit. The subject deliberately engages in it.

(b) Action understanding

Action observation constitutes another instance of simulation. Why does this happen? About 10 years ago a class of premotor neurons was discovered in the macaque monkey brain that discharged not only when the monkey executed goal-related hand actions but also when observing other individuals (monkeys or humans) executing similar actions. We called these neurons 'mirror neurons' (Gallese et al. 1996, 2002a; Rizzolatti et al. 1996a, 2000, 2001; Gallese 2000a, 2001).

In order to be activated by visual stimuli, mirror neurons require an interaction between the agent (be it a human being or a monkey) and its target object. The visual presentation of objects does not evoke any response. Similarly, actions that, although achieving the same goal and looking similar to those performed by the experimenter's hand, are made with tools such as pliers or pincers have little effect on the response of mirror neurons (Gallese et al. 1996). Neurons with similar properties were later discovered in a sector of the posterior parietal cortex reciprocally connected with area F5, area PF or 7b (PF mirror neurons; see Gallese et al. 2002b).

The discovery of mirror neurons has changed our views on the neural mechanisms at the basis of action understanding. The observation of an action leads to the activation of the same neural network active during its actual execution: action observation causes in the observer the automatic simulated re-enactment of the same action. It was proposed that this mechanism could be at the basis of an implicit form of action understanding (Gallese *et al.* 1996, 2002*a*,*b*; Rizzolatti *et al.* 1996*a*; Gallese 2000*a*, 2003*b*).

The relationship between action understanding and action simulation is even more evident in the light of the results of two more recent studies. In the first series of experiments, F5 mirror neurons were tested in two conditions: in the first condition the monkey could see the entire action (e.g. a hand grasping action); in the second condition the same action was presented, but its final critical part, that is the hand–object interaction, was hidden. Therefore, in the hidden condition the monkey only 'knew' that the target object was present behind the occluder. The results showed that more than half of the recorded neurons responded also in the hidden condition (Umiltà *et al.* 2001).

Behavioural data have shown that, like humans, monkeys can also infer the goal of an action even when the visual information about it is incomplete (Filion *et al.* 1996). Data from myself and colleagues reveal the probable neural mechanism at the basis of this cognitive capacity. The inference concerning the goals of the behaviour of others appears to be mediated by the activity of motor neurons coding the goal of the same action in the observer's brain. Out of sight is not 'out of mind' just because, by simulating the action, the gap can be filled.

Some transitive actions are characteristically accompanied by a sound. Imagine hearing the sound produced by your doorbell. This sound will induce you to think that someone is standing in front of the door, waiting to be let into your apartment. That particular sound enables you to understand what is going on even if you have no visual information about what is currently happening outside your closed door. The doorbell sound has the capacity to make an invisible action inferred, and therefore present and understood.

A recent series of experiments were aimed specifically at investigating the neural mechanism possibly underpinning this capacity. F5 mirror neurons were recorded from two monkeys under four different experimental conditions: when the monkey executed noisy actions (e.g. breaking peanuts, tearing sheets of paper apart, and similar actions); when the monkey saw and heard, or just saw or just heard the same actions performed by another individual. The results showed that a consistent percentage of the tested mirror neurons fired when the monkey *executed* the action, just *observed* or just *heard* the same action performed by another agent (see Kohler *et al.* 2001, 2002).

These 'audio-visual mirror neurons' not only responded to the sound of actions, but also discriminated between the sounds of different actions. The actions whose sounds were preferred were also the actions producing the strongest responses when observed or executed. It did not matter at all for the activity of this neural network if the actions were specified at the motor, visual or auditory level. The activation of the premotor neural network controlling the execution of action A in the presence of sensory information related to the same action A, can be characterized as simulating action A.

The multimodal-driven simulation of action goals instantiated by neurons situated in the ventral premotor cortex of the monkey instantiates properties that are strikingly similar to the symbolic properties so characteristic of human thought. The similarity to conceptual content is quite appealing: the same conceptual content ('the goal of action A') results from a multiplicity of states subsuming it: sounds, observed and executed actions. These states, in turn, are subsumed by differently triggered patterns of activations within a population of 'audio-visual mirror neurons'.

The *action simulation* embodied by audio-visual mirror neurons is indeed similar to the use of predicates: the verb 'to break' is used to convey a meaning that can be used in different contexts: 'Seeing someone breaking a peanut', 'Hearing someone breaking a peanut', 'Breaking a peanut'. The predicate, similarly to the responses in audiovisual mirror neurons, does not change depending on the context to which it applies, nor depending on the subject/agent performing the action. All that changes is the context the predicate refers to.

The general picture conveyed by these results is that the sensorimotor integration supported by the premotor-parietal F5-PF mirror-matching system instantiates simulations of actions utilized not only to generate and control goal-related behaviours, but also to provide a meaningful account of the goals and purposes of others' actions, by means of their simulation.

What is the importance of these data for our understanding of human social cognition? Several studies using different experimental methodologies and techniques have also demonstrated the existence of a similar mirror system in humans, matching action observation and execution (see Fadiga *et al.* 1995; Grafton *et al.* 1996; Rizzolatti *et al.* 1996*b*; Decety *et al.* 1997; Cochin *et al.* 1998; Hari *et al.* 1998; Iacoboni *et al.* 1999; Buccino *et al.* 2001). In particular, it is interesting to note that brain imaging experiments in humans have shown that during action observation there is a strong activation of premotor and parietal areas, the likely human homologue of the monkey areas in which mirror neurons were originally described (Grafton *et al.* 1996; Rizzolatti *et al.* 1996*b*; Decety *et al.* 1997; Decety and Grèzes 1999; Iacoboni *et al.* 1999; Buccino *et al.* 2001).

In humans, as in monkeys, action observation constitutes a form of action simulation. As anticipated above, this kind of simulation, however, is different from the simulation processes occurring during visual and motor imagery. Action observation *automatically triggers action simulation*. In mental imagery, as we have seen, the simulation process is triggered by a deliberate act of the will: one purposely decides to imagine oneself observing something or doing something.

An empirical validation of this difference comes from brain imaging experiments. If we compare the motor centres activated by action observation with those activated during action imagery, we will notice that only the latter leads to the activation of pre-SMA and of the primary motor cortex.

That said, it appears nonetheless that both mental imagery and action observation are kinds of simulation. The main difference is what triggers the simulation process: an internal event in the case of mental imagery, and an external event in the case of action observation. This difference leads to slightly different patterns of brain activation. However, both conditions share a common mechanism: the simulation of actions by means of the activation of parietal-premotor cortical networks. This process of automatic simulation constitutes also a level of understanding, a level that does not entail the explicit use of any theory or symbolic representation.

(c) Imitation

The neural bases of human imitation have just begun to be unravelled with the aid of the new brain imaging techniques. The first study showing which parts of the brain are activated during observation and actual, *non-deferred* imitation of the same motor behaviour was published only three years ago (Iacoboni *et al.* 1999). In their study, Iacoboni *et al.* contrasted conditions in which subjects observed hand movements (finger lifting), with conditions in which the subject had to imitate the observed movement. The results showed a cortical network active during both observation and imitation, with greater activation during the second condition. This circuit comprises the ventral premotor cortex, the posterior parietal cortex and the posterior region of the STS.

An interesting and unexpected result of the study of Iacoboni *et al.* (1999) was that the STS region, traditionally considered a purely sensory area, was more activated during imitation than during action observation. If the function of the STS were solely to provide a visual description of the observed action, it is hard to explain why it should be more active during imitation, since the imitated action was identical to that observed.

A possible explanation is that the activation of the STS during action imitation reflected the expected visual consequence of the imitated action, in other words the neural correlate of the activation of the forward model of the action, *simulating the sensory consequences of the action to be imitated*.

The results of a second fMRI study by the same authors corroborated this hypothesis (Iacoboni *et al.* 2001). In this second study, subjects were required to observe and imitate hand actions in two different configurations. During the *specular* configuration, subjects had to observe or imitate with their right hand a left-hand action. During the *anatomical* configuration, subjects had to observe or imitate with their right hand a right-hand action. The results showed that: (i) in the observation condition, STS activation was stronger when the observed hand was the right one; (ii) in the imitation condition, STS activation was stronger when the imitated hand was the left. A straightforward interpretation of these results holds that in order to imitate the observed action, the internal model of the action predicts *via simulation* the sensory consequences of the impending imitative action, thus allowing the possibility of establishing a match with the action to be imitated, and eventually bringing about corrections, if needed to attain a better match.

It appears therefore that actual imitation of observed actions involves a network of brain areas whose activation can be accounted for in terms of simulation.

(d) Empathy

As proposed by Damasio (1994, 1999), one of the mechanisms enabling feelings of emotion to emerge is probably the activation of neural '*as if* body loops'. These automatic, implicit and non-reflexive simulation mechanisms, bypassing the body proper through the *internal* activation of sensory body maps, create a representation of emotion-driven body-related changes.

As anticipated above, my proposal is that the activation of these '*as if* body loops' can probably also be triggered by the observation of the behaviour of other individuals (see Adolphs *et al.* 2000; Goldman and Gallese 2000; Gallese 2001).

Preliminary evidence suggests that the same neural structures that are active during the experience of sensations and emotions are also active when the same sensations and emotions are to be detected in others. I take this type of externally driven activation to be a further instance of simulation. A whole range of different 'mirror-matching mechanisms' instantiating simulation routines might therefore be present in our brain. What does this preliminary evidence look like?

Hutchison *et al.* (1999) studied pain-related neurons in the human cingulate cortex, by investigating whether neurons in the anterior cingulate cortex of locally anaesthetized but awake patients responded to painful stimuli. These authors reported that neurons responded not only to noxious mechanical stimulation applied to the patient's hand, but also when the patient watched pinpricks being applied to the examiner's fingers. Both applied and observed painful stimuli elicited the same response in the same neurons. *Simulated* painful experience activates the same neurons normally active during actual painful experience.

Calder *et al.* (2000) showed that a patient who suffered a stroke damaging various cortical and sub-cortical structures such as the insula and the putamen was selectively impaired in detecting disgust in many different modalities (e.g. facial expressions, non-verbal emotional sounds and emotional prosody). The same patient was also selectively impaired in subjectively experiencing disgust and therefore in reacting appropriately to it. These results seem to suggest that once the capacity to *experience* and *express* a given emotion is lost, the same emotion cannot be easily *represented* and *detected* in others.

As we have learned from developmental psychology, emotions constitute one of the earliest ways available to the individual to acquire knowledge about its situation, thus enabling him to reorganize this knowledge in the light of the relations with others. This points to a strong interaction between emotion and action. The coordinated activity of sensorimotor and affective neural systems results in the simplification and automatization of the behavioural responses that living organisms have to produce in order to survive.

The strict coupling between affect and sensorimotor integration is highlighted by a recent study by Adolphs *et al.* (2000), where over 100 brain-damaged patients were reviewed. Among other results, this study showed that the patients who suffered damage to the amygdala and to the sensorimotor cortices were also those who scored worst when asked to rate or name facial emotions displayed by human faces.

A further empirical support to the theory put forward here, of a tight link between simulation and empathy, comes from a recent fMRI study by Iacoboni and coworkers on healthy participants (Carr *et al.* 2001). This study shows that both observation and imitation of facial emotions activate the same restricted group of brain structures, including the premotor cortex, the insula and the amygdala. It is possible to speculate that such a double activation pattern during observation and imitation of emotions could be due to the activity of a neural mirror-matching mechanism, constituting another kind of embodied simulation.

My theory also predicts the existence of 'somatosensory mirror neurons' giving us the capacity to map different body locations when observing the bodies of others, and to refer them to equivalent locations of our body. Experiments are currently underway in the laboratory to test this theory.

To summarize, motor imagery, action observation, imitation and empathy all share the same basic mechanism, the mechanism of embodied simulation: simulation of actions, simulation of emotions, simulation of feelings and sensations. Embodied simulation enables models of real or imaginary worlds to be created. These models are the only way we have to establish a meaningful relationship with these worlds, because these worlds are never objectively given, but always recreated by means of simulated models. In Section 7.8 I provide a multilayered account of simulation that will allow me to describe different forms of interpersonal relations within a unitary framework.

7.8 The shared manifold

I have suggested that the establishment of self–other identity is a driving force for the cognitive development of more articulated and sophisticated forms of interpersonal relations. It is this identity relation that enables us to understand others' behaviour, to imitate it, to share the sensations and emotions that others experience.

What I propose is to characterize an identity relation orthogonal to all the dimensions of our social cognition in terms of a 'shared manifold'. It is by means of the shared manifold that we recognize other human beings as similar to us that intersubjective communication, social imitation and the ascription of intentions become possible. The shared manifold can be described at three different levels: (i) a phenomenological level; (ii) a functional level; and (iii) a sub-personal level.

The *phenomenological level* is responsible for the sense of similarity, of being individuals within a larger social community of people like us, which we experience whenever we confront other human beings. It could be defined as the *empathic* level, provided that empathy is characterized as broadly as I do here. Actions, emotions and sensations experienced by others become meaningful to us because we can *share* their underlying basic format with others.

The *functional level* is characterized in terms of embodied simulation routines, '*as if*' modes of interaction enabling models of self/other to be created. The same functional logic at work during self-control operates also during the understanding of others' behaviour. Both instances are *models of interaction*, which map their referents on identical relational functional nodes. All modes of interaction share a relational character. At the functional level of description of the shared manifold, the relational logic of operation produces the self/other identity by enabling the system to detect coherence, regularity and predictability, independently from their situated source.

The *sub-personal level* is instantiated as the level of activity of a series of mirror-matching neural circuits. The activity of these neural circuits is, in turn, tightly coupled with multilevel changes within body states. *Mirror neurons instantiate at the sub-personal level the multimodal intentional shared space.* These are the shared spaces that allow us to appreciate, experience and understand the actions we observe, the emotions and the sensations we take others to experience.

There is one further important point that needs to be clarified. The shared manifold of intersubjectivity, as I conceive it, does not entail our experiencing others *as* we experience ourselves. The shared manifold simply enables and bootstraps mutual intelligibility. Of course, self–other identity constitutes only one aspect of intersubjectivity. As highlighted by Husserl (1989; see also Zahavi 2001), it is the otherness (*alterity*) of the other that provides the objective character of reality. The quality of our lived experience (*erlebnis*) of the 'external world' and its content are constrained by the presence of other subjects that are intelligible, while preserving their otherness.

We can recognize the otherness of the other at the sub-personal level also, as this is instantiated by the different neural networks that come into play when *I* act as opposed to when *others* act.

7.9 Conclusions

In this paper I have examined three fundamental aspects of interpersonal relations: imitation, empathy and the ascription of intentions, or mind reading.

I have suggested that all these different levels and modes of interaction share a common basic mechanism defining a shared interpersonal space: embodied simulation. I have also suggested that this mechanism is automatic, pre-reflexive and unconscious. Embodied simulation, according to the characterization I provide, is a distinctive functional feature of the brain–body system, its role being that of modelling the interactions between a situated organism and its environment. According to this characterization of simulation, our understanding of interpersonal relations relies on the basic capacity to model the behaviour of other individuals by employing the same resources used to model our own behaviour.

As shown by an impressive amount of converging neuroscientific data, there is a *basic level* of our interpersonal interactions that does not make explicit use of propositional attitudes. This basic level consists of embodied simulation processes that enable the constitution of a shared meaningful interpersonal space.

This shared space relies heavily on action and action imitation, but is not confined to the domain of action. It covers a more global dimension, comprising all aspects defining a life form, from its particular body to its particular affect. This manifold shared space defines the broad range of implicit certainties we entertain about other individuals. Self and other relate to each other, because they both represent opposite extensions of the same correlative and reversible *we-centric* space. The observer and the observed are part of a dynamic system governed by reversible rules.

The shared intersubjective space in which we live from birth continues to constitute a substantial part of our semantic space. When we observe other acting individuals, and face their full range of *expressive* power (the way they act, the emotions and feelings they display), a meaningful embodied interpersonal link is automatically established by means of simulation.

Another interesting source of data that demonstrates the importance of embodied simulation is provided by social psychology. Brandt and Stark (1997) showed that subjects, while listening to syllogisms containing the words 'left' and 'right', moved their eyes prevalently in the horizontal dimension, while tending to move their eyes vertically when listening to sentences containing the words 'above' and 'below'. Spivey *et al.* (2000) showed that when listening to vignettes describing the top of a skyscraper subjects tended to gaze systematically upward, whereas they tended to look downward when the vignette was describing the bottom of a canyon. All these studies and several more (for a comprehensive review, see Barsalou *et al.* 2003) show that humans tend to accompany their understanding of sentences or their imaginative activities with body reactions that simulate real experiences. The triggering stimulus, regardless of its external or internal nature, induces a congruent embodied simulation as a default automatic reaction. These studies show a striking relationship between different aspects of higher cognition, such as sentence processing and embodied simulation.

To what extent embodied simulation explains the sophisticated, and unique, human capacity to interpret the inner world of others is an empirical issue to be addressed by future research.

This work was supported by MIURST and ESF.

References

Adolphs, R., Damasio, H., Tranel, D., Cooper, G. and Damasio, A. R. (2000). A role for somatosensory cortices in the visual recognition of emotion as revealed by three-dimensional lesion mapping. *J. Neurosci.* **20**, 2683–90.

Baron-Cohen, S. (1995). *Minblindness. An essay on autism and theory of mind.* Cambridge, MA: MIT Press.

Barsalou, L. W., Niedenthal, P. M., Barbey, A. K. and Ruppert, J. A. (2003). Social embodiment. In *The psychology of learning and motivation*, vol. 43 (ed. B. H. Ross). San Diego, CA: Academic Press.

Brandt, S. A. and Stark, L. W. (1997). Spontaneous eye movements during visual imagery reflect the content of the visual scene. *J. Cogn. Neurosci.* **9**, 27–38.

Buccino, G., Binkofski, F., Fink, G. R., Fadiga, L., Fogassi, L., Gallese, V., *et al.* (2001). Action observation activates premotor and parietal areas in a somatotopic manner: an fMRI study. *Eur. J. Neurosci.* **13**, 400–4.

Byrne, R. W. (1995). *The thinking ape. Evolutionary origins of intelligence.* Oxford: Oxford University Press.

Calder, A. J., Keane, J., Manes, F., Antoun, N. and Young, A. W. (2000). Impaired recognition and experience of disgust following brain injury. *Nature Neurosci.* **3**, 1077–8.

Carr, L., Iacoboni, M., Dubeau, M.-C. Mazziotta, J. C. and Lenzi, G. L. (2001). Observing and imitating emotion: implications for the neurological correlates of empathy. Paper presented at the *First Int. Conf. of Social Cognitive Neuroscience, Los Angeles, 24–6 April 2001.*

Carruthers, P. and Smith, P. K. (eds) (1996). *Theories of theories of mind.* New York: Cambridge University Press.

Cochin, S., Barthelemy, C., Lejeune, B., Roux, S. and Martineau, J. (1998). Perception of motion and qEEG activity in human adults. *Electroenceph. Clin. Neurophysiol.* **107**, 287–95.

Damasio, A. R. (1994). *Descartes' error.* New York: G. P. Putnam's Sons.

Damasio, A. R. (1999). *The feeling of what happens: body and emotion in the making of consciousness.* New York: Harcourt Brace.

Decety, J. and Grèzes, J. (1999). Neural mechanisms subserving the perception of human actions. *Trends Cogn. Sci.* **3**, 172–8.

Decety, J., Jeannerod, M. and Prablanc, C. (1989). The timing of mentally represented actions. *Behav. Brain Res.* **34**, 35–42.

Decety, J., Sjoholm, H., Ryding, E., Stenberg, G. and Ingvar, D. (1990). The cerebellum participates in cognitive activity: tomographic measurements of regional cerebral blood flow. *Brain Res.* **535**, 313–7.

Decety, J., Jeannerod, M., Germain, M. and Pastene, J. (1991). Vegetative response during imagined movement is proportional to mental effort. Behav. *Brain Res.* **34**, 35–42.

Decety, J., Grèzes, J., Costes, N., Perani, D., Jeannerod, M., Procyk, E., *et al.* (1997). Brain activity during observation of actions. Influence of action content and subject's strategy. *Brain* **120**, 1763–77.

Fadiga, L., Fogassi, L., Pavesi, G. and Rizzolatti, G. (1995). Motor facilitation during action observation: a magnetic stimulation study. *J. Neurophysiol.* **73**, 2608–11.

Farah, M. J. (1989). The neural basis of mental imagery. *Trends Neurosci.* **12**, 395–9.

Farah, M. J. (2000). The neural bases of mental imagery. In *The cognitive neurosciences*, 2nd edn (ed. M. S. Gazzaniga), pp. 965–74. Cambridge, MA: MIT Press.

Filion, C. M., Washburn, D. A. and Gulledge, J. P. (1996). Can monkeys (*Macaca mulatta*) represent invisible displacement? *J. Comp. Psychol.* **110**, 386–95.

Fodor, J. (1992). A theory of the child's theory of mind. *Cognition* **44**, 283–96.

Fodor, J. (1994). *The elm and the expert: mentalese and its semantics*. Cambridge, MA: MIT Press.

Fox, P., Pardo, J., Petersen, S. and Raichle, M. (1987). Supplementary motor and premotor responses to actual and imagined hand movements with positron emission tomography. *Soc. Neurosci. Abstr.* **13**, 1433.

Gallese, V. (2000*a*). The acting subject: towards the neural basis of social cognition. In *Neural correlates of consciousness. Empirical and conceptual questions* (ed. T. Metzinger), pp. 325–33. Cambridge, MA: MIT Press.

Gallese, V. (2000*b*). The inner sense of action: agency and motor representations. *J. Consc. Stud.* **7**, 23–40.

Gallese, V. (2001). The 'shared manifold' hypothesis: from mirror neurons to empathy. *J. Consc. Stud.* **8**, 33–50.

Gallese, V. (2003*a*). A neuroscientific grasp of concepts: from control to representation. *Phil. Trans. R. Soc. Lond.* B **358**. (In the press.)

Gallese, V. (2003*b*). The roots of empathy: the shared manifold hypothesis and the neural basis of intersubjectivity. *Psychopathology*. (In the press.)

Gallese, V. and Goldman, A. (1998). Mirror neurons and the simulation theory of mind-reading. *Trends Cogn. Sci.* **12**, 493–501.

Gallese, V., Fadiga, L., Fogassi, L. and Rizzolatti, G. (1996). Action recognition in the premotor cortex. *Brain* **119**, 593–609.

Gallese, V., Ferrari, P. F., Kohler, E. and Fogassi, L. (2002*a*). The eyes, the hand, and the mind: behavioral and neurophysiological aspects of social cognition. In *The cognitive animal* (ed. M. Bekoff, C. Allen and G. Burghardt), pp. 451–61. Cambridge, MA: MIT Press.

Gallese, V., Fogassi, L., Fadiga, L. and Rizzolatti, G. (2002*b*). Action representation and the inferior parietal lobule. In *Attention and performance*, vol. XIX (ed. W. Prinz and B. Hommel), pp. 247–66. Oxford: Oxford University Press.

Goldman, A. (1989). Interpretation psychologized. *Mind Lang.* **4**, 161–85.

Goldman, A. (1992). In defense of the simulation theory. *Mind Lang.* **7**, 104–19.

Goldman, A. (1993a). The psychology of folk psychology. *Behav. Brain Sci.* **16**, 15–28.

Goldman, A. (1993*b*). *Philosophical applications of cognitive science*. Boulder, CO: Westview Press.

Goldman, A. (2000). The mentalizing folk. In *Metarepresentation* (ed. D. Sperber), pp. 171–96. Oxford: Oxford University Press.

Goldman, A. and Gallese, V. (2000). Reply to Schulkin. *Trends Cogn. Sci.* **4**, 255–6.

Gopnik, A. and Meltzoff, A. N. (1997). *Words, thoughts, and theories*. Cambridge, MA: MIT Press.

Gordon, R. (1986). Folk psychology as simulation. *Mind Lang.* **1**, 158–71.

Grafton, S. T., Arbib, M. A., Fadiga, L. and Rizzolatti, G. (1996). Localization of grasp representations in humans by PET: 2. Observation compared with imagination. *Exp. Brain Res.* **112**, 103–11.

Hari, R., Forss, N., Avikainen, S., Kirveskari, S., Salenius, S. and Rizzolatti, G. (1998). Activation of human primary motor cortex during action observation: a neuromagnetic study. *Proc. Natl Acad. Sci. USA* **95**, 15061–5.

Harris, P. (1989). *Children and emotion*. Oxford: Blackwell Scientific.

Hayes, C. M. (1998). Theory of mind in nonhuman primates. *Behav. Brain Sci.* **21**, 101–48.

Humphrey, N. K. (1976). The social function of intellect. In *Growing points in ethology* (ed. P. Bateson and R. A. Hinde), pp. 303–21. Cambridge: Cambridge University Press.

Humphrey, N. K. (1978). Nature's psychologists. *New Scient.*, 29 June.

Humphrey, N. K. (1980). Nature's psychologists. In *Consciousness and the physical world* (ed. B. D. Josephson and V. S. Ramachandran), pp. 57–75. Oxford: Pergamon.

Husserl, E. (1989). *Ideas pertaining to a pure phenomenology and to a phenomenological philosophy, second book: studies in the phenomenology of constitution*. Dordrecht, The Netherlands: Kluwer.

Hutchison, W. D., Davis, K. D., Lozano, A. M., Taskev, R. R. and Dostrovsky, J. O. (1999). Pain related neurons in the human cingulate cortex. *Nature Neurosci.* **2**, 403–5.

Iacoboni, M., Woods, R. P., Brass, M., Bekkering, H., Mazziotta, J. C. and Rizzolatti, G. (1999). Cortical mechanisms of human imitation. *Science* **286**, 2526–8.

Iacoboni, M., Koski, L. M., Brass, M., Bekkering, H., Woods, R. P., Dubeau, M. C., *et al.* (2001). Reafferent copies of imitated actions in the right superior temporal cortex. *Proc. Natl Acad. Sci. USA* **98**, 13995–9.

Jeannerod, M. (1994). The representing brain: neural correlates of motor intention and imagery. *Behav. Brain Sci.* **17**, 187–245.

Kohler, E., Umiltà, M. A., Keysers, C., Gallese, V., Fogassi, L. and Rizzolatti, G. (2001). Auditory mirror neurons in the ventral premotor cortex of the monkey. *Soc. Neurosci. Abstr.* **27**, 129.9.

Kohler, E., Keysers, C., Umiltà, M. A., Fogassi, L., Gallese, V. and Rizzolatti, G. (2002). Hearing sounds, understanding actions: action representation in mirror neurons. *Science* **297**, 846–8.

Kosslyn, S. M. (1994). *Image and brain: the resolution of the imagery debate*. Cambridge, MA: MIT Press.

Kosslyn, S. M. and Thompson, W. L. (2000). Shared mechanisms in visual imagery and visual perception: insights from cognitive science. In *The cognitive neurosciences*, 2nd edn (ed. M. S. Gazzaniga), pp. 975–85. Cambridge, MA: MIT Press.

Kosslyn, S. M., Ball, T. M. and Reiser, B. J. (1978). Visual images preserve metric spatial information: evidence from studies of image scanning. *J. Exp. Psychol. Hum. Percept. Perform.* **4**, 47–60.

Kosslyn, S. M., Alpert, N. M., Thompson, W. L., Maljkovic, V., Weise, S., Chabris, C., *et al.* (1993). Visual mental imagery activates topographically organized visual cortex: PET investigations. *J. Cogn. Neurosci.* **5**, 263–87.

Le Bihan, D., Turner, R., Zeffiro, T. A., Cuenod, C. A., Jezzard, P. and Bonnerot, V. (1993). Activation of human primary visual cortex during visual recall: a magnetic resonance imaging study. *Proc. Natl Acad. Sci. USA* **90**, 11802–5.

Leslie, A. M. (1987). Pretence and representation. The origins of 'theory of mind'. *Psychol. Rev.* **94**, 412–26.

Lipps, T. (1903). Einfulung, innere nachahmung und organ-enempfindung. In *Arch. F. Ges. Psy.*, vol. I, part 2. Leipzig: W. Engelmann.

Meltzoff, A. N. (2002). Elements of a developmental theory of imitation. In *The imitative mind: development, evolution and brain bases* (ed. W. Prinz and A. Meltzoff), pp. 19–41. New York: Cambridge University Press.

Meltzoff, A. N. and Borton, R. W. (1979). Intermodal matching by human neonates. *Nature* **282**, 403–5.

Meltzoff, A. N. and Moore, M. K. (1977). Imitation of facial and manual gestures by human neonates. *Science* **198**, 75–8.

Meltzoff, A. N. and Moore, M. K. (1997). Explaining facial imitation: a theoretical model. *Early Dev. Parent.* **6**, 179–92.

Parsons, L., Fox, P., Downs, J., Glass, T., Hirsch, T., Martin, C., *et al.* (1995). Use of implicit motor imagery for visual shape discrimination as revealed by PET. *Nature* **375**, 54–8.

Porro, C. A., Francescato, M. P., Cettolo, V., Diamond, M. E., Baraldi, P., Zuiani, C., *et al.* (1996). Primary motor and sensory cortex activation during motor performance and motor imagery. A functional magnetic resonance study. *J. Neurosci.* **16**, 7688–98.

Povinelli, D. J., Bering, J. M. and Giambrone, S. (2000). Toward a science of other minds: escaping the argument by analogy. *Cogn. Sci.* **24**, 509–41.

Premack, D. and Woodruff, G. (1978). Does the chimpanzee have a theory of mind? *Behav. Brain Sci.* **1**, 515–26.

Prigman, G. W. (1995). Freud and the history of empathy. *Int. J. Psycho-Anal.* **76**, 237–52.

Rizzolatti, G., Fadiga, L., Gallese, V. and Fogassi, L. (1996*a*). Premotor cortex and the recognition of motor actions. *Cogn. Brain Res.* **3**, 131–41.

Rizzolatti, G., Fadiga, L., Matelli, M., Bettinardi, V., Paulesu, E., Perani, D., *et al.* (1996*b*). Localization of grasp representations in humans by PET: 1. Observation versus execution. *Exp. Brain Res.* **111**, 246–52.

Rizzolatti, G., Fogassi, L. and Gallese, V. (2000). Cortical mechanisms subserving object grasping and action recognition: a new view on the cortical motor functions. In *The cognitive neurosciences*, 2nd edn (ed. M. S. Gazzaniga), pp. 539–52. Cambridge, MA: MIT Press.

Rizzolatti, G., Fogassi, L. and Gallese, V. (2001). Neurophysiological mechanisms underlying the understanding and imitation of action. *Nature Neurosci. Rev.* **2**, 661–70.

Roland, P., Larsen, B., Lassen, N. and Skinhoj, E. (1980). Supplementary motor area and other cortical areas in organization of voluntary movements in man. *J. Neurophysiol.* **43**, 118–36.

Romano, G. (2002). La mente mimetica: riflessioni e prospettive sulla teoria della simulazione mentale. PhD thesis, Cognitive Sciences, University of Siena, Italy.

Roth, M., Decety, J., Raybaudi, M., Massarelli, R., Delon-Martin, C., Segebarth, C., *et al.* (1996). Possible involvement of primary motor cortex in mentally simulated movement: a functional magnetic resonance imaging study. *NeuroReport* **7**, 1280–4.

Schnitzler, A., Salenius, S., Salmelin, R., Jousmaki, V. and Hari, R. (1997). Involvement of primary motor cortex in motor imagery: a neuromagnetic study. *NeuroImage* **6**, 201–8.

Spivey, M., Tyler, M., Richardson, D. and Young, E. (2000). Eye movements during comprehension of spoken scene descriptions. In *Proc. 22nd A. Conf. Cogn. Sci. Soc.*, pp. 487–92. Mahwah, NJ: Erlbaum.

Stern, D. N. (1985). *The interpersonal world of the infant*. London: Karnac Books.

Tomasello, M. and Call, J. (1997). *Primate cognition*. New York: Oxford University Press.

Umiltà, M. A., Kohler, E., Gallese, V., Fogassi, L., Fadiga, L., Keysers, C., *et al.* (2001). 'I know what you are doing': a neurophysiological study. *Neuron* **32**, 91–101.

Visalberghi, E. and Fragaszy, D. (1990). Do monkeys ape? In *'Language' and intelligence in monkeys and apes* (ed. S. T. Parker and K. R. Gibson), pp. 247–73. Cambridge, MA: Cambridge University Press.

Visalberghi, E. and Fragaszy, D. (2001). Do monkeys ape? Ten years after. In *Imitation in animals and artifacts* (ed. K. Dautenhahn and C. Nehaniv). Boston, MA: MIT Press.

Whiten, A. and Byrne, R. W. (1997). *Machiavellian intelligence 2: evaluations and extensions*. Cambridge: Cambridge University Press.

Whiten, A. and Custance, D. (1996). Studies of imitation in chimpanzees and children. In *Social learning in animals: the roots of culture* (ed. C. M. Hayes and B. G. Galef), pp. 291–318. London: Academic Press.

Yue, G. and Cole, K. (1992). Strength increases from the motor program: comparison of training with maximal voluntary and imagined muscle contractions. *J. Neurophysiol.* **67**, 1114–23.

Zahavi, D. (2001). Beyond empathy. Phenomenological approaches to intersubjectivity. *J. Consc. Stud.* **8**, 151–67.

Glossary

AIM: active intermodal mapping
fMRI: functional magnetic resonance imaging
SMA: supplementary motor area
STS: superior temporal sulcus
ToM: theory of mind
TT: theory–theory

8

Imitation as behaviour parsing

R. W. Byrne

Non-human great apes appear to be able to acquire elaborate skills partly by imitation, raising the possibility of the transfer of skill by imitation in animals that have only rudimentary mentalizing capacities: in contrast to the frequent assumption that imitation depends on prior understanding of others' intentions. Attempts to understand the apes' behaviour have led to the development of a purely mechanistic model of imitation, the 'behaviour parsing' model, in which the statistical regularities that are inevitable in planned behaviour are used to decipher the organization of another agent's behaviour, and thence to imitate parts of it. Behaviour can thereby be *understood statistically* in terms of its correlations (circumstances of use, effects on the environment) without understanding of intentions or the everyday physics of cause-and-effect. Thus, imitation of complex, novel behaviour may not require mentalizing, but conversely behaviour parsing may be a necessary preliminary to attributing intention and cause.

Keywords: great apes; segmentation; hierarchical organization; statistical regularities; intentionality; causality

8.1 Introduction

Imitation has fascinated behavioural scientists for more than 100 years (Thorndike 1898), and over this period has acquired many shades of meaning. At the core, however, lie two enigmas.

(i) How is it possible for *actions as seen* to be matched with *actions as imitated*? (the 'correspondence' problem).
(ii) How is it possible for *novel, complex behaviours* to be acquired by observation? (the 'transfer of skill' problem).

Much of the thrust of imitation research in animal behaviour and developmental psychology has focused on the first of these problems, implicitly treating the second as more straightforward.

When attention is restricted to human imitation, this appears at first sight a good strategy. The young child will later develop into an adult who will certainly be able to learn new, highly structured and flexible skills in other ways, including: experimentation and practice, mental planning, explicit teaching or a combination of all three. It is therefore tempting to treat the planning and organizational issues as much the same in imitated and non-imitated behaviour, thus focusing attention on the problem of recognizing correspondence between actions as seen and actions as done. For less sophisticated animals, that becomes a sleight of hand. The ability to organize complex behaviour cannot be assumed for a non-human animal (hereafter, 'animal'), and indeed this may be a greater difficulty even than recognizing correspondence. Moreover, when the two issues are confronted together, a greater challenge emerges: to understand how the underlying organization of novel, complex behaviour can be perceived, and how what is perceived can be used to guide new learning. This paper will offer some steps towards an eventual solution to this larger problem: how do we detect the organizational structure of observed behaviour in other agents (and consequently acquire new skills by imitation), and how did we acquire this ability?

The long history of imitation research in comparative psychology has, however, bequeathed a useful legacy of terminology, and illustrated that quite effective social learning may be achieved *without* the capacity to imitate. Profiting from this experience can allow several other phenomena to be set aside, allowing clearer focus on the main task.

(a) Stimulus enhancement, response facilitation and emulation

In the early history of psychology, persisting today in lay parlance, imitation could refer to almost any case of actions matching in form. E. L. Thorndike's original definition 'learning to do an act from seeing it done' drew attention to the key role which *observation* plays, ruling out cases in which prior observation is unnecessary for behavioural matching to occur (Thorndike 1898). The behaviourist K. W. Spence showed further that rather simple and general behavioural tendencies could aid learning in social contexts. He introduced the notion of *stimulus enhancement*, in which seeing some act done in a particular place or to some particular object would increase the observer's probability of going to that place or interacting with that object (Spence 1937). As he noted, once behavioural exploration is concentrated upon a narrowed range of stimuli, chance discovery of the means of achieving the goal is made much more likely. Numerous cases of social learning, once claimed to show imitation, have proved to be explicable as stimulus enhancement (Galef 1988). Research on animal imitation therefore contracted again, to cases where the form of action matched more or less precisely what was seen. Efforts were thenceforth made to separate out direct behavioural copying from learning about other aspects of the physical situation.

Not all behavioural copying, however, implies that the observer has learned by imitation. A simpler possibility is that a pre-existing response may be facilitated (i.e. made more available) by seeing it done, causing a higher probability of the response occurring subsequently: *response facilitation* (Byrne 1994;

Byrne and Russon 1998). Response facilitation involves one of the enigmas of imitation, the correspondence problem, but not the other, the transfer of skill by observation, because to be 'facilitated' the behaviour must exist already within the individual's repertoire. The relationship of response facilitation to stimulus enhancement is evidently close, although here it is a voluntary act that is enhanced or facilitated. Response facilitation and stimulus enhancement may indeed be two manifestations of the same phenomenon: *priming* of neural correlates (Byrne 1994, 1998*b*). Priming neural correlates of aspects of the social situation and environment results in stimulus enhancement; priming neural correlates of action patterns in the current repertoire results in response facilitation. Part of the neural mechanism of response facilitation has apparently been identified, in the mirror neurons found in premotor cortex of rhesus monkeys, *Macaca mulatta* (Gallese *et al.* 1996; Rizzolatti *et al.* 1996, 2002). These cells respond equally to simple, goal-directed manual actions whether made by the monkey itself or an individual it is watching. An experimental paradigm, the two-action method (Dawson and Foss 1965), has shown that facilitation of recently seen, simple manual actions that are part of the observer's normal repertoire does occur in several primate species (e.g. marmosets (Bugnyar and Huber 1997); capuchin monkeys (Custance *et al.* 1999); gorillas (Stoinski *et al.* 2001); and chimpanzees (Whiten *et al.* 1996)). Confusingly, because of the near-exclusive focus on the correspondence problem, this same evidence has been claimed to be the only convincing evidence of imitative capability in animals (see, for example, Heyes 1993, p. 1000). Certainly, the existence of cells that generalize over action-as-seen and action-as-done shows that even monkeys *can* solve this particular correspondence problem. Because manual manipulations are distal to the body the visual appearance of the action will be quite similar, however, and in two-action experiments there is no evidence of learning new skills by anything other than rewarded trial and error. By contrast, compare human neonatal imitation (Meltzoff and Moore 1977; Meltzoff *et al.* 1991) which cannot be accounted for by response facilitation but is thought to function in social bonding rather than skill learning. The possibility that imitation has evolved twice in the human lineage, under quite independent selective pressures for (respectively) social mimicry and skill learning, has even been suggested (Byrne and Russon 1998).

Finally, it has been proposed that an animal watching another individual's actions may more readily or simply learn properties of the physical situation, by *emulation* (Tomasello 1990, 1998), than learn the actions themselves by imitation. For instance, seeing a nut broken may reveal the facts that it is hard, brittle and contains edible material, encouraging rapid future learning of nut-cracking. However, the term emulation has been used with various meanings (Byrne 1998*a*), ranging from simple associative learning (e.g. nut equals food) to acquisition of cognitively complex ideas such as containment. The more complex—and therefore more powerful—of these proposed learning mechanisms may be harder to explain computationally than is imitation itself. A recent meta-analysis of developmental studies could find no clear evidence that children under 5 years old were able to emulate, although they imitated readily (Want and Harris 2002). Moreover, although emulation has been used as a 'null hypothesis' for detecting imitation in great apes, the ability of nonhuman apes to emulate has been doubted (Byrne and Russon 1998; Byrne 2002*a*). For these reasons, the concept of emulation may not prove useful in understanding the social learning of complex skills in animals or young children.

It is now clear that most animal social learning does not need imitation to explain it, and there is at present no clear experimental demonstration of imitation in any animal, in the full sense of imitation: observational learning of a novel and complex skill, requiring more than priming of actions in the existing repertoire. However, a great deal of observational evidence indicates that at least the great apes have some ability to learn skills by imitation, as well as by other social and non-social learning mechanisms.

(b) Imitation in great apes

Socially mediated traditions of behaviour, although known in many species of animal (see, for example, Galef 1980, 1990; Roper 1983; Terkel 1994; Reader and Laland 2000; Rendell and Whitehead 2001), are particularly striking in the chimpanzee *Pan troglodytes* (Whiten *et al.* 1999), and the variation among the tools made and used by different chimpanzee populations is so rich that it has been studied as 'material culture' (McGrew 1992). Although all such variation can be challenged as reflecting subtle and unknown ecological influences (Tomasello 1990), some striking 'incompetences' are more readily understood if imitative learning is sometimes a necessary part of normal acquisition. Thus, it would otherwise be puzzling that chimpanzees in East Africa do not exploit the hard nuts available to them at many sites, which in West Africa are obtained by nut-cracking with stones (Sugiyama and Koman 1979; Boesch and Boesch 1990); and that chimpanzees at some sites discard carefully prepared insect-fishing tools when they become blunted in use, whereas at others the tools are re-sharpened or simply reversed (McGrew *et al.* 1979; McGrew 1998). Mountain gorillas *Gorilla beringei* do not use tools, but their plant preparation shows behavioural organization just as elaborate as chimpanzee tool use, involving several ordered stages, bimanual coordination and manual role differentiation, hierarchical organization of component subroutines, and the flexible omission or substitution of routines according to external circumstances (Byrne and Byrne 1991, 1993; Byrne *et al.* 2001*a*,*b*). As with the chimpanzee data, it is difficult to prove that learning these elaborate skills requires imitation, but two aspects are not easily explained otherwise: (i) although the low-level organization and choice of action is highly variable and idiosyncratic, the overall behavioural programme is highly standardized within the population (Byrne and Byrne 1993), giving rise to the term 'program-level imitation' for the likely process of acquisition (Byrne 1994); and (ii) even in the case of severe maiming in infancy (an unfortunate consequence of young apes' tendency to explore snares set for other animals), the affected individuals nevertheless acquire the normal technique, i.e. that of their mothers, rather than devise a novel method better suited to their hands' residual competence (Stokes and Byrne 2001; Byrne and Stokes 2002). If there were only one obvious way to consume the plants these observations would be trivial, but in fact there are very many methods, some more obvious to human observers and often attempted by young animals. The standardization to a local population norm and its resistance to change even with severe disability therefore suggests the 'conservative' influence of imitation. Although fewer data are available for the orangutan, the strongest observational evidence of imitative capacity comes from this species: individuals under rehabilitation to the wild after illegal captivity copy a range of complex and elaborate human activities, including some that are strongly discouraged (Russon and Galdikas 1993; Russon 1996). In the forest, orangutans also acquire hierarchically organized action plans (Russon 1998), and one population has been found to possess traditions of tool use very like those of chimpanzees (Van Schaik *et al.* 1996; Fox *et al.* 1999). Given the benefits that this population apparently gains from tool use, the lack of it more generally in orangutans has been attributed to their solitary ranging behaviour, making social transmission of skill inefficient (Van Schaik *et al.* 1999); by contrast, the complete lack of tool using in wild gorillas and bonobos, *Pan paniscus*, may reflect the lack of ecological advantage they stand to gain by using tools (McGrew 1989).

(c) Imitation without intentionality

Thus a picture emerges of great apes being able to acquire complex and elaborate local traditions of food acquisition, some of them involving tool use; and it seems highly probable that apes' ability to imitate, so conspicuous under the artificial conditions of human captivity, has its functional origin in efficient food acquisition (Byrne 1997). At the same time, evidence for mentalizing abilities in great apes is much more limited (e.g. Tomasello and Call 1994, 1997; although see Byrne 1995; Suddendorf and Whiten 2001). Therefore, in developing a possible model of the kind of imitation that serves to facilitate skill acquisition, a priority was to eschew mental states as explanatory variables, 'imitation without intentionality' (Byrne 1999*a*), rather than treating an understanding of the model's purposes and understanding of the situation as an early and fundamental part of the process (e.g. cf. Tomasello *et al.* 1993).

The aim has been to develop a purely mechanistic account, meshing where possible with known neural mechanisms, and specified in a sufficiently definite fashion to make future machine implementation a possibility. As an explanatory aid, I will consider the model as applied to one of the complex food preparation tasks of mountain gorillas, beginning with a description of the behaviour and in particular aspects that would gain most from acquisition by imitation. Then, an essential preliminary stage is advanced, that of segmenting observed behaviour into a vocabulary of elements. This ability seems much more widespread than the capacity to imitate, and may have evolved for other functions altogether. The 'behaviour parsing' model (Byrne 2002b), operating on strings of behavioural elements, is hypothesized to extract the statistical regularities that specifically correlate with organizational structure, and so enable subsequent copying without an understanding of intentions or causal logic. Finally, speculations are advanced about the relationship of these processes to cognition in general.

8.2 An illustrative task

Nettles, *Laportea alatipes*, are an important food of mountain gorillas in Rwanda (Watts 1984), rich in protein and low in secondary compounds and structural carbohydrate (Waterman *et al*. 1983). Unfortunately for the gorillas, this plant is 'defended' by powerful stinging hairs, especially dense on the stem, petioles and leaf-edges. All gorillas in the local population process nettles in broadly the same way, a technique that minimizes contact of stinging hairs with their hands and lips (Byrne and Byrne 1991; Fig. 8.1). A series of small transformations is made to plant material: stripping leaves off stems, accumulating larger bundles of leaves, detachment of petioles, picking out unwanted debris, and finally folding a package of leaf blades within a single leaf before ingestion. The means by which each small change is made are idiosyncratic and variable with context (Byrne and Byrne 1993), thus presumably best learned by individual experience. However, the overall sequence of five discrete stages in the process is standardized and appears to be essential for efficiency (Byrne *et al*. 2001a). The same applies to the precise bimanual coordination between the hands, in which each hand performs a different role but in temporal and spatial conjunction (manual role differentiation (Elliott and Connolly 1974)). Imitative learning of the *sequence* and the pattern of *bimanual coordination* would therefore be highly beneficial, if not essential for timely acquisition before the young gorilla is weaned and must forage independently at 3–4 years old. Manual laterality is high in almost every individual, often to the point of exclusive hand use, suggesting that the task is a challenging one, and there is a significant population bias towards right-handedness for delicate manipulations (Byrne and Byrne 1991; McGrew and Marchant 1996). However, there is no tendency for an individual's hand preference to match that of its mother (Byrne and Byrne 1991), so this aspect is clearly not imitated. Like other complex feeding tasks in great apes, preparing nettles is a hierarchically organized skill, showing considerable flexibility: stages that are occasionally unnecessary are omitted, and sections of the process (of one or several ordered stages) are often repeated iteratively to a

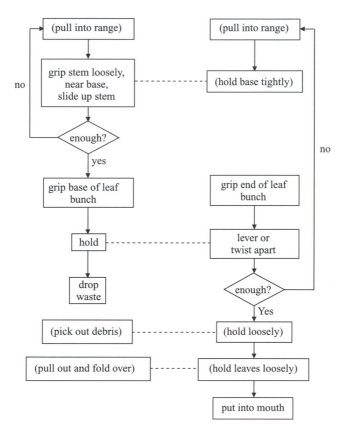

Fig. 8.1 Flow diagram that summarizes the processing sequences used by a right-handed mountain gorilla when preparing bundles of nettle leaves to eat. The process starts at the top of the diagram with acquisition of a nettle plant and ends at bottom right when a folded handful of leaves is put into the mouth. Actions are shown in square boxes; optional actions are in brackets; position of actions to left and right of the figure show where hand preference is significantly lateralized; horizontal dotted lines indicate that the actions of the two hands must be accurately coordinated.

criterion apparently based on an adequate size of food bundle (Byrne and Russon 1998). As noted above, that young gorillas can discern and thereby imitate the hierarchical organization of efficient processing is suggested by the standardization of these aspects in the local population; and their inability to compute novel hierarchical organization even when it would pay is suggested by the lack of any such response to severe, permanent hand injury. Clearly, a good model of imitative learning would include the *hierarchical structure* of the task.

I propose that these cardinal aspects of program-level imitation—sequence, bimanual coordination and hierarchical structure—are extracted from statistical regularities in repeated action. For this parsing process to operate, a preliminary requirement is that the fluid movements of skilled action are 'seen' as composed of strings of *elements*. This segmentation process is considered next.

8.3 Segmenting action into elements

To be used as building blocks in effective planning, elements of action discerned in another's behaviour must meet one simple principle: each element should *already* be within the repertoire of the observer. By contrast, the 'size' of an element is irrelevant. Under different circumstances, a particular movement of a single finger and an elaborate sequence of bimanual movements might both properly be seen as single elements, if each was a pattern already in the observer's repertoire. When watching an entirely unfamiliar process, the level at which elements were familiar might be that of finger movements; when watching a slight variant of a complex but already familiar activity, the basic elements might themselves be complex processes. Most commonly perhaps, the level at which observed behaviour matches the existing repertoire would be neither of these, but rather simple and highly practised movements that produce visible effects on environmental objects: that is, simple, goal-directed movements.

The mirror neuron system, noted already as capable of explaining response facilitation (Byrne 2002c; Rizzolatti *et al.* 2002), responds to precisely this class of actions. The cardinal property of mirror neurons is that they detect simple, goal-directed movements in the observing monkey's own repertoire, whether the movement is performed by the monkey itself or by another agent that it is watching. It is unlikely that mirror neurons have any role in imitation in monkeys, simply because monkeys have repeatedly failed to show evidence of imitative capacity (Visalberghi and Fragaszy 1990). Rather, it is thought that the evolutionary origin of mirror neurons is related to social sophistication: i.e. that the system functions in revealing the demeanour and likely future actions of conspecifics, by reference to actions the observer monkey might itself have done (Rizzolatti *et al.* 2002). (These qualities are sometimes called 'intentions', though without any implication of mentalizing.)

Despite the apparent lack of imitative ability in monkeys, mirror neurons may be *part* of the process of imitation in some other species. By responding to movement patterns that correspond to actions that the observer can already perform, the mirror neuron system could convert a continuous flow of observed movements into a string of recognized, familiar actions. If seeing a string of familiar actions also allows construction of links between them, then 'action-level' imitation can occur (Byrne and Russon 1998). In action-level imitation, a linear sequence of actions are copied without recognition of any higher-order organization that may be present: the organization is 'flat'. Chimpanzees have been reported to copy the order of actions, even though the sequence was entirely arbitrary and unrelated to success (Whiten 1998), and a detailed learning model has been developed to account for action-level imitation in animals (Heyes and Ray 2000).

The question is, can this sort of 'bottom up', mechanistic analysis go beyond action-level imitation, and explain how behavioural organization can also be copied, i.e. program-level imitation? For arbitrary, random actions or behaviour that is genuinely linear in structure (e.g. the 'fixed action patterns' described by early ethologists), there will be no difference between action-level and program-level copying. However, most human action, and arguably also much of the behaviour of other great apes, is constructed in such a way that aspects of the organization are planned and relate to intended effects during execution. Can this planning be 'seen' in the behaviour of another?

8.4 Parsing strings of actions to reveal organization

Every execution of a motor act, however familiar and well-practised, will differ slightly from others. Nevertheless, this variation is constrained because if certain characteristics are missing or stray too far from their canonical form the act will fail to achieve its purpose. Watching a single performance will not betray these underlying constraints, but the statistical regularities of repeated, goal-directed action can serve to reveal the organizational structure that lies behind it.

Consider how this might work for an infant gorilla learning about nettle processing. Unweaned great apes spend most of each day within a few feet of their mothers, and (as their main nutrition still comes from milk) they have almost full-time leisure to watch any nearby activities, as well as learn about the structure of plants by their own exploration. A young gorilla first begins to process a nettle plant at the late age of about 2 years because the stinging hairs discourage earlier attempts. At that time they will have watched many hundreds of plants being processed expertly by the mother. Suppose her behaviour is seen by the infant as a string of elements, each of which is already familiar (i.e. a mirror neuron exists for the element). At this time, the young gorilla's repertoire of familiar elements of action derives from its innate manual capacities, many hours of playing with plants and discarded debris of the mother's feeding, and from its own feeding on other, perhaps simpler plants. The string of elements that it sees when watching its mother eat nettles will differ each time, although her starting point is always a growing, intact nettle stem, and—because she is expert at this task—the final stage is always the same: popping a neatly folded package of nettle leaves into the mouth.

With repeated watching, other regularities begin to become apparent: the mother always uses one hand to fold a bundle of leaf-blades protruding from the other hand, and holds down this folded bundle with her thumb; she always

makes a twisting movement of the hands against each other, and immediately
drops several leaf-petioles (which she does not eat) onto the ground; she
always makes a sweeping movement of one hand, held around a nettle stem
which is sometimes held in the other hand even though the plant is still
attached to the ground, and this leaves a leafless stem protruding from the
ground (see Fig. 8.2 for a visual representation of this process). Moreover,
these stages always occur in exactly the same order each time: the reverse
order to that in which they have been mentioned here. Statistical regularities
thereby separate the minimal set of *essential actions* from the many others
that occur during nettle eating but which are not crucial to success, and
reveal the correct order in which they must be arranged. (The ability of human
babies as young as eight months to detect statistical regularities in spoken
strings of nonsense words shows that just such sensitivity to repeated
orderings is active early in human development (Saffran *et al.* 1996).) The
usefulness of detecting regularities applies not only to the linear sequence of
movements of each hand, but also the hands' operation together: stages that
crucially depend on the hands' close temporal and spatial coordination while
doing different jobs will recur in every string, whereas other coincidental
conjunctions will not.

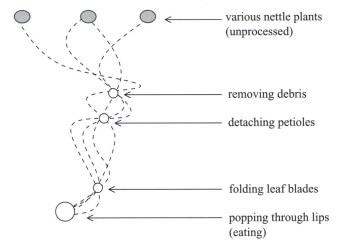

Fig. 8.2 Nettle processing may be viewed as paths through a two-dimensional space
of transformations, where each transformation is an action that may be applied.
Because each plant is potentially unique in form, each is represented as a different
starting point. The manual operations that are applied will vary on each occasion, so
no paths overlap perfectly. However, certain operations are critical for success, and
these are represented as points where all paths converge. These convergence points
define the *essential* actions that must always be performed for eventual success,
and may allow them to be recognized among the many inessential, idiosyncratic
movements in a typical real sequence.

Other statistical regularities relate to modular organization and hierarchical organization (see Fig. 8.3). Although not present in every string, whenever the operation of removing debris is performed (by opening the hand that holds nettle leaf-blades, and delicately picking out debris with the other hand), it occurs at the same place in the string. Also, on some occasions but not others, a section of the entire string is repeated twice or several times. For instance, the process of 'pulling a nettle plant into range, stripping leaves from its stem in a bimanually coordinated movement, then detaching and dropping the leaf-petioles', may be repeated several times before the mother continues to remove debris and fold the leaf-blades before eating. (Already-processed leaf-blades are transferred to the lower fingers of one hand for retention during the process of acquiring more, an ability that shows that gorillas are able to control individual digits independently.) Subsections of the string of actions that are marked out in this way may be single elements, or as in this example a string of several elements. Both omission and repetition signal that some parts of the string are more tightly bound together than others, i.e. that they function as *modules*. Optional stages, like cleaning debris, occur between but not within modules. Moreover, repetition of a substring gives evidence of a module used as a subroutine, in this case iterated several times to accumulate a larger handful. Further clues to modular structure are likely to be given by the distribution of pauses (occurring between but not within modules), and the possibility of smooth recovery from interruptions that occur between modules. Gorillas often pause for several seconds during the processing of a handful of plant material,

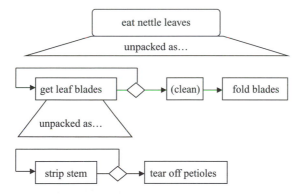

Fig. 8.3 Hierarchical organization of nettle leaf processing must, on current observational evidence, be at least as elaborate as this diagram. The modules 'get leaf blades' and 'fold blades' are known to be independent, because they may on occasion be separated by the optional action, 'clean'. In addition, 'get leaf blades' may or may not be iterated, again implying that this is a distinct module. However, 'get leaf blades' is itself a routine composed of at least two component modules: the evidence that 'strip stem' and 'tear off petioles' are separate modules is that 'strip stem' may or may not be iterated.

to monitor the movements and actions of other individuals. Finally, a different module entirely may be substituted for part of the usual sequence (e.g. if one hand is required for postural support, then a normally bimanual process may need to be performed unimanually), and if this module is recognized as an already-familiar sequence its substitution again reveals structure; eventually, it may be that a taxonomy of substitutable methods are built up.

This example has been developed as a heuristic exercise, but in fact the existence of statistical regularities that reveal underlying structure is known in this case, because they are precisely the regularities that enabled the scientists to discover the hierarchical structure of nettle processing by adult gorillas (Byrne and Byrne 1993; Byrne and Russon 1998; Byrne 1999b). What is proposed in the behaviour parsing model is that the same information can be extracted and used by the apes themselves, and that this ability is what enables a young ape to perceive and copy the sequential, bimanually coordinated, hierarchical organization of complex skills from repeated watching of another. This claim has further implications for how imitation relates to other cognitive activities.

8.5 Potential implications

Just as mirror neurons may be regarded as much more than devices for copying familiar actions (i.e. response facilitation), but as mechanisms for discerning the future behavioural dispositions of other animals, so behaviour parsing may be seen as more than simply part of programlevel imitation. Because behaviour parsing reveals the organization of behaviour in other individuals, in terms of actions that the observer can (if it so desires) perform itself, the consequence is that behaviour can better be interpreted in terms of its function and mechanism of operation. In effect, behaviour can be *understood statistically* in terms of its correlations—under what circumstances is a particular organization seen, and what are its normal effects on the environment—without prior knowledge of intentions in the mind of the observed agent, or any understanding of the everyday physics of cause-and-effect relationships between action and consequence. Copying a novel, complex organization of behaviour, and so acquiring a new skill by imitation, may only be a spin-off from a more fundamental ability to understand the world of action. If behaviour parsing enables an agent to 'see through' the surface form of behaviour to an underlying deep structure of actions, then it is perhaps only a small step to perceiving the plans and intentions that lie behind these structures.

The implications of following these speculations are twofold. First, activities that have been claimed to rely on perceiving the intentions of others (as has been argued for learning by imitation (e.g. Whiten and Byrne 1991; Tomasello *et al.* 1993)), may in fact be possible in a more straightforward, mechanistic fashion. This would ramify the position argued by Bargh and Chartrand (1999), that much more of everyday human action than is currently recognized relies on fast, mechanistic, low-level processes, rather than on elaborate, rational thought processes and deeply intentional understanding. Moreover, if the same competence is discovered in non-human animals, as appears to be increasingly the case, this need not raise awkward questions of non-verbal mentalizing and consciousness. Rather, mentalizing ability may have different and more recent evolutionary origins, functioning to construe actions in various ways (e.g. rationalizing our own and others' actions whose real cause we do not understand, or deliberately misconstruing those actions for our own ends), and be intimately tied to linguistic ability (see Karmiloff-Smith (1993) and Povinelli (2000) for closely related perspectives). The second implication is that, although imitation of novel behaviour and other complex cognitive activity may not require mentalizing, mentalizing may require behaviour parsing as part of the process. The evolution of the ability to parse the behaviour of others, which on current evidence evolved at least as long ago as the shared ancestors of humans and other great apes around 12 Myr ago, may therefore have been a necessary preliminary to the later development exclusively in humans of the ability to mentalize: to attribute intentions and causes to observed actions. Behaviour parsing may still be part of the everyday process of doing so.

References

Bargh, J. A. and Chartrand, T. L. (1999). The unbearable automaticity of being. *Am. Psychol.* **54**, 462–79.

Boesch, C. and Boesch, H. (1990). Tool use and tool making in wild chimpanzees. *Folia Primatologica* **54**, 86–99.

Bugnyar, T. and Huber, L. (1997). Push or pull: an experimental study of imitation in marmosets. *Anim. Behav.* **54**, 817–31.

Byrne, R. W. (1994). The evolution of intelligence. In *Behaviour and evolution* (ed. P. J. B. Slater and T. R. Halliday), pp. 223–65. Cambridge: Cambridge University Press.

Byrne, R. W. (1995). *The thinking ape: evolutionary origins of intelligence.* Oxford: Oxford University Press.

Byrne, R. W. (1997). The technical intelligence hypothesis: an additional evolutionary stimulus to intelligence? In *Machiavellian intelligence. II. Extensions and evaluations* (ed. A. Whiten and R. W. Byrne), pp. 289–311. Cambridge: Cambridge University Press.

Byrne, R. W. (1998*a*). Comments on C. Boesch and M. Tomasello 'Chimpanzee and human cultures'. *Curr. Anthropol.* **39**, 604–5.

Byrne, R. W. (1998*b*). Imitation: the contributions of priming and program-level copying. In *Intersubjective communication and emotion in early ontogeny* (ed. S. Braten), pp. 228–44. Cambridge: Cambridge University Press.

Byrne, R. W. (1999*a*). Imitation without intentionality. Using string parsing to copy the organization of behaviour. *Anim. Cogn.* **2**, 63–72.

Byrne, R. W. (1999*b*). Object manipulation and skill organization in the complex food preparation of mountain gorillas. In *The mentality of gorillas and orangutans* (ed. S. T. Parker, R. W. Mitchell and H. L. Miles), pp. 147–59. Cambridge: Cambridge University Press.

Byrne, R. W. (2002*a*). Emulation in apes: verdict 'not proven'. *Devl. Sci.* **5**, 20–2.

Byrne, R. W. (2002*b*). Imitation of complex novel actions: what does the evidence from animals mean? *Adv. Study Behav.* **31**, 77–105.

Byrne, R. W. (2002*c*). Seeing actions as hierarchically organized structures. Great ape manual skills. In *The imitative mind: development, evolution, and brain bases* (ed. A. Meltzoff and W. Prinz), pp. 122–40. New York: Cambridge University Press.

Byrne, R. W. and Byrne, J. M. E. (1991). Hand preferences in the skilled gathering tasks of mountain gorillas (*Gorilla g. beringei*). *Cortex* **27**, 521–46.

Byrne, R. W. and Byrne, J. M. E. (1993). Complex leaf-gathering skills of mountain gorillas (*Gorilla g. beringei*): variability and standardization. *Am. J. Primatol.* **31**, 241–61.

Byrne, R. W. and Russon, A. E. (1998). Learning by imitation: a hierarchical approach. *Behav. Brain Sci.* **21**, 667–721.

Byrne, R. W. and Stokes, E. J. (2002). Effects of manual disability on feeding skills in gorillas and chimpanzees: a cognitive analysis. *Int. J. Primatol.* **23**, 539–54.

Byrne, R. W., Corp, N. and Byrne, J. M. (2001*a*). Manual dexterity in the gorilla: bimanual and digit role differentiation in a natural task. *Anim. Cogn.* **4**, 347–61.

Byrne, R. W., Corp, N. and Byrne, J. M. E. (2001*b*). Estimating the complexity of animal behaviour: how mountain gorillas eat thistles. *Behaviour* **138**, 525–57.

Custance, D., Whiten, A. and Fredman, T. (1999). Social learning of an artificial fruit task in capuchin monkeys (*Cebus apella*). *J. Comp. Psychol.* **113**, 13–23.

Dawson, B. V. and Foss, B. M. (1965). Observational learning in budgerigars. *Anim. Behav.* **13**, 470–4.

Elliott, J. and Connolly, K. (1974). Hierarchical structure in skill development. In *The growth of competence* (ed. K. Connolly and K. Bruner), pp. 135–68. London: Academic Press.

Fox, E., Sitompul, A. and Van Schaik, C. P. (1999). Intelligent tool use in wild Sumatran orangutans. In *The mentality of gorillas and orangutans* (ed. S. T. Parker, H. L. Miles and R. W. Mitchell), pp. 99–116. Cambridge: Cambridge University Press.

Galef, B. G. (1980). Diving for food: analysis of a possible case of social learning in wild rats (*Rattus norvegicus*). *J. Comp. Physiol. Psychol.* **94**, 416–25.

Galef, B. G. (1988). Imitation in animals: history, definitions, and interpretation of data from the psychological laboratory. In *Social learning: psychological and biological perspectives* (ed. T. Zentall and B. G. Galef Jr), pp. 3–28. Hillsdale, NJ: Erlbaum.

Galef, B. G. (1990). Tradition in animals: field observations and laboratory analyses. In *Interpretations and explanations in the study of behaviour: comparative perspectives* (ed. M. Bekoff and D. Jamieson), pp. 74–95. Boulder, CO: Westview Press.

Gallese, V., Fadiga, L., Fogassi, L. and Rizzolatti, G. (1996). Action recognition in the premotor cortex. *Brain* **119**, 593–609.

Heyes, C. M. (1993). Imitation, culture, and cognition. *Anim. Behav.* **46**, 999–1010.

Heyes, C. M. and Ray, E. D. (2000). What is the significance of imitation in animals? *Adv. Study Behav.* **29**, 215–45.

Karmiloff-Smith, A. (1993). *Beyond modularity: a developmental perspective on cognitive science*. Cambridge, MA: Bradford/MIT Press.

McGrew, W. C. (1989). Why is ape tool use so confusing? In *Comparative socioecology: the behavioural ecology of humans and other mammals* (ed. V. Standen and R. A. Foley), pp. 457–72. Oxford: Blackwell Scientific.

McGrew, W. C. (1992). *Chimpanzee material culture: implications for human evolution*. Cambridge: Cambridge University Press.

McGrew, W. C. (1998). Culture in nonhuman primates? *A. Rev. Anthropol.* **27**, 301–28.

McGrew, W. C. and Marchant, L. F. (1996). On which side of the apes? Ethological study of laterality of hand use. In *Great ape societies* (ed. W. C. McGrew, L. F. Marchant and T. Nishida), pp. 255–72. Cambridge: Cambridge University Press.

McGrew, W. C., Tutin, C. E. G. and Baldwin, P. J. (1979). Chimpanzees, tools, and termites: cross cultural comparison of Senegal, Tanzania and Rio Muni. *Man* **14**, 185–214.

Meltzoff, A. N. and Moore, M. K. (1977). Imitation of facial and manual gestures by human neonates. *Science* **198**, 75–8.

Meltzoff, A. N., Kuhl, P. K. and Moore, M. K. (1991). Perception, representation, and the control of action in newborns and young infants: towards a new synthesis. In *Newborn attention: biological constraints and the influence of experience* (ed. M. J. Weiss and P. R. Zelazo), pp. 377–411. Norwood, NJ: Ablex Press.

Povinelli, D. (2000). *Folk physics for apes*. Oxford: Oxford University Press.

Reader, S. and Laland, K. (2000). Diffusion of foraging innovations in the guppy. *Anim. Behav.* **60**, 175–80.

Rendell, L. and Whitehead, H. (2001). Culture in whales and dolphins. *Behav. Brain Sci.* **24**, 309–82.

Rizzolatti, G., Fadiga, L., Fogassi, L. and Gallese, V. (1996). Premotor cortex and the recognition of motor actions. *Brain Res.* **3**, 131–41.

Rizzolatti, G., Fadiga, L., Fogassi, L. and Gallese, V. (2002). From mirror neurons to imitation: facts and speculations. In *The imitative mind: development, evolution, and brain bases* (ed. A. Meltzoff and W. Prinz), pp. 247–66. New York: Cambridge University Press.

Roper, T. J. (1983). Learning as a biological phenomenon. In *Animal behaviour, vol. 3. Genes, development and learning* (ed. T. R. Halliday and P. J. B. Slater), pp. 178–212. Oxford: Blackwell Scientific.

Russon, A. E. (1996). Imitation in everyday use: matching and rehearsal in the spontaneous imitation of rehabilitant orangutans (*Pongo pygmaeus*). In *Reaching into thought: the minds of the great apes* (ed. A. E. Russon, K. A. Bard and S. T. Parker), pp. 152–76. Cambridge: Cambridge University Press.

Russon, A. E. (1998). The nature and evolution of intelligence in orangutans (*Pongo pygmaeus*). *Primates* **39**, 485–503.

Russon, A. E. and Galdikas, B. M. F. (1993). Imitation in free-ranging rehabilitant orangutans. *J. Comp. Psychol.* **107**, 147–61.

Saffran, J. R., Aslin, R. N. and Newport, E. L. (1996). Statistical learning by 8-month-old infants. *Science* **274**, 1926–8.

Spence, K. W. (1937). Experimental studies of learning and higher mental processes in infra-human primates. *Psychol. Bull.* **34**, 806–50.

Stoinski, T. S., Wrate, J. L., Ure, N. and Whiten, A. (2001). Imitative learning by captive western lowland gorillas (*Gorilla gorilla gorilla*) in a simulated food-processing task. *J. Comp. Psychol.* **115**, 272–81.

Stokes, E. J. and Byrne, R. W. (2001). Cognitive capacities for behavioural flexibility in wild chimpanzees (*Pan troglodytes*): the effect of snare injury on complex manual food processing. *Anim. Cogn.* **4**, 11–28.

Suddendorf, T. and Whiten, A. (2001). Mental evolution and development: evidence for secondary representation in children, great apes, and other animals. *Psychol. Bull.* **127**, 629–50.

Sugiyama, Y. and Koman, J. (1979). Tool-using and tool-making behaviour in wild chimpanzees at Bossou, Guinea. *Primates* **20**, 513–24.

Terkel, J. (1994). Social transmission of pine cone feeding behaviour in the black rat. In *Behavioural aspects of feeding* (ed. B. G. J. Galef, M. Mainardi and P. Valsecchi), pp. 229–56. London: Harwood Academic.

Thorndike, E. L. (1898). Animal intelligence: an experimental study of the associative process in animals. *Psychol. Rev. Monogr.* **2**, 551–3.

Tomasello, M. (1990). Cultural transmission in the tool use and communicatory signaling of chimpanzees? In *'Language' and intelligence in monkeys and apes* (ed. S. T. Parker and K. R. Gibson), pp. 274–311. Cambridge: Cambridge University Press.

Tomasello, M. (1998). Emulation learning and cultural learning. *Behav. Brain Sci.* **21**, 703–4.

Tomasello, M. and Call, J. (1994). Social cognition of monkeys and apes. *Yearbook Phys. Anthropol.* **37**, 273–305.

Tomasello, M. and Call, J. (1997). *Primate cognition.* New York: Oxford University Press.

Tomasello, M., Kruger, A. C. and Ratner, H. H. (1993). Cultural learning. *Behav. Brain Sci.* **16**, 495–552.

Van Schaik, C. P., Fox, E. A. and Sitompul, A. F. (1996). Manufacture and use of tools in wild Sumatran orangutans. Implications for human evolution. *Naturwissenschaften* **83**, 186–8.

Van Schaik, C. P., Deaner, R. O. and Merrill, M. Y. (1999). The conditions for tool-use in primates: implications for the evolution of material culture. *J. Hum. Evol.* **36**, 719–41.

Visalberghi, E. and Fragaszy, D. M. (1990). Do monkeys ape? In *'Language' and intelligence in monkeys and apes* (ed. S. T. Parker and K. R. Gibson), pp. 247–73. Cambridge: Cambridge University Press.

Want, S. C. and Harris, P. L. (2002). How do children ape? Applying concepts from the study of non-human primates to the developmental study of 'imitation' in children. *Devl. Sci.* **5**, 1–13.

Waterman, P. G., Choo, G. M., Vedder, A. L. and Watts, D. (1983). Digestibility, digestion-inhibitors and nutrients and herbaceous foliage and green stems from an African montane flora and comparison with other tropical flora. *Oecologia* **60**, 244–9.

Watts, D. P. (1984). Composition and variability of mountain gorilla diets in the central Virungas. *Am. J. Primatol.* **7**, 323–56.

Whiten, A. (1998). Imitation of the sequential structure of actions by chimpanzees (*Pan troglodytes*). *J. Comp. Psychol.* **112**, 270–81.

Whiten, A. and Byrne, R. W. (1991). The emergence of metarepresentation in human ontogeny and primate phylogeny. In *Natural theories of mind: evolution, development and simulation of everyday mindreading* (ed. A. Whiten), pp. 267–81. Oxford: Blackwell.

Whiten, A., Custance, D.M., Gomez, J.-C., Teixidor, P. and Bard, K. A. (1996). Imitative learning of artificial fruit processing in children (*Homo sapiens*) and chimpanzees (*Pan troglodytes*). *J. Comp. Psychol.* **110**, 3–14.

Whiten, A., Goodall, J., McGrew, W. C., Nishida, T., Reynolds, V., Sugiyama, Y., *et al.* (1999). Cultures in chimpanzees. *Nature* **399**, 682–5.

9

Computational approaches to motor learning by imitation

Stefan Schaal, Auke Ijspeert, and Aude Billard

Movement imitation requires a complex set of mechanisms that map an observed movement of a teacher onto one's own movement apparatus. Relevant problems include movement recognition, pose estimation, pose tracking, body correspondence, coordinate transformation from external to egocentric space, matching of observed against previously learned movement, resolution of redundant degrees-of-freedom that are unconstrained by the observation, suitable movement representations for imitation, modularization of motor control, etc. All of these topics by themselves are active research problems in computational and neurobiological sciences, such that their combination into a complete imitation system remains a daunting undertaking—indeed, one could argue that we need to understand the complete perception-action loop. As a strategy to untangle the complexity of imitation, this paper will examine imitation purely from a computational point of view, i.e. we will review statistical and mathematical approaches that have been suggested for tackling parts of the imitation problem, and discuss their merits, disadvantages and underlying principles. Given the focus on action recognition of other contributions in this special issue, this paper will primarily emphasize the motor side of imitation, assuming that a perceptual system has already identified important features of a demonstrated movement and created their corresponding spatial information. Based on the formalization of motor control in terms of control policies and their associated performance criteria, useful taxonomies of imitation learning can be generated that clarify different approaches and future research directions.

Keywords: imitation; motor control; duality of movement generation and movement recognition; motor primitives

9.1 Introduction

Movement imitation is familiar to everybody from daily experience: a teacher demonstrates[1] a movement, and immediately the student is capable of approximately repeating it. In addition to a variety of social, cultural and cognitive implications that the ability to imitate entails (cf. reviews in Piaget 1951; Tomasello *et al.* 1993; Meltzoff and Moore 1994; Byrne and Russon 1998; Rizzolatti and Arbib 1998; Dautenhahn and Nehaniv 2002), from the viewpoint of learning, a teacher's demonstration as the starting point of one's own learning can significantly speed up the learning process, as imitation usually drastically reduces the amount of trial-and-error that is needed to accomplish the movement goal by providing a good example of a successful movement (Schaal 1999). Thus, from a computational point of view, it is important to understand the detailed principles, algorithms and metrics that subserve imitation, starting from the visual perception of the teacher up to issuing motor commands that move the limbs of the student.

Fig. 9.1 sketches the major ingredients of a conceptual imitation learning system (Schaal 1999). Visual sensory information needs to be parsed into information about objects and their spatial location in an internal or external coordinate system; the depicted organization is largely inspired by the dorsal (what) and ventral (where) stream as discovered in neuroscientific research (Van Essen and Maunsell 1983). As a result, some form of postural information of the movement of the teacher and/or 3D object information about the manipulated object (if an object is involved) should become available. Subsequently, one of the major questions revolves around how such information can be converted into action. For this purpose, Fig. 9.1 alludes to the concept of

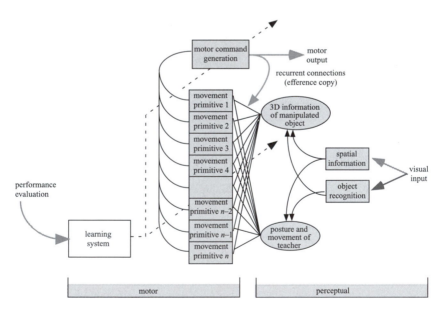

Fig. 9.1 Conceptual sketch of an imitation learning system. The right-hand side contains primarily perceptual elements and indicates how visual information is transformed into spatial and object information. The left-hand side focuses on motor elements, illustrating how a set of movement primitives competes for a demonstrated behaviour. Motor commands are generated from input of the most appropriate primitive. Learning can adjust both movement primitives and the motor-command generator.

movement primitives, also called 'movement schemas', 'basis behaviours', 'units of action', 'macro actions', etc. (e.g. Arbib 1981; Sternad and Schaal 1999; Sutton *et al.* 1999; Dautenhahn and Nehaniv 2002). Movement primitives are sequences of action that accomplish a complete goaldirected behaviour. They could be as simple as an elementary action of an actuator, e.g. 'go forward', 'go backward', etc., but, as discussed in Schaal (1999), such low-level representations do not scale well to learning in systems with many degrees of freedom. Thus, it is useful for a movement primitive to code complete temporal behaviours, like 'grasping a cup', 'walking', 'a tennis serve', etc. Fig. 9.1 assumes that the perceived action of the teacher is mapped onto a set of existing primitives in an assimilation phase, also suggested in Demiris and Hayes (2002) and Chapter 14, this volume. This mapping process also needs to resolve the correspondence problem concerning a mismatch between the teacher's body and the student's body (Dautenhahn and Nehaniv 2002). Subsequently, the most appropriate primitive is adjusted by learning to improve the performance in an accommodation phase. Figure 1 indicates such a process by highlighting the better-matching primitives with increasing linewidths. If no existing primitive is a good match for the observed behaviour, a new primitive must be generated. After an initial imitation phase, self-improvement, e.g. with the help of a reinforcement-based performance evaluation criterion (Sutton and Barto 1998), can refine both movement primitives and an assumed stage of motor-command generation (see Section 9.2b) until a desired level of motor performance is achieved.

In Sections 9.2 and 9.3, we will attempt to formalize the conceptual picture of Fig. 9.1 in the context of previous work on computational approaches to imitation. Given that Chapter 4 already concentrates on the perceptual part of imitation in this issue, our review will focus on the motor side in Fig. 9.1.

9.2 Computational imitation learning

Initially, at the beginning of the 1980s, computational imitation learning found the strongest research interest in the field of manipulator robotics, as it seemed to be a promising route to automate the tedious manual programming of these machines. Inspired by the ideas of artificial intelligence, symbolic reasoning was the common choice to approach imitation, mostly by parsing a demonstrated movement into some form of 'if–then' rules that, when chained together, created a finite state machine controller (e.g. Lozano-Pérez 1982; Dufay and Latombe 1984; Levas and Selfridge 1984; Segre and DeJong 1985; Segre 1988). Given the reduced computational power available at this time, a demonstration normally consisted of manually 'pushing' the robot through a movement sequence and using the proprioceptive information that the robot sensed during this guided movement as basis to extract the if–then rules. In essence, many recent robotics approaches to imitation learning have remained closely related to this strategy. New elements include the use of visual input from the teacher and movement segmentation derived from computer vision algorithms (Kuniyoshi *et al.* 1989, 1994; Ikeuchi *et al.* 1993). Other projects used data gloves or marker-based observation systems as input for imitation learning (Tung and Kak 1995).

More recently, research on imitation learning has been influenced increasingly by non-symbolic learning tools, for instance artificial neural networks, fuzzy logic, statistical learning, etc. (Pook and Ballard 1993; Dillmann *et al.* 1995; Hovland *et al.* 1996). An even more recent trend takes inspiration of the known behavioural and neuroscientific processes of animal imitation to develop algorithms for robot programming by demonstration (e.g. Arbib *et al.* 2000; Billard 2000; Oztop and Arbib 2002) with the goal of developing a more general and less task-specific theory of imitation learning. It is these neural computation techniques that we will focus on in this review, as they offer the most to both biologically inspired modelling of imitation and technological realizations of imitation in artificial intelligence systems.

(a) A computational formalization of imitation learning

Successful motor control requires issuing motor commands for all the actuators of a movement system at the right time and of correct magnitude in response to internal and external sensations and a given behavioural goal. Thus, the problem of motor control can generally be formalized as finding a task-specific *control policy* π

$$u(t) = \pi(z(t),t,\alpha), \tag{2.1}$$

where u denotes the vector of motor commands, z the vector of all relevant internal states of the movement system and external states of the environment, t represents the time parameter, and α stands for the vector of open parameters that need to be adjusted during learning, e.g. the weights of a neural network (Dyer and McReynolds 1970). We will denote a policy that explicitly uses a dependence on time as a *nonautonomous* policy, whereas a policy without explicit time dependence, i.e. $u(t) = \pi(z(t),\alpha)$, will be called *autonomous*. The formulation in equation (2.1) is very general and can be applied to any level of analysis, like a detailed neuronal level or a more abstract joint angular level. If the function π were known, the task goal could be achieved from every state z of the movement system. This theoretical view allows us to reformulate imitation learning in terms of the more formal question of how control policies, which we also call movement primitives, can be learned (or bootstrapped) by watching a demonstration.

Crucial to the issue of imitation is a second formal element, an evaluation criterion that creates a metric of the level of success of imitation

$$J = g(z(t),u(t),t). \tag{2.2}$$

Without any loss of generality, we will assume that the cost J should be minimized; particular instantiations of J will be discussed in the following paragraphs. In general, J can be any kind of cost function, defined as an accumulative cost over a longer time horizon as is needed for minimizing energy, or only over one instant of time, e.g. as needed when trying to reach a particular goal state. Moreover, J can be defined on variables based in any coordinate system, e.g. external, internal or a mixed set of coordinates. The different ways of creating control policies and metrics will prove to be a useful taxonomy of previous approaches to imitation learning and the problem of imitation in general.

Defining the cost J for an imitation task is a complex problem. In an ideal scenario, J should capture the task goal and the quality of imitation in achieving the task goal. For instance, the task goal could be to reach for a cup, which could be formalized as a cost that penalizes the squared distance between the hand and the cup. The teacher's demonstration, however, may have chosen a particular form of reaching for the cup, e.g. in a strangely curved hand trajectory. Thus, faithful imitation may require adding an additional term to the cost J that penalizes deviations from the trajectory the teacher demonstrated, depending on whether the objective of imitation is solely focused on the task or also on how to move to perform the task. Hence, the cost J quickly becomes a complex, hybrid criterion defined over various objectives. In biological research, it is often difficult to discover what kind of metric the student applied when imitating (Mataric and Pomplun 1998; Nehaniv and Dautenhahn 1999).

(b) Imitation by direct policy learning

The demonstrated behaviour can be used to learn the appropriate control policy directly by supervised learning of the parameters α of the policy (cf. equation (2.1)), i.e. a nonlinear map $z \rightarrow u$, employing an *autonomous* policy and using as evaluation criterion (cf. equation (2.2)) simply the squared error of reproducing u in a given state z. For this purpose, the state z and the action u of the teacher need to be observable and identifiable, and they must be meaningful for the student, i.e. match the student's kinematic and dynamic structure (cf. Dautenhahn and Nehaniv 2002). This prerequisite of observability, shared by all forms of imitation learning, imposes a serious constraint since, normally, motor commands, i.e. kinetic variables, and internal variables of the teacher are hidden from the observer. Although statistical learning has methods to uncover hidden states, e.g. by Hidden Markov Models, Kalman filters or more advanced methods (Arulampalam *et al.* 2002), we are not aware that such techniques have been applied to imitation yet.

Thus, to instantiate a movement primitive from a demonstration, the primitive needs to be defined in variables that can be perceived, leaving only kinematic variables as potential candidates, e.g. positions, velocities and accelerations. Given that the output of a movement primitive has to be interpreted as some

form of a command to the motor system, usually implying a desired change
of state, movement primitives that output a desired velocity or acceleration
can be useful, i.e. a 'desired time-derivative' of the state information[2] that is
used to represent the teacher's movement. Our generic formulation of a policy
in equation (2.1) can, therefore, be written more suitably as

$$\dot{z}(t) = \pi(z)(t),t,\boldsymbol{\alpha}). \tag{2.3}$$

From a control theoretical point of view, this line of reasoning requires that
motor control be modular, i.e. has at least separate processes for movement
planning (i.e. generating the right kinematics) and execution (i.e. generating
the right dynamics) (Wolpert 1997; Wolpert and Kawato 1998).

Fig. 9.2 illustrates two classical examples (e.g. Craig 1986) of modular
control in the context of imitation learning and motor primitives. In Fig. 9.2*a*,
the demonstrated behaviour is mapped onto a movement primitive that is
defined in internal coordinates of the student: joint angular coordinates θ are
a good candidate as they can be extracted from visual information, a problem
addressed under the name of pose estimation in computer vision (Deutscher
et al. 2000; Chapter 4 this volume). Such internal coordinates can directly
serve as desired input to a motor-command execution stage (see Fig. 9.1), here
assumed to be composed of a feedback and a feed-forward control block
(Kawato 1999).

Alternatively, Fig. 9.2*b* illustrates the subtle but important change when
movement primitives are represented in external coordinates, i.e. a task-level representation (Saltzman and Kelso 1987; Aboaf *et al.* 1989). For instance, the
acceleration of the fingertip in the task of pole balancing would be interpreted as
a task-level command issued by the movement primitive in external coordinates,

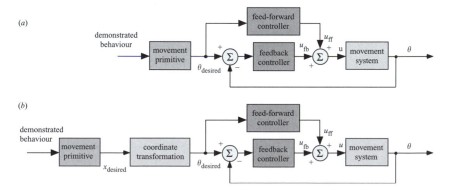

Fig. 9.2 Modular motor control with movement primitives, using (*a*) a movement
primitive defined in internal coordinates, and (*b*) a movement primitive defined in
external coordinates.

by contrast to joint angular accelerations of the entire arm and body that would be issued by a movement primitive in internal coordinates. Most often, task-level representations are easier to extract from a demonstration, and have a more compact representation. Task-level representations can also cope with a mismatch in dynamic and/or kinematic structure between the teacher and the student—only the task state is represented, not the state of motor system that performs the task. Task-level imitation requires prior knowledge of how a task-level command can be converted into a command in internal coordinates, a classic problem in control theory treated under the name of inverse kinematics (Baillieul and Martin 1990), but which has found several elegant solutions in neural computation in the recent years (Bullock *et al.* 1993; Guenther and Barreca 1997; D'Souza *et al.* 2001).

In summary, movement primitives for imitation learning seem to be the most useful if expressed in kinematic coordinates, either in internal (e.g. joint, muscle) space

$$\dot{\theta}(t) = \pi(z(t), t, \boldsymbol{\alpha}) \tag{2.4}$$

or in external (task) space

$$\dot{x}(t) = \pi(z(t), t, \boldsymbol{\alpha}). \tag{2.5}$$

Note that the formulations in equations (2.4) and (2.5) intentionally use z, the variable that represents all possible state information about the movement system and the environment as input, but only output a variable that is the desired change of state of the student in the selected coordinate system, i.e., $\dot{x}$ in external space, and $\dot{\theta}$ in internal space. By dropping the explicit time dependence on the right-hand sides of equations (2.4) and (2.5), both policy formulations can be made to be autonomous.

Direct policy learning from imitation can now be reviewed more precisely in the context of the discussions of the previous paragraphs and figure 2. Direct policy learning in task space was conducted for the task of pole balancing with a computer-simulated pole (Widrow and Smith 1964; Nechyba and Xu 1995). For this purpose, a supervised neural network was trained on task-level data recorded from a human demonstration. Similarly, several mobile robotics groups adopted imitation by direct policy learning using a 'robot teacher' (Lin 1991; Hayes and Demiris 1994; Dautenhahn 1995; Grudic and Lawrence 1996). For example, the 'robot student' followed the 'robot teacher's' movements in a specific environment, mimicked its kinematic, task-oriented actions, and learned to associate which action to choose in which state. Afterwards, the robot student had the same competence as the teacher in this environment. An impressive application of direct policy learning in a rather complex control system, a flight simulator, was demonstrated by Sammut *et al.* (1992). Kinematic control actions from several human subjects were recorded and an inductive machine learning algorithm was trained to represent the control with decision trees. Subsequently, the system was able to autonomously perform various flight manoeuvres.

In all these direct policy-learning approaches, there is no need for the student to know the task goal of the teacher, i.e. equation (2.2) has only imitation-specific criteria, but no task-specific criteria. Imitation learning is greatly simplified in this manner. However, the student will not be able to undergo self-improvement unless an explicit reward signal, usually generated from a task-specific optimization criterion, is provided to the student, as in approaches discussed in the following section. Another problem with direct policy learning is that there is no guarantee that the imitated behaviour is stable, i.e. can reach the (implicit) behavioural goal from all start configurations. Lastly, imitation by direct policy learning usually generates policies that cannot be re-used for a slightly modified behavioural goal. For instance, if reaching for a specific target was learned by direct policy learning, and the target location changes, the commands issued by the learned policy are wrong for the new target location. Such a form of imitation of is often called 'indiscriminate imitation' or 'mimicking' as it just repeats an observed action pattern without knowledge about how to modify it for a new behavioural context.

(c) Imitation by learning policies from demonstrated trajectories

A teacher's demonstration usually provides a rather limited amount of data, best described as 'sample trajectories'. Various projects investigated how a stable policy can be instantiated from such small amount of information. As a crucial difference with respect to direct policy learning, it is now assumed that the task goal is known (see the following examples), and the demonstrated movement is only used as a seed for an initial policy, to be optimized by a self-improvement process. This self-learning adjusts the imitated movement to kinematic and dynamic discrepancies between the student and the teacher, and additionally ensures behavioural stability.

The idea of learning from trajectories was explored with an anthropomorphic robot arm for dynamic manipulation tasks, for instance learning a tennis forehand and the game of kendama ('ball-in-the-cup') (Miyamoto *et al.* 1996; Miyamoto and Kawato 1998). At the outset, a human demonstrated the task, and his/her movement trajectory was recorded with marker-based optical recording equipment (OptoTrack). This process resulted in spatio-temporal data about the movement of the manipulated object in Cartesian coordinates, as well as the movement of the actuator (arm) in terms of joint angle coordinates. For imitation learning, a hybrid internal/external evaluation criterion was chosen. Initially, the robot aimed at indiscriminate imitation of the demonstrated trajectory in task space based on position data of the endeffector, while trying to use an arm posture as similar as possible to the demonstrated posture of the teacher (cf. D'Souza *et al.* 2001). This approximation process corrected for kinematic differences between the teacher and the robot and resulted in a desired trajectory for the robot's motion—a desired trajectory can also be conceived of as a nonautonomous policy (Schaal *et al.* 2000). Afterwards, using manually provided knowledge of the task goal in form of an optimization criterion, the robot's performance improved by trial and error learning until the task was accomplished. For this purpose, the desired endeffector trajectory of the robot was approximated by splines, and the spline nodes, called via-points, were adjusted in space and time by optimization techniques (e.g. Dyer and McReynolds 1970) until the task was fulfilled. Using this method, the robot learned to manipulate a stochastic, dynamic environment within a few trials.

A spline-based encoding of a control policy is nonautonomous, because the via-points defining the splines are parameterized explicitly in time. There are two drawbacks in using such nonautonomous movement primitives. First, modifying the policy for a different behavioural context, e.g. a change of target in reaching or a change of timing and amplitude in a locomotion pattern, requires more complex computations in terms of scaling laws of the viapoints (Kawamura and Fukao 1994). Second, and more severely, nonautonomous policies are not very robust in coping with unforeseen perturbations of the movement. For instance, when abruptly holding the arm of a tennis player during a forehand swing, a nonautonomous policy would continue creating desired values for the movement system, and, owing to the explicit time dependency, these desired values would increasingly more open a large gap between the current position and the desired position. This gap can potentially cause huge motor commands that fight the advert perturbation, and, if the arm were released, it would 'jump' to catch up with the target trajectory; a behaviour that is undesirable in any motor system as it leads to potential damage. By contrast, autonomous movement primitives can avoid this behaviour as the output of the policy is solely state and not time dependent, and perturbations can create inhibitive terms in the policy that ensure that the planned movement of the policy will never deviate too much from the actual position. In this vein, Ijspeert *et al.* (2002*a,b*) suggested the use of autonomous dynamical systems as an alternative to spline-based imitation learning, realizing that equations (2.4) and (2.5) are nothing but nonlinear differential equations. In their approach, a demonstrated trajectory is encoded by learning the transformation from a simple canonical attractor system to a new nonlinear attractor landscape that has the demonstrated trajectory as its unique attractor. Both limit cycle or point attractors could be realized, corresponding to rhythmic or discrete movement primitives. The evaluation criterion for imitation was the deviation of the reproduced trajectory from the demonstrated one, either in internal or external space—reaching the target of the movement, i.e. either a point or a limit cycle, is automatically guaranteed by shaping the attractor landscape appropriately. The dynamic systems policies were designed to provide a spatial and temporal invariant, i.e. a qualitatively similar movement will always lead to a similarly parameterized movement primitive, irrespective of the timing of the movement and the target to which the movement was executed. Coupling terms to the differential equations allowed natural robustness towards external perturbations (see also Hatsopoulos (1996)). The effectiveness of imitation learning with these dynamic systems primitives was successfully demonstrated on a humanoid robot that learned a series of movements

(*a*)   (*b*)

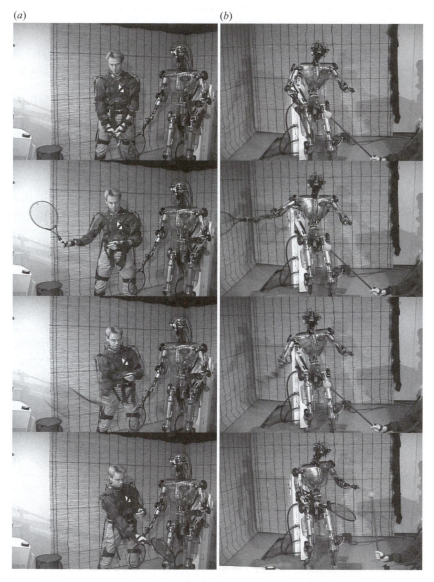

Fig. 9.3   Four frames of a tennis swing over time, progressing from the top downwards. (*a*) Teacher demonstration of a tennis swing; (*b*) imitated movement by the humanoid robot.

such as tennis forehand, tennis backhand and drumming sequences from a human teacher (Fig. 9.3), and that was subsequently able to re-use the learned movement in modified behavioural contexts.

Another, more biologically inspired, dynamic systems approach to imitation was pursued by Billard and colleagues (Billard 2000; Billard and Mataric 2001; Billard and Schaal 2001). Joint angular trajectories, recorded from human demonstrations, were segmented using zero velocity points. The policy approximated the segment for each joint movement by a second-order differential equation that activated a pair of antagonistic muscles, modelled as spring– damper systems (Lacquaniti and Soechting 1986). Owing to the dynamic properties of muscles, this policy generates joint angle trajectories with a bell-shaped velocity profile similarly to human motion; the initial flexion or extension force determines entirely the trajectory and is computed using the initial acceleration of the demonstrated trajectory segment. After acquiring this movement, primitive imitation learning is used to combine joint trajectory segments to produce whole body motion. For this purpose, a time-delay recurrent neural network is trained to reproduce the sequential activation of each joint, similar to methods of associative memory (Schwenker *et al.* 1996). Both speed and amplitude of movement that can be modulated by adjusting appropriate parameters in the network. This imitation system can generate complex movement sequences (Fig. 9.4) and even 'improvise' movement by randomly activating nodes in the associative memory.

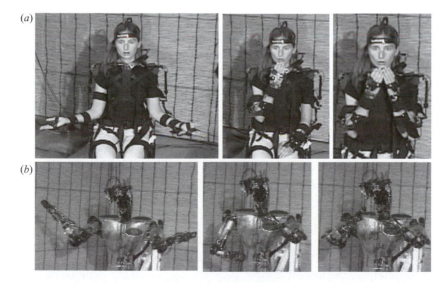

Fig. 9.4 Learning of movement sequences by imitation. (*a*) Teacher demonstrates movement sequence; (*b*) imitated movement by the humanoid robot.

(d) Imitation by model-based policy learning

A third approach to learning a policy from imitation employs model-based learning (Atkeson and Schaal 1997*a*; Schaal 1997). From the demonstrated behaviour, not the policy but a predictive model of the task dynamics is approximated (cf. Wolpert *et al.* 1998). Given knowledge of the task goal, the task-level policy of the movement primitive can be computed with reinforcement learning procedures based on the learned model. For example, Atkeson and Schaal (Atkeson and Schaal 1997*a*,*b*; Schaal 1997) showed how the model-based approach allowed an anthropomorphic robot arm to learn the task of pole-balancing in just a single trial, and the task of a 'pendulum swing-up' in only three to four trials. These authors also demonstrated that task-level imitation based on direct policy learning, augmented with subsequent self-learning, can be rather fragile and does not necessarily provide significant learning speed improvement over pure trial-and-error learning without a demonstration.

(e) Matching of demonstrated behaviour against existing movement primitives

The approaches discussed in the previous sections illustrated some computational ideas for how *novel* behaviours can be learned by imitation. Interesting insights into these methods can be gained by analysing the process of how a perceived behaviour is mapped onto a set of existing primitives. Two major questions (Meltzoff and Moore 1997) are: what is the matching criterion for recognizing a behaviour; and in which coordinate frame does matching take place?

(i) Matching based on policies with kinetic outputs

If only a kinetic control policy of the movement primitive exists (cf. equation (2.1)), finding a matching criterion becomes difficult because kinetic outputs such as forces or torques cannot be observed from demonstrations. One solution would be to execute a primitive, observe its outcome in either internal or external kinematic space, and generate in the chosen coordinate frame a performance criterion based on the similarity between the executed and the teacher's behaviour, e.g. the squared difference of state variables over time or distance to a goal at the end of the movement. This procedure needs to be repeated for every primitive in the repertoire and is thus quite inefficient. Given that kinetic policies are also not very useful for learning novel movements by imitation (see Section 9.2b), kinetic policies seem to be of little use in imitation learning.

(ii) Matching based on policies with kinematic outputs

If the primitive outputs observable variables, e.g. kinematic commands as in equations (2.4) and (2.5), matching is highly simplified because the output of the primitive can be compared directly with the teacher's performance. Such kinematic matching assumes that the motor execution stage of Fig. 9.2 creates motor commands that faithfully realize the kinematic plans of the primitive, i.e. that motor-command generation approximately inverts the dynamics of the movement system (Kawato 1999). At least two forms of matching mechanisms are possible.

One matching mechanism simply treats the demonstrated movement as a candidate for a *new* movement primitive and fits the parameterization of this primitive. The parameters are subsequently compared with the parameters of all previously learned primitives, and the best matching one in memory is chosen as the winner. For this method to work, the parameterization of the movement primitive should have suitable invariances towards variations of a movement, e.g. temporal and spatial scale invariance. The via-point method of Miyamoto *et al.* (1996) can easily be adapted for such movement recognition, as via-points represent a parsimonious parameterization of a movement that is easily used in classification algorithms, e.g. nearest neighbour methods (Wada and Kawato 1995). Similarly, the dynamic systems approach to motor primitives of Ijspeert *et al.* (2002*b*) creates a movement parameterization that affords classification in parameter space—indeed, the in-built scale and time invariances of this technique adds significant robustness to movement recognition in comparison to methods.

The second matching paradigm is based on the idea of predictive forward models (Miall and Wolpert 1996; Schaal 1997; Atkeson and Schaal 1997*a*; Wolpert *et al.* 1998; Chapter 14 this volume, Demiris and Hayes 2002). While observing the teacher, each movement primitive can try to predict the temporal evolution of the observed movement based on the current state z of the teacher. The primitive with the best prediction abilities will be selected as the best match. If, as mentioned above, the motor execution stage of the control circuit (Fig. 9.2) faithfully realizes the movement plan issued by a movement primitive, the primitive can act itself as a forward model, i.e. it can predict a change in state z of the teacher (cf. equations (2.4) and (2.5)). Alternatively, it is also possible to include prediction over the entire dynamics of the movement system. For this purpose, the output of the movement primitive is fed to the motor-command execution stage, whose output is subsequently passed through a predictive forward model of the dynamics of the student's movement system (see Demiris and Hayes 2002; Chapter 14 this volume), thus predicting the change of state of movement without actually performing it. This technique will work even when the motor execution stage is less accurate in realizing desired movement kinematics, but it comes at the cost of two more levels of signal processing, i.e. the simulated motorcommand generation and the need for a forward model of the motor system. Demiris and Hayes (2002) realized such an imitation system in a simulated humanoid.

What is particularly noteworthy in these approaches to movement recognition is the suggested bi-directional interaction between perception and action: movement recognition is directly accomplished with the movement-generating mechanism. This concept is compatible with the concept of mirror neurons in neurobiology (Rizzolatti *et al.* 1996; Rizzolatti and Arbib 1998), with the simulation theory of mind reading (Gallese and Goldman 1998), and it also ties into other research projects that emphasize the bi-directional interaction of generative and recognition models (Dayan *et al.* 1995; Kawato 1996) in unsupervised learning. Such bi-directional theories enjoy an increasing popularity in theoretical models to perception and action as they provide useful constraints for explaining the autonomous development of such system.

(iii) Matching based on other criteria

Exploiting the literature on computer vision and statistical classification, a large variety of alternative approaches to movement recognition can be developed, mostly without taking into account mutuality criteria between movement generation and movement recognition. Chapter 4 provides an overview of techniques in this vein.

(f) The correspondence problem

An important topic of imitation learning concerns how to map the external and internal space of the teacher to the student, often called the 'correspondence problem' (Alissandrakis *et al.* 2002; Chapter 8 this volume). Solving correspondence in external space is usually simplified, as external coordinates (or task coordinates) are mostly independent of the kinematic and dynamic structure of the teacher. For instance, if pole balancing could be demonstrated by a dolphin, a human student could imitate despite the mismatch in body structure if only task-level imitation is attempted—the only transformation needed is a mapping from the teacher's body-centred external space to the student's body-centred external space, which is just a linear transformation. Correspondence in internal space is a more complex problem. Even when teacher and student have the same degrees of freedom, as it is the case with human-to-human or human-to-humanoid-robot imitation, the bodies of student and teacher are bound to differ in many ways, including in their ranges of motion, in their exact kinematics, and their dynamics. The mapping is even more difficult when the teacher and student have dissimilar bodies. In that case, the student can only imitate approximately, reproducing only sub-goals or substates of the demonstrated motion. The correspondence problem consists of defining which sub-states of the motion *can* and/or *should* be reproduced. Dautenhahn and Nehaniv (2002) proposed a general mathematical framework to express such a mapping function in terms of transfer functions across different spaces. Alissandrakis *et al.* (2002) implement this framework to solve the correspondence problem in a chess game case study. The movement of two chess pieces (e.g. queen and knight) are directed by very different rules such that the two pieces cannot replicate each other's move in just one time step. For the knight to replicate the trajectory followed by the queen, it must define several sub-goals (positions on the chessboard) through which the queen has travelled and that the knight can reach using its own movement capacities. The best strategy to define the sub-goals depends on the metric applied to measure the imitation performance. The authors compare metrics that minimize either the total number of moves required for the reproduction, or the space covered during the reproduction by the motion.

(g) Imitation of complex movement sequences

One final issue concerns the imitation of complex motor acts that involve learning a sequence of primitives and when to switch between them. In this context, Fagg and Arbib (1998) provided a model of reaching and grasping based on the known anatomy of the fronto-parietal circuits, including the mirror neuron system. Essentially, their model employed a recurrent neural network that sequenced and switched between motor schemas based on sensory cues. The work of Billard and colleagues (Billard 2000; Billard and Mataric 2001; Billard and Schaal 2001; Section 9.2c) follows a similar vein, just at a higher level of biological abstraction and more suitable for the control of real, complex robotic systems. In a robotic study, Pook and Ballard (1993) used hidden Markov models to learn appropriate sequencing from demonstrated behaviour for a dexterous manipulation task. There is also large body of literature in the field of time-series segmentation (Cacciatore and Nowlan 1994; Weigend *et al*. 1995; Pawelzik *et al*. 1996) that employed competitive learning and forward models for recognition and sequencing in a way that is easily adapted for imitation learning as illustrated in Fig. 9.1.

9.3 Summary

Using the formalization of motor control in terms of generating control policies under a chosen performance criterion, we discussed computational imitation learning as methodology to bootstrap a student's control policy from a teacher's demonstration. Different methods of imitation were classified according to which variables were assumed observable for the student, whether variables were of kinetic or kinematic nature, whether internal, external coordinates, or both were used during demonstration, and whether the task goal was explicitly known to the student or not. Additional insights could be obtained by discussing how a demonstrated movement can be mapped onto a set of existing movement primitives. Important topics in computational imitation concerned the formation of motor primitives, their representation, their sequencing, the reciprocal interaction of movement recognition and movement generation, and the correspondence problem. At the current stage of research, all these issues have been modelled in various ways, demonstrating an increasingly growing formal understanding of how imitation learning can be accomplished. Among the most crucial missing points to be addressed in imitation is presumably a formalization of extracting the intent of a demonstrated movement. Billard and Schaal (2002) suggested some initial ideas towards this goal by modelling the probability distribution over manipulated objects by the teacher, which triggered appropriate imitation behaviour in a humanoid robot. However, a more abstract representation of task goals, perhaps as a set of generic goal taxonomies, is needed to make further progress in this area.

This work was made possible by awards, nos. 9710312/0010312 and 0082995, of the National Science Foundation, award AC no. 98-516 by NASA, an AFOSR grant on Intelligent Control, the ERATO Kawato Dynamic Brain Project funded by the Japanese Science and Technology Agency, and the ATR Human Information Processing Research Laboratories.

Endnotes

1. For this paper, only visually mediated imitation will be considered, although, at least in humans, verbal communication can supply important additional information.
2. Note that instead of a formulation as a differential equation, we would also choose a difference equation, i.e. where a desired 'next state' is the output of the policy, not a desired change of state.

References

Aboaf, E. W., Drucker, S. M. and Atkeson, C. G. (1989). Tasklevel robot learing: juggling a tennis ball more accurately. In *Proc. IEEE Int. Conf. Robotics Automation, Scottsdale, AZ, 14–19 May*, pp. 331–48. Piscataway, NJ: IEEE.

Alissandrakis, A., Nehaniv, C. L. and Dautenhahn, K. (2002). Imitating with ALICE: learning to imitate corresponding actions across dissimilar embodiments. *IEEE Transact. Systems, Man and Cybernetics, Part A: Systems Hum.* **32**, 482–96.

Arbib, M. A. (1981). Perceptual structures and distributed motor control. In *Handbook of physiology*, section 2: *The nervous system*, vol. II, *Motor control*, part 1 (ed. V. B. Brooks), pp. 1449–80. Bethesda, MD: American Physiological Society.

Arbib, M. A., Billard, A., Iacoboni, M. and Oztop, E. (2000). Synthetic brain imaging: grasping, mirror neurons and imitation. *Neural Networks* **13**, 975–97.

Arulampalam, S., Maskell, S., Gordon, N. and Clapp, T. (2002). A tutorial on particle filters for on-line non-linear/non-Gaussian Bayesian tracking. *IEEE Trans. Signal Processing* **50**, 174–88.

Atkeson, C. G. and Schaal, S. (1997*a*). Learning tasks from a single demonstration. In *IEEE Int. Conf. Robotics Automation (ICRA97), Albuquerque, NM, 20–25 April 1997*, vol. 2, pp. 1706–12. Piscataway, NJ: IEEE.

Atkeson, C. G. and Schaal, S. (1997*b*). Robot learning from demonstration. In *Machine learning: Proc. 14th Int. Conf. (ICML '97), Nashville, TN, 8–12 July 1997* (ed. D. H. Fisher Jr), pp. 12–20. San Mateo, CA: Morgan Kaufmann.

Baillieul, J. and Martin, D. P. (1990). Resolution of kinematic redundancy. In *Proc. Symp. Appl. Math., San Diego, CA, May 1990*, vol. 41, pp. 49–89. Providence, RI: American Mathematical Society.

Billard, A. (2000). Learning motor skills by imitation: a biologically inspired robotic model. *Cybern. Systems* **32**, 155–93.

Billard, A. and Mataric, M. (2001). Learning human arm movements by imitation: evaluation of a biologically-inspired architecture. *Robotics Autonomous Systems* **941**, 1–16.

Billard, A. and Schaal, S. (2001). A connectionist model for online robot learning by imitation. In *IEEE Int. Conf. Intell. Robots Systems (IROS 2001), Maui, Hawaii, 29 October–3 November 2001*.

Billard, A. and Schaal, S. (2002). Computational elements of robot learning by imitation. In *Am. Math. Soc. Central Section Meeting, Madison, WI, 12–13 October 2002*. Providence, RI: American Mathematical Society.

Bullock, D., Grossberg, S. and Guenther, F. H. (1993). A selforganizing neural model of motor equivalent reaching and tool use by a multijoint arm. *J. Cogn. Neurosci.* **5**, 408–35.

Byrne, R. W. (2003). Imitation as behavior parsing. *Phil. Trans. R. Soc. Lond.* B **358**, 529–36. (DOI 10.1098/rstb.2002. 1219.)

Cacciatore, T. W. and Nowlan, S. J. (1994). Mixtures of controllers for jump linear and non-linear plants. In *Advances in neural information processing systems 6* (ed. J. D. Cowen, G. Tesauro and J. Alspector), pp. 719–26. San Mateo, CA: Morgan Kaufmann.

Craig, J. J. (1986). *Introduction to robotics*. Reading, MA: Addison-Wesley.

D'Souza, A., Vijayakumar, S. and Schaal, S. (2001). Learning inverse kinematics. In *IEEE Int. Conf. Intell. Robots Systems (IROS 2001), Hilton Head Island, SC, 13–15 June 2000*.

Dautenhahn, K. (1995). Getting to know each other—artificial social intelligence for autonomous robots. *Robotics Autonomous Systems* **16**, 333–56.

Dautenhahn, K. and Nehaniv, C. L. (eds) (2002). *Imitation in animals and artifacts*. Cambridge, MA: MIT Press.

Dayan, P., Hinton, G. E., Neal, R. M. and Zemel, R. S. (1995). The Helmholtz machine. *Neural Comput.* **7**, 889–904.

Demiris, J. and Hayes, G. (2002). Imitation as a dual-route process featuring predictive and learning components: a biologically plausible computational model. In *Imitation in animals and artifacts* (ed. K. Dautenhahn and C. L. Nehaniv), pp. 327–61. Cambridge, MA: MIT Press.

Deutscher, J., Blake, A. and Reid, I. (2000). Articulated body motion capture by annealed particle filtering. In *IEEE Comput. Vision Pattern Recognition (CVPR 2000)*. Piscataway, NJ: IEEE.

Dillmann, R., Kaiser, M. and Ude, A. (1995). Acquisition of elementary robot skills from human demonstration. In *Int. Symp. Intell. Robotic Systems (SIRS'95), 10–14 July 1999, Pisa, Italy*, pp. 1–38.

Dufay, B. and Latombe, J. C. (1984). An approach to automatic robot programming based on inductive learning. *Int. J. Robot. Res.* **3**, 3–20.

Dyer, P. and McReynolds, S. R. (1970). *The computation and theory of optimal control*. New York: Academic Press.

Fagg, A. H. and Arbib, M. A. (1998). Modeling parietal-premotor interactions in primate control of grasping. *Neural Networks* **11**, 1277–303.

Gallese, V. and Goldman, A. (1998). Mirror neurons and the simulation theory of mind-reading. *Trends Cogn. Sci.* **2**, 493–501.

Grudic, G. Z. and Lawrence, P. D. (1996). Human-to-robot skill transfer using the SPORE approximation. In *Int. Conf. Robotics Automation, Minneapolis, MN, April 1996*, pp. 2962–7. Piscataway, NJ: IEEE.

Guenther, F. H. and Barreca, D. M. (1997). Neural models for flexible control of redundant systems. In *Self-organization, computational maps, and motor control* (ed. P. Morasso and V. Sanguineti), pp. 102–8. Amsterdam: Elsevier.

Hatsopoulos, N. G. (1996). Coupling the neural and physical dynamics in rhythmic movements. *Neural Comput.* **8**, 567–81.

Hayes, G. and Demiris, J. (1994). A robot controller using learning by imitation. In *Proc. 2nd Int. Symp. Intell. Robotic Systems, Grenoble, France, July 1994* (ed. A. Borkowski and J. L. Crowley), pp. 198–204. Grenoble, France: LIFTA-IMAG.

Hovland, G. E., Sikka, P. and McCarragher, B. J. (1996). Skill acquisition from human demonstration using a hidden Markov Model. In *IEEE Int. Conf. Robotics Automation, Minneapolis, MN, April 1996*, pp. 2706–11. Piscataway, NJ: IEEE.

Ijspeert, J. A., Nakanishi, J. and Schaal, S. (2002*a*). Learning rhythmic movements by demonstration using nonlinear oscillators. In *IEEE Int. Conf. Intell. Robots Systems (IROS 2002), Lausanne, 30 September–4 October 2002*. Piscataway, NJ: IEEE.

Ijspeert, J. A., Nakanishi, J. and Schaal, S. (2002*b*). Movement imitation with nonlinear dynamical systems in humanoid robots. In *Int. Conf. Robotics Automation (ICRA2002), Washington, DC, 11–15 May 2002*. Piscataway, NJ: IEEE.

Ikeuchi, K., Kawade, M. and Suehiro, T. (1993). Assembly task recognition with planar, curved and mechanical contacts. In *Proc. IEEE Int. Conf. Robotics Automation, Atlanta, GA, May 1993*, vol. 2, pp. 688–93. Piscataway, NJ: IEEE.

Kawamura, S. and Fukao, N. (1994). Interpolation for input torque patterns obtained through learning control. In *Int. Conf. Automation, Robotics Computer Vis. (ICARCV '94), Singapore, November 1994*, pp. 183–91.

Kawato, M. (1996). Bi-directional theory approach to integration. In *Attention and performance XVI* (ed. J. Konczak and E. Thelen), pp. 335–67. Cambridge, MA: MIT Press.

Kawato, M. (1999). Internal models for motor control and trajectory planning. *Curr. Opin. Neurobiol.* **9**, 718–27.

Kuniyoshi, Y., Inaba, M. and Inoue, H. (1989). Teaching by showing: generating robot programs by visual observation of human performance. In *Proc. Int. Symp. Industrial Robots, Tokyo, Japan, 4–6 October 1989*, pp. 119–26.

Kuniyoshi, Y., Inaba, M. and Inoue, H. (1994). Learning by watching: extracting reusable task knowledge from visual observation of human performance. *IEEE Trans. Robotics Automation* **10**, 799–822.

Lacquaniti, F. and Soechting, J. F. (1986). Simulation studies on the control of posture and movement in a multi-jointed limb. *Biol. Cybern.* **54**, 367–78.

Levas, A. and Selfridge, M. (1984). A user-friendly high-level robot teaching system. In *Int. Conf. Robotics, Atlanta, GA, March 1984*, pp. 413–16. Piscataway, NJ: IEEE.

Lin, L.-J. (1991). Programming robots using reinforcement learning and teaching. In *Proc. 9th Natl Conf. Artificial Intell., Anaheim, CA, 14–19 July 1991*, vol. 2, pp. 781–6. Menlo Park, CA: AAAI.

Lozano-Pérez, T. (1982). Task-Planning. In *Robot motion: planning and control* (ed. M. Brady, J. M. Hollerbach, T. L. Johnson, T. Lozano-Pérez and M. T. Mason), pp. 473–98. Cambridge, MA: MIT Press.

Mataric, M. J. and Pomplun, M. (1998). Fixation behavior in observation and imitation of human movement. *Cogn. Brain Res.* **7**, 191–202.

Meltzoff, A. N. and Moore, M. K. (1994). Imitation, memory, and the representation of persons. *Infant Behav. Dev.* **17**, 83–99.

Meltzoff, A. N. and Moore, M. K. (1997). Explaining facial imitation: a theoretical model. *Early Dev. Parenting* **6**, 179–92.

Miall, R. C. and Wolpert, D. M. (1996). Forward models for physiological motor control. *Neural Networks* **9**, 1265–85.

Miyamoto, H. and Kawato, M. (1998). A tennis serve and upswing learning robot based on bi-directional theory. *Neural Networks* **11**, 1331–44.

Miyamoto, H., Schaal, S., Gandolfo, F., Koike, Y., Osu, R., Nakano, E., *et al.* (1996). A Kendama learning robot based on bi-directional theory. *Neural Networks* **9**, 1281–302.

Nechyba, M. C. and Xu, Y. (1995). Human skill transfer: neural networks as learners and teachers. In *IEEE/RSJ Int. Conf. Intell. Robots Systems, Pittsburgh, PA, 5–9 August 1995*, vol. 3, pp. 314–19. Piscataway, NJ: IEEE.

Nehaniv, C. L. and Dautenhahn, K. (1999). Of hummingbirds and helicopters: an algebraic framework for interdisciplinary studies of imitation and its applications. In *Learning robots: an interdisciplinary approach* (ed. J. Demiris and A. Birk). Singapore: World Scientific.

Oztop, E. and Arbib, M. A. (2002). Schema design and implementation of the grasp-related mirror neuron system. *Biol. Cybern.* **87**, 116–40.

Pawelzik, K., Kohlmorgen, J. and Müller, K. R. (1996). Annealed competition of experts for a segmentation and classification of switching dynamics. *Neural Comput.* **8**, 340–56.

Piaget, J. (1951). *Play, dreams, and imitation in childhood*. New York: Norton.

Pook, P. K. and Ballard, D. H. (1993). Recognizing teleoperated manipulations. In *Proc. IEEE Int. Conf. Robotics Automation, Atlanta, GA, May 1993*, vol. 3, pp. 913–18. Piscataway, NJ: IEEE.

Rizzolatti, G. and Arbib, M. A. (1998). Language within our grasp. *Trends Neurosci.* **21**, 188–94.

Rizzolatti, G., Fadiga, L., Gallese, V. and Fogassi, L. (1996). Premotor cortex and the recognition of motor actions. *Cogn. Brain Res.* **3**, 131–41.

Saltzman, E. and Kelso, S. J. A. (1987). Skilled actions: a taskdynamic approach. *Psychol. Rev.* **94**, 84–106.

Sammut, C., Hurst, S., Kedzier, D. and Michie, D. (1992). Learning to fly. In *Proc. 9th Int. Machine Learning Conf. (ML'92), Aberdeen, Scotland, 1–3 July 1992* (ed. D. Sleeman and P. Edwards), pp. 385–93. San Mateo, CA: Morgan Kaufmann.

Schaal, S. (1997). Learning from demonstration. In *Advances in neural information processing systems 9* (ed. M. C. Mozer, M. Jordan and T. Petsche), pp. 1040–6. Cambridge, MA: MIT Press.

Schaal, S. (1999). Is imitation learning the route to humanoid robots? *Trends Cogn. Sci.* **3**, 233–42.

Schaal, S., Sternad, D., Dean, W., Kotoska, S., Osu, R. and Kawato, M. (2000). Reciprocal excitation between biological and robotic research. In *Sensor fusion and decentralized control in robotic systems* III, *Proc. of SPIE, Boston, MA, 5–8 November 1992*, vol. 4196, pp. 30–40.

Schwenker, F., Sommer, F. T. and Palm, G. (1996). Iterative retrieval of sparsely coded associative memory patterns. *Neural Networks* **9**, 445–55.

Segre, A. B. and DeJong, G. (1985). Explanation-based manipulator learning: acquisition of planning ability through observation. In *IEEE Conf. Robotics Automation, St Louis, MO, March 1985*, pp. 555–60. Piscataway, NJ: IEEE.

Segre, A. M. (1988). *Machine learning of robot assembly plans*. Kluwer International Series in Engineering and Computer Science. Knowledge representation, learning, and expert systems. Boston, MA: Kluwer.

Sternad, D. and Schaal, D. (1999). Segmentation of endpoint trajectories does not imply segmented control. *Exp. Brain Res.* **124**, 118–36.

Sutton, R. S. and Barto, A. G. (1998). *Reinforcement learning: an introduction. Adaptive computation and machine learning*. Cambridge, MA: MIT Press.

Sutton, R. S., Singh, S., Precup, D. and Ravindran, B. (1999). Improved switching among temporally abstract actions. In *Advances in neural information processing systems*, vol. 11. Cambridge, MA: MIT Press.

Tomasello, M., Savage-Rumbaugh, S. and Kruger, A. C. (1993). Imitative learning of actions on objects by children, chimpanzees, and enculturated chimpanzees. *Child Dev.* **64**, 1688–705.

Tung, C. P. and Kak, A. C. (1995). Automatic learning of assembly task using a DataGlove system. In *IEEE/RSJ Int. Conf. Intell. Robots Systems, Pittsburgh, PA*, vol. 1, pp. 1–8.

Van Essen, D. C. and Maunsell, J. M. R. (1983). Hierachical organization and functional streams in the visual cortex. *Trends Neurosci.* **6**, 370–5.

Wada, Y. and Kawato, M. (1995). A theory for cursive handwriting based on the minimization principle. *Biol. Cybern.* **73**, 3–13.

Weigend, A. S., Mangeas, M. and Srivastava, A. N. (1995). Nonlinear gated experts for time series: discovering regimes and avoiding overfitting. *Int. J. Neural Systems* **6**, 373–99.

Widrow, B. and Smith, F. W. (1964). Pattern recognizing control systems. In *1963 Comput. Inform. Sci. (COINS) Symp. Proc.*, pp. 288–317. Spartan.

Wolpert, D. M. (1997). Computational approaches to motor control. *Trends Cogn. Sci.* **1**, 209–16.

Wolpert, D. M. and Kawato, M. (1998). Multiple paired forward and inverse models for motor control. *Neural Networks* **11**, 1317–29.

Wolpert, D. M., Miall, R. C. and Kawato, M. (1998). Internal models in the cerebellum. *Trends Cogn. Sci.* **2**, 338–47.

10

Detecting agents

Susan C. Johnson

This paper reviews a recent set of behavioural studies that examine the scope and nature of the representational system underlying theory-of-mind development. Studies with typically developing infants, adults and children with autism all converge on the claim that there is a specialized input system that uses not only morphological cues, but also behavioural cues to categorize novel objects as agents. Evidence is reviewed in which 12- to 15-month-old infants treat certain non-human objects as if they have perceptual/attentional abilities, communicative abilities and goal-directed behaviour. They will follow the attentional orientation of an amorphously shaped novel object if it interacts contingently with them or with another person. They also seem to use a novel object's environmentally directed behaviour to determine its perceptual/attentional orientation and object-oriented goals. Results from adults and children with autism are strikingly similar, despite adults' contradictory beliefs about the objects in question and the failure of children with autism to ultimately develop more advanced theory-of-mind reasoning. The implications for a general theory-of-mind development are discussed.

Keywords: agency; infancy; self-propelled motion; intentionality; theory of mind; autism

10.1 Mentalism in infancy: people as agents

One commonly held position in the study of infant social cognition is that:

(i) infants distinguish between people and non-people; and
(ii) infants' earliest understanding of other minds maps directly onto this distinction.

Although the first claim has been well-documented, the second has been largely taken for granted (see Legerstee 1992, 1994; Wellman 1993; Meltzoff 1995; Poulin-Dubois 1999; Johnson 2000 for related reviews). This second point can be broken down into two related questions: when do children first attribute mental states to others and when they do, whom do they attribute mental states to? The answer to these questions may well provide insight into the nature of the representational systems underlying mentalistic reasoning. This paper will review a line of research designed to do just that.

Mental states are unobservable constructs that must be inferred by observers rather than perceived directly. They are distinguished from other sorts of unobservables or internal states by the specific kind of relationship they hold with the world. That is, mental states are *directed at* the world; they are *about* things (Lycan 1999). Other commonplace, commonsense unobservables (e.g. life, essences, atoms, etc.), although presumed by lay thinkers to exist in the world, are not presumed to be about the world. The ability to construe ourselves and others as agents with mental states such as perceptions, attention, desires and beliefs is critical. With this mentalizing ability we can communicate referentially, predict and explain others' behaviours, and manipulate both our own and others' mental states for the purposes of complex problem-solving and learning, not to mention deception. Mentalizing is so critical in fact, that its absence is thought by some to be a central cause of autism (Baron-Cohen *et al.* 1993; Baron-Cohen 1995).

Garnering evidence sufficient to demonstrate mentalizing is difficult, however. Many behaviours that could potentially serve as indices of mentalizing (e.g. gaze-following, pointing, goal imitation) can typically be interpreted in both mentalistic and non-mentalistic ways. Non-mentalistic explanations based on signal releasers, attentional enhancement and object affordances have all been proposed to explain the variety of behaviours produced by prelinguistic infants (Butterworth and Jarrett 1991; Gerwitz and Pelaez-Nogueras 1992; Moore and Corkum 1994; Hood *et al.* 1998). The interpretative problems are particularly acute for the attribution of mental states that are correlated with reality (e.g. perception or goals) and can thus be mimicked by conditioned or reality-driven behaviours (Dennett 1978).

Although the point is well taken, it does not mean that infants do not attribute mental states to agents; only that sufficient evidence for such a claim is difficult to generate. It does mean, however, that as long as the agents used to test infants' competency are highly familiar to infants, as are people, non-mentalistic explanations are difficult, if not impossible, to rule out. Much of the work in this area has none the less presupposed the role of people in infants' attributions of mental states. Certainly, between the ages of 9 and 18 months, infants have begun to interact with people as though they believe people have minds. They produce communicative gestures such as points, requests and displays for other people (see Bates *et al.* 1975; Leung and Rheingold 1981; Bretherton *et al.* 1981; Butterworth and Grover 1988); they follow adults' gazes (Scaife and Bruner 1975; Lempers 1979; Butterworth and Jarrett 1991; D'Entremont *et al.* 1997; Corkum and Moore 1998) and they guide their own behaviour towards objects on the basis of other people's emotional and goal-directed behaviour towards those objects (Meltzoff 1995; Baldwin and Moses 1996; Repacholi and Gopnik 1997; Woodward 1998; Moses *et al.* 2001; see also Johnson 2000, for a recent review.)

The emphasis on humans as the target of infants' mentalizing is not accidental. A great deal of evidence has accumulated showing that very young infants can and do *distinguish* between humans and non-humans. At birth, infants preferentially track the movement of faces (Morton and Johnson 1991) and imitate the facial and hand gestures of people (Meltzoff and Moore 1977, 1983; Field *et al.* 1982) but not inanimate objects (Legerstee 1991). From 3 months to a year, infants smile, vocalize and gesture more in the presence of people than inanimate objects, while visually fixating and reaching more towards animals or inanimate objects, even when the inanimate objects resemble people in very salient ways both perceptually and behaviourally such as dolls, interactive robots and animals (see Legerstee *et al.* 1987; Ellsworth *et al.* 1993; Ricard and Allard 1993; Legerstee 1994, 1997; Poulin-Dubois *et al.* 1996; but see Frye *et al.* 1983 for contradictory results).

The ability to *discriminate* people from non-people, however, is no more sufficient evidence of mentalizing abilities than any of those described in the previous paragraph. It is possible that person discrimination could develop in support of important social and cognitive processes that are independent of mental state attributions (e.g. attachment and/or observational learning). Neither is person discrimination logically necessary for mentalizing abilities. That is, object recognition processes for identifying mentalistic agents need not be isomorphic with the processes for identifying people.

Given these two concerns:

(i) the problem of interpreting infants' behaviour in the context of highly familiar agents like people; and
(ii) the still underspecified function of the person/non-person distinction in infancy, it may be time to look more closely at infants' interpretation of non-humans.

It is particularly important to do so using measures that are closely associated with mentalizing abilities, such as communicative behaviours, joint attention behaviours, and so on.

In fact, several largely untested theoretical proposals have been offered about the cues that lay thinkers may use to identify mentalistic agents, human or otherwise. The features proposed fall into several overlapping classes: morphological features such as faces and eyes (Carey and Spelke 1994, 1996; Baron-Cohen 1995); asymmetry along one axis (Premack 1990, 1991; Baron-Cohen 1995); non-rigid transformation (Gibson *et al.* 1978); self-propulsion (Premack 1990, 1991; Leslie 1994, 1995; Baron-Cohen 1995); and the ability to engage in contingent and reciprocal interactions with other agents (Premack 1990, 1991; Spelke *et al.* 1995).

The remainder of this paper will review work done by this author and colleagues on the role of these cues in eliciting mentalistic interpretations in both infants and adults. Initial work focused on the relationship between the infant's agent category and the infant's person category. More recent work has begun to test the limits on exactly what sorts of non-human objects infants are willing to attribute mental states to and the sorts of assumptions infants seem to make when doing so. Additional work examining the parallels between infant and adult attributions and their implications will be discussed. Finally, some preliminary results from autism will be discussed.

10.2 The attribution of perception/attention to non-human agents: morphological and behavioural cues

Johnson *et al.* (1998) was the first study of this series to examine whether any of the putative cues of agency would elicit mentalistic attributions in infants. To do this we created a small novel object that could be introduced to infants as the actor in a standard gaze-following method (Scaife and Bruner 1975). The object embodied many of the proposed cues for mentalistic agents, without being person-like. The size of a small beach ball, it was made of natural-looking fuzzy brown fur and had a naturalistic shape that was symmetrical along only one axis with a small cone-shaped bulge at one end (see Fig. 10.1). It was designed to vary in two dimensions: the presence or absence of facial features and the quality of its behaviour—specifically, whether or not its behaviour was contingently interactive with the infant or not. Its 'behaviour' was generated via a small remote-controlled beeper and incandescent light hidden inside it. Thus, it was possible to control the object from a hidden vantage point such that when the infant babbled, the object beeped back and when the infant moved, the internal light flashed in response.

Infants received a brief (60 s) familiarization period in which either the object reacted contingently to the infant's own behaviour, or the infant saw equivalent amounts of apparently self-generated beeping and flashing, but in a sequence that was random with the infant's own behaviour. After this familiarization, the object made a final attention-grabbing beep and turned to orient itself towards one of two targets placed on either edge of the setup (see Fig. 10.2). Infants were found to follow the orientation of the object by shifting their own attention (as indexed by eye movements) in the same direction as the object's turn significantly more often than in the opposite direction in three out of the four familiarization conditions; if the object had a face; if, when the infant babbled or moved, the object beeped back and flashed lights; or, both of these characteristics together (see Fig. 10.3).

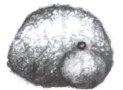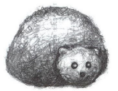

Fig. 10.1   The novel object from Johnson *et al.* (1998). Both versions could make noises and flash an internal light.

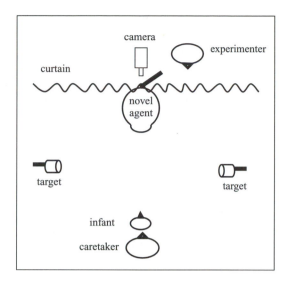

Fig. 10.2   The setup from Johnson *et al.* (1998).

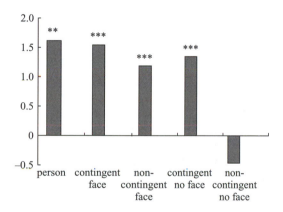

Fig. 10.3   Data from Johnson *et al.* (1998). The score on the *y*-axis equals the total number of looks in the predicted direction minus the total number of looks in the unpredicted direction. **$p < 0.01$, ***$p < 0.005$.

Importantly, the object in the non-contingent, faceless condition embodied the same shape and movement cues as it did in the other conditions, but infants showed no reliable sign of following its orientation. This finding rules out the possibility that very general, perceptual information triggered shifts in the infants' attention without regard to the object's identity.

Finally, a comparison condition with unfamiliar adults taking the place of the object indicated that infants were no more likely to follow the gaze of a contingently interacting person than a contingently interacting fuzzy brown object with a face. Thus, these results seem to show that infants use relatively selective cues to decide when an object does or does not have a mind to perceive or attend with, specifically the presence of a face, or the propensity to interact contingently.

Taken alone, these findings might be interpreted as a generalization of previously conditioned behaviour from people to other objects that share some relevant but non-mentalistically interpreted feature such as eyes or interactive behaviour (though, interestingly, not self-generated behaviour). Why infants would generalize on some dimensions (i.e. interaction), but not others (i.e. self-movement) would then become an important question that a non-mentalistic account would have to address. None the less, as previously discussed, non-mentalistic accounts are difficult to rule out entirely.

10.3 The attribution of goals to non-human agents: morphological and behavioural cues

There is one prediction that non-mentalistic accounts of individual behaviours give rise to that is not made by the mentalism account. Under non-mentalistic accounts, the scope of the putative agent category should vary across different behavioural contexts (e.g. attentional following, communication, imitation). For instance, a conditioning account of attentional following would not predict that the same set of object features would elicit both headturns in attentional following contexts and object manipulation in imitation contexts. Similarly, when behavioural contexts differ, signal-releaser accounts should predict different behavioural responses based on the existence of independent, evolutionarily specified mechanisms.

Conversely, converging (putative) attributions of agency to the same class of novel entities across a variety of diverse behaviours and contexts would indicate a common underlying representation. This would be evidence against disparate non-mentalistic interpretations. It is therefore all the more important to re-examine the person/non-person distinction in infancy, using as wide a variety of candidate mentalizing behaviours as possible.

With this in mind, Johnson *et al.* (2001) adapted two additional behavioural methods in such a way that infants could be introduced to a novel, contingently interacting agent and then given the opportunity to:

(i) re-enact the agent's unseen goals (Meltzoff 1995); and
(ii) interact communicatively with the agent by directing greetings, object requests and object displays at the agent.

In the method of Meltzoff (1995), 18-month-old infants were shown to re-enact the object-related goals of human actors (e.g. dropping a string of beads into a cup). When a human actor tried but failed to accomplish his goal, 18-month-old infants re-enacted the *inferred, unseen goal* rather than the spatio-temporally witnessed event. Meltzoff (1995) argued that the infants' performance could not be motivated purely by the spatio-temporal information in the action itself. In a condition in which the human actor was replaced by a mechanical set of pincers performing the same spatio-temporal actions, infants failed to re-enact any unseen actions. Meltzoff (1995) attributed this differential behaviour to an early naive psychology, based on and restricted to the infants' knowledge of people.

Johnson *et al.* (2001) challenged the extent to which infants, in fact, restrict their attribution of goals to human actors. We reasoned that unlike the novel object used in the gaze-following study of Johnson *et al.* (1998), the mechanical pincers of Meltzoff (1995) failed to embody any of the characteristics thought to imply a mind, and certainly had neither a face nor the ability to engage in contingent interactions. Therefore, we replicated the design and procedure of Meltzoff (1995), replacing the human actor with an animated stuffed orangutan that had a face and hands, the ability to move on its own, and the ability to interact contingently with the infant.

At 15 months of age, the infants tested in this study were somewhat younger than those tested by Meltzoff. None the less, the results revealed the same patterns seen in the original re-enactment method of Meltzoff (1995). Not only were infants able to reproduce the same literal outcomes of a series of actions produced by a non-human agent on objects (52% of the time), they were also able to produce the same target outcomes even when the agent tried but failed to produce them itself (37%). Both of the experimental conditions produced more target actions than infants produced spontaneously (only 10% of the time). As argued by Meltzoff (1995), this pattern indicates that the infants interpreted the agent's actions in terms of the agent's goals, rather than the spatio-temporal characteristics of the movements themselves, thus confirming the prediction that infants attribute goals (and mentalism) more broadly than previously thought.

10.4 The attribution of communication to non-human agents: morphological and behavioural cues

In Johnson *et al.* (2001) we reasoned that if imitation of goals reflects an interpretation of the orangutan as an agent, that interpretation might be manifested in other ways as well. Communicative gestures such as showing, requesting and waving are all behaviours reflecting putative mentalistic attributions of agents. Informal coding of the infants in the goal re-enactment study revealed that most infants in all three conditions directed some sort of social/communicative behaviour at the agent at least once, including waving, showing or giving objects, requesting objects or alternating attention between the agent's face and a toy.

We ran a further study to rule out the possibility that the infants were simply taking their cues from the experimenter either by imitating the experimenter's gestures directly or by more generally imitating the experimenter's stance toward the agent. To do this, we built another novel object out of a common table lamp that was matched to the orangutan as closely as possible for visual interest without actually having any intrinsically agentive features of its own. It had comparable shape, colour patterns and moving parts. The experimenter then deliberately tried to induce in the infant a mentalistic stance towards the lamp on the basis of the experimenter's behaviour alone. The experimenter talked to the lamp, called it by name ('Bob'), and invited infants to communicate with the lamp by giving and requesting objects. Despite these direct attempts to induce the mentalistic stance infants were quite reluctant to treat it as an agent themselves. Though they waved to the orangutan, showed it objects, offered it objects, requested objects from it and actually withdrew physically from the orangutan, these behaviours were rarely used with the lamp.

10.5 Preliminary summary

These three distinct infant behaviours, attentional following, imitation/ goal-re-enactment and communicative gestures, have traditionally been thought to be the unique province of infant–adult interactions. These data now show that each can be elicited by non-human objects if those objects look or behave as agents themselves. The remainder of this paper will review two distinct lines of work that follow on from these original findings. The first addresses how the changes or lack of changes in these attribution patterns over development can inform our understanding of the representational systems involved. The second tests the power of behaviour alone to elicit mentalistic attributions from infants in the absence of supporting morphological cues. I will then conclude with some preliminary work on autism.

10.6 The revisability of the agent category

Some theorists (Fodor 1983; Leslie 1994, 1995; Baron-Cohen 1995; Carey and Spelke 1996; Johnson 2000; Scholl and Tremoulet 2000) have suggested that the selective use of low-level spatio-temporal information of the sort epitomized in temporally contingent interactions and facial configurations is characteristic of 'hardwired' object recognition processes. In addition, there is ample evidence now that infants can detect both faces and contingency information within the first weeks of life, while experience is still quite limited (faces: Morton and Johnson 1991; Slater *et al.* 2000; Slater and Quinn 2001; contingency: Watson 1972, 1979; Rovee-Collier *et al.* 1989).

One consequence of hardwired processes is incorrigibility in the face of counter-evidence, both over time developmentally and in real-time processing as seen in the case of familiar perceptual illusions. Illusions, such as the Mueller-Lyer illusion in which two lines of objectively equal length are made to look subjectively unequal by adding either inverted or everted arrows to their ends, are found throughout the processes responsible for the detection of 3D physical objects (Rock 1983). For real illusions, no amount of counter-evidence or insight into the reality of the situation will eliminate the perception.

Conversely, revisability is considered a characteristic of constructed concepts (Gopnik and Wellman 1994; Carey and Spelke 1996; Gopnik and Meltzoff 1997). Consider for instance, whether markings on a piece of paper are recognized as art. The answer can vary from culture to culture, generation to generation, person to person, and most importantly for present purposes, even over time within the same person. There appear to be no universal, hardwired 'art recognition' processes that yield the same output for all viewers regardless of past experience or beliefs.

This distinction between incorrigible and revisable representational systems and the resulting potential for illusions indicates a possible point of leverage into processes underlying infants' responses to the novel agent of Johnson *et al.* (1998). Even in its most animated states, the novel agent presented ample evidence *against* a categorization as an agent. To an adult, it would clearly be an artefact made of synthetic materials with an electromechanical noise generator and mechanically driven movement. If, despite this obvious counter-evidence, it elicited a psychological interpretation in adults, the argument that agent recognition is grounded in a hardwired system would be supported. Furthermore, this would indicate that the system is functional by at least 12 months as reflected in the infants' behaviour in Johnson *et al.* (1998).

Empirical evidence indicates that adults do experience illusions of mentalistic agency based on certain types of movement cue (e.g. the work of Heider and Simmel (1944)). Less work has been done on the role of contingent interactivity in adults' mentalistic attributions. Bassili (1976) showed adults 2D animations similar to those of Heider and Simmel (1944), except that temporal contingency and directional information were both carefully manipulated. He found that adults were sensitive to both types of information when interpreting the behaviour of unknown objects. Interestingly, participants seemed to use an object's contingent behaviour to categorize it as intentional and the direction of its movement to identify the content of its intention (i.e. its goal).

Given these considerations—the existence of hardwired object recognition processes in general and the probable existence of an 'illusion of psychological agency' in adulthood—whether the features that elicit attentional following in infants are themselves part of a dedicated system for recognizing agents bears consideration. If so, they should elicit parallel attributions in adults, despite adults' undeniable *beliefs* to the contrary. The results by Bassili (1976) suggest that they would, but given the considerable differences in stimuli and methods between the infant and adult work, additional studies seem merited.

S. C. Johnson (unpublished data) presented adults with a series of studies based on the attentional-following studies with infants described in Johnson *et al.* (1998). Adults were introduced to the same novel object under the same conditions—whether it had facial features and whether it interacted contingently to another agent. The proven verbal method used in the work of Heider and Simmel (1944) was adopted, rather than attentional following owing to the seeming potential for conscious, overt suppression of voluntary eye movements by adults. Participants' implicit impressions of the objects would be expressed in their verbal descriptions, which could then be coded for the use of mentalistic language.

The parallels between the adults' attributions and those found previously with infants were striking. Adults used mentalistic language to describe the behaviour of the object in just those conditions that infants followed the object's directional orientation with their gaze. If the object had a face or if it was faceless, but interacted contingently with another agent, adults described it as 'wanting' something, 'looking' for something, 'trying' to do something, and so on. If, however, it did not have a face and acted only randomly, adults rarely if ever used mentalistic language to describe its behaviour. This result held regardless of whether the object's behaviour was instantiated auditorily (via contingent or random beeping) or visually (via contingent or random wiggling).

10.7 Directly experienced versus observed interaction

One important difference characterized the contingent behaviours in the study with adults and the original study with infants. Infants interacted with the object themselves and thus experienced the contingency directly. Adults, however, were not expected to babble spontaneously, nor respond to the object if it acted. Therefore the interactivity of the object was modelled for the adults by a confederate. Using a standard script, the confederate engaged in 'small talk' with the object for 60 s before leaving the subject alone with it. In the contingent conditions, when the confederate spoke to the object, the object beeped or wiggled in response. To ensure that this change did not affect infants' ability to perceive the interactivity of the object, we ran a further infant condition in which they also observed the object interact with a confederate. Like the adults, and the infants before them, they followed the directional orientation of the contingently interacting object, but not the object that beeped randomly.

Some might worry that the data collected under these conditions could reflect attributions by the infant based on cues extrinsic to the object, such as the modelled 'intentional stance' of the confederate. Indeed, a further study with adults showed that some, though not all, of adults' attributions could be accounted for by just such an extrinsic cue. Such an explanation of infants' behaviours would warrant a different theoretical account than the one offered here. Two points argue against this possibility. First, data already discussed suggest that infants of this age are not yet able to exploit that sort of information. In Johnson *et al.* (2001; discussed in Section 10.4) we deliberately tried and failed to elicit mentalistic attributions from 15-month-old infants on the basis of the experimenter's behaviour alone. Without the accompanying mentalistic cues from the object itself, infants failed to make the mentalistic attributions.

Second, although infants certainly have the ability by this age to imitate the intentions of an adult (or an animated, stuffed orangutan), even among more commonplace contexts, infants' imitation abilities are constrained by their ability to make sense of the intention. For example, 11-month-old infants are happy to imitate an adult putting a bird to bed 'to sleep'. They will, however, resist putting a car to bed 'to sleep' even after seeing an adult do so (McDonough and Mandler 1998). The implication is that infants imitate things they can make sense of. It appears that the overt mentalistic attributions of an adult towards another object only makes sense when that other object is already construed as an agent by a child of this age. When and how infants acquire the ability to use only another's stance towards a novel object to categorize it is still an open question.

10.8 The attribution of perception/attention to morphologically ambiguous objects: reasoning from behavioural cues alone

The work described so far indicates that infants can use either morphological or behavioural information to categorize a novel object as an agent. The evidence for either as an entirely sufficient cue in its own right has not yet been shown. In each case in which infants seemed to have made a mentalistic attribution a combination of cues were present. For instance, in the attentional-following studies of Johnson *et al.* (1998), neither the presence of a face nor the ability to interact contingently was necessary to elicit following from infants—either cue could elicit the behaviour without the other. However, in all cases the object was also animated and had familiar animal-like, if not human, morphology. A face stencilled onto an inert plastic blob might not be a convincing agent, neither might a faceless, plastic blob even if it were animated in appropriately mentalistic ways.

In the following studies we have concentrated on the ability of just one of these cues—behaviour—to elicit mentalistic attributions on its own. Are infants willing to categorize a novel object as an agent even if it bears no perceptual similarity to any familiar agent? To address this issue, we created a new novel object that was intended to be as perceptually unlike any familiar agent as we could make it. The object was the approximate size and shape of an adult's shoe, draped in bright green fibrefill. It could make beeping noises and move on its own around a large black table. It was symmetrical both front to back and side to side and had no distinguishing marks anywhere on its surface. Unlike the original furry brown agent, adults never spontaneously label this 'agent' as anything other than an inanimate object. Anecdotally when shown the object sitting inactive on the table, adults typically describe it as a slipper, lint, cotton candy, etc. (see Fig. 10.4).

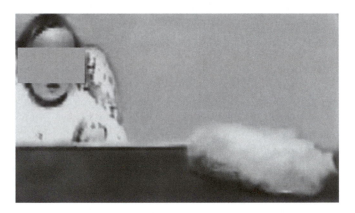

Fig. 10.4   The green blob. This object could move around and make noise on its own. (From Johnson *et al.* 2003.) See Plate 5 of the Plate Section, at the centre of this book.

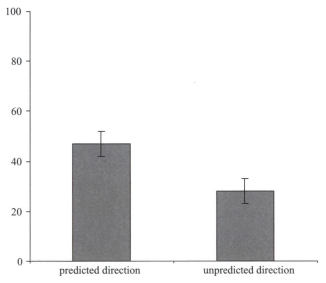

Fig. 10.5   Results from first green blob attentional-following study of Johnson *et al.* (2003). The score on the *y*-axis equals the average percentage of first looks in a given direction across all trials.

In our first study with this object (Johnson *et al.* 2003), 14-month-old infants were seated in front of the experimental display and shown the location of two toy target objects at each front corner. Infants then observed an adult confederate engage the object in small talk as before. After the confederate left the room, the infant watched as the object turned to one side or the other. Again, infants' responses were coded as either in the predicted or unpredicted direction. If infants' responses to the original agent were owing to its similarity to familiar animals, looks in this condition, with a very un-animal like object, should be evenly split in the two directions. Fig. 10.5 shows the relative percentages of infants' first looks in each direction. As in the case with the original furry brown agent, infants looked significantly more often in the direction in which the object turned, even though the agent in this case was more perceptually reminiscent of a shoe than an animal.

10.9 Assigning perceptual/attentional orientation

Although the results described in Section 10.8 were predicted on the assumption of the importance of behaviour in the categorization of agents, they did pose a puzzle of sorts. By stripping the object of any recognizable facial or body features, we also stripped the object of a distinctive front and back. It is one thing to realize that an unfamiliar object is an agent with the ability to perceive the world, it is possibly a separate thing altogether to determine that agent's perceptual orientation. That is, in the absence of eyes and the absence of any relevant asymmetry in the object's shape, how did the infants know which end was the front? Put another way, owing to the object's symmetry and rigidity, a single clockwise rotation of the object could be interpreted by an observer as either the end proximal (or nearest to the observer) turning to the observer's left or as the distal end turning to the observer's right. Regardless of the interpretation, the objective spatio-temporal event witnessed by the observer would be the same. None the less, infants were able to make a systematic judgement about this, without which they would not have produced systematic behaviours.

Given the absence of any detectable facial or head-like features, we proposed that infants would use the apparent ability of the object to *perceive* the confederate and targets to disambiguate its front from its back. That is, they would assume that the side facing the confederate and targets was the front, independent of their own orientation. Of course this prediction holds only on the assumption that infants do categorize the object as an agent—that is, as an object whose behaviour is directed at the world. Importantly, this prediction is agnostic with respect to which specific modality, if any, infants assume the perception is embedded in (i.e. vision, audition, electromagnetic sensors, etc.).

If this hypothesis is correct, we should be able to control which end infants designate as the object's 'front', and thus which direction they look, by manipulating the location of the confederate and the targets during the interaction.

Again, such a result would imply that infants interpreted the behaviour of the object in terms of its *inferred relationship with the world*—a notion at the heart of agency—rather than simply responding to non-relational characteristics of its appearance or movement.

Fourteen-month-old infants participated in one of two conditions (Johnson *et al.* 2003). In both conditions the infants were first shown the targets. They then observed a human confederate engage the agent in the same scripted 'conversation' used before. The two conditions varied only in where the confederate stood during her conversation with the agent and where the targets were placed on the platform. In one condition the confederate stood next to the seated infant, facing the proximal end of the agent. In the other the confederate stood across the table from the infant, facing the distal end of the agent (see Fig. 10.6). The targets were placed on the same side as the confederate. After interacting for around 60 s, the confederate left the room and the agent executed four test trials in which it first beeped loudly then rotated around 45° in one direction or the other.

In the proximal condition (Fig. 10.6*a*) significantly more of infants' first looks away from the object were in the same direction that the proximal end of the object turned than predicted by chance. This replicated the results shown in the previous study. The interesting question is what they did in the distal condition. The observed test event was exactly the same. However, if infants were categorizing the object as an agent with a distinct front through which it perceived the world, the inferred event should have been reversed. That is, infants should now preferentially look in the same direction as the end of the object most distal to themselves.

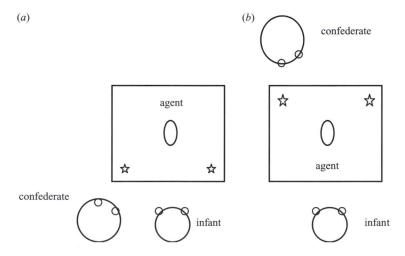

Fig. 10.6 A bird's-eye view of the setup in the orientation assignment study of Johnson *et al.* (2003). (*a*) Proximal condition, (*b*) distal condition.

That is what they did. Infants in the distal condition (Fig. 10.6*b*) reversed their looking behaviour relative to infants in the proximal condition. Significantly more of the first looks away from the object were in the direction of the distal end, rather than the canonical proximal end. In effect, infants behaved as though they were watching an agent from behind. These results are remarkable not only because infants in this context did not need facial features to cue their looking, but they were also able to override any potential prepotent egocentric tendencies to treat the side facing them as the front. How exactly infants accomplished this and how they represented the hidden 'face' to themselves, remains to be seen.

Based on these results we can tentatively conclude that around the end of the first year, infants are able to categorize a completely novel object as a mentalistic agent on the basis of its behaviour alone. In the studies described so far they seem to be reasoning not only about the ability of the object to perceive or attend to the world, but the actual geometric orientation of the object that would make that most plausible.

10.10 The attribution of goals to morphologically ambiguous objects: reasoning from behavioural cues alone

Returning again to our original empirical strategy, we hoped to test whether infants would attribute other putative mental states to the novel green blob using different behavioural measures from those involved in attentional following. As before, we chose the attribution of goals as an important test. Previously we showed that infants would attribute goals to an agent that looked in many ways like a human. The current study was designed to test whether they would also attribute goals to an agent that was entirely unlike any agent the infant was likely to have seen.

Importantly, the orangutan agent in the previous goal study (Johnson *et al*. 2001) had articulated hands. This had two advantages not available in the current study. First, the hands allowed the agent to manipulate objects in a variety of ways. This provided a wide range of possible object-directed goals for testing purposes. In contrast, the current agent has no articulated parts of any sort. This restricted the possible object manipulations to varieties of pushing actions, thereby limiting the overall attractiveness of the method.

Second, with the possession of an articulated set of hands, the mapping between actions the infant observed and actions the infant needed to produce was (relatively) straightforward. In contrast, an infant observing the green blob act on objects would gain little information about how to produce the same outcomes with their own, very different, body. This lack of correspondence has important task demand implications for us. To the extent that infants observe goals that are achieved through means—actions that cannot be easily mapped onto their own action patterns, a failure to imitate is difficult to interpret.

To avoid these issues we sought a methodology that would be both sensitive to goal attributions and also appropriate for use with infants of this age given this agent. The work by Woodward (1998) provides such a method. This used the visual habituation method to test whether infants encode human actions as the goals of the actor, or solely as the spatio-temporal movements involved. One group of infants were habituated to a hand approaching one of two toys on a stage. In the test events, one of two things changed, either (i) the spatio-temporal path of the hand, or (ii) its target object. Woodward reasoned that if infants encoded the hand's action as *goal*-directed (reflecting an agent–world relationship), test trials in which the goal changed should be more novel, and therefore more interesting, than those in which the path changed. Indeed, infants less than a year old dishabituated to the change in the hand's target relative to the change in the hand's path. A separate group of infants habituated and tested on identical events in which the 'agent' was a rod instead of a hand, exhibited quite different patterns. These infants did not dishabituate to the change in the target object of the rod, indicating that they had not encoded the *relationship* between the rod and the object as an important aspect of the event.

The results of Woodward (1998) indicate that even before the end of the first year, infants recognize that:

(i) the behaviour of some (but not all) entities is directed at the world; and
(ii) the identity of the entity's target is relevant, i.e. the content of the relationship is represented.

We can therefore say that infants attribute an intentional relationship between the object and the world (i.e. one based on content).

Like Meltzoff (1995); Woodward (1998) argued that infants' reasoning about goals and mental states is restricted to their reasoning about humans. However, like Meltzoff (1995), Woodward (1998) showed that infants exclude some objects from their agent category, not that they include only humans. Like the non-agentive pincers of Meltzoff (1995), the rod of Woodward (1998), though grossly similar to a human arm and hand, shows none of the specific putative behaviour or morphology of agents. To adequately demonstrate a person-only reasoning domain, infants need to be tested with more theoretically motivated non-human 'agents'.

Shimizu and Johnson (2003) tested these claims by showing 12-month-old infants the novel green blob in a procedure based on the dishabituation method of Woodward (1998) that compared changes in spatio-temporal path to changes in target object. To make the behavioural test as strong as possible, two groups of infants were tested with the same green blob. The only difference between the two groups was the behaviour of the novel object in the introduction and habituation phases of the study. In an agent condition, infants were introduced to the object with our now-standard confederate conversation. The confederate talked to the object and the object beeped back. In the non-agent condition the confederate remained silent while the object beeped its way through the same script (thus appearing random). In addition, at the beginning of each habituation trial, the agentive blob began its action facing the 'non-goal' object, thus requiring a deliberate 'choice' to turn toward the 'goal' before beginning its approach. In comparison the non-agentive blob simply began each habituation trial facing in the same direction that it ultimately moved—towards the target object.

Infants in both conditions saw exactly the same test events—one in which the green blob's trajectory was changed, but its target object was not, and one in which the blob's target object was changed, but the trajectory itself remained unchanged. Unlike in the habituation trials, in the test trials, the green blob always began its action oriented in the direction it moved, regardless of condition.

None the less, these two conditions, the interactive, choice-making agent versus the non-interactive mechanical-like non-agent, yielded quite different interpretations from the infants. Infants in the non-agent condition treated the two test outcomes (changes in trajectory versus changes in target) equivalently. Nothing in their behaviour indicated that they selectively attended to the relationship between the blob and the objects in its immediate world. Infants in the agent condition acted quite differently however. They looked significantly longer at the test events in which the target of the blob's action changed compared with those events in which the trajectory of the blob's action changed. As in the studies of Woodward (1998), this indicates that infants coded the relationship between the blob's actions and a specific object in the world to the exclusion of other more superficial or perceptual aspects of the events that they could have attended to. Thus, we can conclude that infants considered the interactive, choice-making blob to be an agent, just like a human. The fact that infants in the other condition did not reach that conclusion when they observed the very same object behave in non-agentive ways strengthens the case that it is the behaviour, not the appearance of the object, that infants used in making their interpretations.

10.11 The relationship between agency and metarepresentations: the case of autism

It is tempting to predict that people with autism, now famous for their inability to read minds (Baron-Cohen *et al*. 1985, 1993; Baron-Cohen 1995), would be incapable of detecting or following the attentional orientation of the novel objects described in this chapter. It is, after all, well documented that people with autism do not spontaneously follow the gaze of other humans (e.g. Leekam *et al*. 1997). Preliminary results from our laboratory, however, indicate that this prediction is premature (Giovanelli and Johnson 2003). A group of older autistic children and adolescents were introduced to the faceless furry brown agent in the same manner used with typical adults and infants—a confederate engaged the agent in a brief conversation and then left the room. When the agent then turned away from participants, the participants turned reliably and spontaneously to look in the direction of its turn. In a non-interactive control condition, participants did not follow the turns.

These results lead to immediate further questions about the development of theory of mind both in general and in autism specifically. In general, additional experiences and/or cognitive mechanisms than those discussed here must clearly be involved in typical development. The additional pieces of the developmental puzzle could come in the form of other specialized mechanisms (see, for instance, the multi-mechanism accounts of theory of mind by both Baron-Cohen (1995) and Leslie (1994, 1995)). Alternatively, further development could depend on more general theory-building abilities (see, for instance, Gopnik and Wellman (1994) and Perner (1991)).

In addition, although it is now well documented that people with autism have difficulty reasoning about other people's higher-order mental states such as beliefs, is this difficulty uniform across the agent domain? Do people with autism also fail to attribute false beliefs to non-humans, e.g. dogs? Although there is scant existing evidence about autistics' conceptions of animals, at least one recent study suggests that their social aversion is restricted to people. In direct contrast to an atypical preference for inanimates over people, tests of their preferences for animals did not differ from typically developing children (Celani 2002). Is the core difficulty therefore with *metarepresentation* in all its manifestations, or with *people* in all their manifestations? These new findings might provide an additional wedge with which to approach the question.

Regardless of how this question is ultimately answered, the results from autism demonstrate that the ability to divide the world into agents and non-agents may be necessary, but is clearly not sufficient for the normal development of theory of mind.

10.12 Conclusions

The studies described here challenge assumptions about the scope and origins of humans' mentalistic reasoning. Twelve- to fifteen-month-old infants were shown to treat novel self-moving objects as though they have both perception/attention, communicative abilities and goals if they either look like an agent (i.e. have a face) or behave in specific ways (e.g. are contingently interactive with other known agents). The infants were able to detect the highly abstract temporal relationship between actors whether they themselves were one of the actors or not. Surprisingly, no evidence has yet been found within these studies to indicate that self-movement alone will elicit this interpretation from infants of this age. Neither did infants of this age appear willing or able to infer an object's agenthood solely on the basis of how an adult treated it. Impressively, it seems that once infants did categorize an object as an agent they actively used the geometric information implicit in its interactions with its environment to infer its perceptual/attentional orientation.

The scope of the agent category implied by these findings is far broader than the category of people. Neither do the findings seem to be easily accounted for by a non-mentalistically interpreted similarity metric with people. Similarity metrics require dimensions. Morphological features, interactivity and self-movement are all possible highly salient dimensions of humans that infants might use to generalize. None the less, infants of this age seem to ignore some morphological features (animal shape, colour and texture) and self-movement as relevant dimensions in their own right for these inferences.

Despite adults' obvious *understanding and beliefs* that the novel objects shown to infants were artefacts and thus not true agents, the objects elicited very similar interpretations in adults to those elicited in infants. This finding suggests that the representational system underlying the infants' attributions is not open to revision. If it were adults would have long since revised it out of existence. By implication then, the system is not a constructed one.

Preliminary evidence tentatively shows that the system typically used to recognize agents is also available in autism. This is consistent with the view that the input system for the social reasoning system is dissociable from other parts of the system, such as the part responsible for handling metarepresentations.

Taken together, the evidence from infants' reasoning about truly ambiguous unfamiliar objects (e.g. novel green blobs) suggests that at least by the age of 1 year, humans have a very abstract representational system for detecting and reasoning about social agents. Whether it is the same system that represents the configural and movement patterns of humans such as described elsewhere in this volume is an open question. Perhaps the human body-centric input system for the social reasoning circuit described in Chapter 3; (STS) is only one of multiple input systems. Alternatively, perhaps STS includes representational abilities that have not yet been described, including the ability to represent temporal relationships between entities independent of their appearance.

The author is supported by a grant from the National Institutes of Health, RO1 HD38361.

References

Baldwin, D. A. and Moses, L. J. (1996). The ontogeny of social information gathering. *Child Dev.* **67**, 1915–39.

Baron-Cohen, S. (1995). *Mindblindness: an essay on autism and theory of mind.* Cambridge, MA: MIT Press.

Baron-Cohen, S., Leslie, A. M. and Frith, U. (1985). Does the autistic child have a 'Theory of Mind'? *Cognition* **21**, 37–46.

Baron-Cohen, S. Tager-Flusberg, H. and Cohen, D. (eds) (1993). *Understanding other minds: perspectives from autism.* Oxford: Oxford University Press.

Bassili, J. N. (1976). Temporal and spatial contingencies in the perception of social events. *J. Personality Soc. Psychol.* **33**, 680–5.

Bates, E., Camaioni, L. and Volterra, V. (1975). The acquisition of performatives prior to speech. *Merrill-Palmer Q.* **21**, 205–26.

Bretherton, I., McNew, S. and Beeghly-Smith, M. (1981). Early person knowledge as expressed in gestural and verbal communications: when do infants acquire a 'theory of mind'? In *Infant social cognition* (ed. M. E. Lamb and L. R. Sherrod), pp. 333–74. Hillsdale, NJ: Lawrence Erlbaum Associates.

Butterworth, G. E. and Grover, L. (1988). The origins of referential communication in human infancy. In *Thought without language* (ed. L. Weiskrantz), pp. 5–24. Oxford: Oxford University Press.

Butterworth, G. and Jarrett, N. (1991). What minds have in common is space: spatial mechanisms serving joint visual attention in infancy. *Br. J. Devl Psychol.* **9**, 55–72.

Carey, S. and Spelke, E. (1994). Domain-specific knowledge and conceptual change. In *Mapping the mind: domain specificity in cognition and culture* (ed. L. A. Hirschfeld and S. A. Gelman), pp. 169–200. New York: Cambridge University Press.

Carey, S. and Spelke, E. (1996). Science and core knowledge. *Phil. Sci.* **63**, 515–33.

Celani, G. (2002). Human beings, animals and inanimate objects: what do people with autism like? *Autism* **6**, 93–102.

Corkum, V. and Moore, C. (1998). The origins of joint visual attention in infants. *Devl Psychol.* **34**, 28–38.

Dennett, D. (1978). Response to Premack, D. and Woodruff, G. Does the chimpanzee have a theory of mind? *Behav. Brain Sci.* **4**, 568–70.

D'Entremont, B., Hains, S. M. J. and Muir, D. W. (1997). A demonstration of gaze following in 3- to 6-month-olds. *Infant Behav. Dev.* **20**, 569–72.

Ellsworth, C., Muir, D. and Hains, S. (1993). Social competence and person–object differentiation: an analysis of the still-face effect. *Devl Psychol.* **29**, 63–73.

Field, T. M., Woodson, R., Greenberg, R. and Cohen, D. (1982). Discrimination and imitation of facial expressions by neonates. *Science* **218**, 179–81.

Fodor, J. A. (1983). *The modularity of mind: an essay on faculty psychology.* Cambridge, MA: MIT Press.

Frye, D., Rawling, P., Moore, C. and Myers, I. (1983). Object–person discrimination and communication at 3 and 10 months. *Devl Psychol.* **19**, 303–9.

Gerwitz, J. L. and Pelaez-Nogueras, M. (1992). Social referencing as a learned process. In *Social referencing and the social construction of reality in infancy* (ed. S. Feinman), pp. 151–73. New York: Plenum Press.

Gibson, E. J., Owsley, C. J. and Johnson, J. (1978). Perception of invariants by 5-month-old infants: differentiation of two types of motion. *Devl Psychol.* **14**, 407–16.

Giovanelli, J. and Johnson, S. C. (2003). The attribution of minds to novel objects by autistic children and adolescents (In preparation.)

Gopnik, A. and Meltzoff, A. (1997). *Words, thoughts, and theories.* Cambridge, MA: MIT Press.

Gopnik, A. and Wellman, H. M. (1994). The theory theory. In *Mapping the mind: domain specificity in cognition and culture* (ed. L. A. Hirschfeld and S. A. Gelman), pp. 257–93. New York: Cambridge University Press.

Heider, F. and Simmel, M. (1944). An experimental study of apparent behavior. *Am. J. Psychol.* **57**, 243–59.

Hood, B. M., Willen, J. D. and Driver, J. (1998). Adults' eyes trigger shifts of visual attention in human infants. *Psychol. Sci.* **9**(2), 131–4.

Johnson, S. C. (2000). The recognition of mentalistic agents in infancy. *Trends Cogn. Sci.* **4**, 22–8.

Johnson, S. C., Slaughter, V. and Carey, S. (1998). Whose gaze will infants follow? Features that elicit gaze-following in 12-month-olds. *Devl Sci.* **1**, 233–8.

Johnson, S. C., Booth, A. and O'Hearn, K. (2001). Inferring the goals of non-human agents. *Cogn. Dev.* **16**, 637–56.

Johnson, S. C., Bolz, M., Carter, E., Mandsangar, J., Teichner, A. and Zettler, P. (2003). Inferring the attentional orientation of morphologically novel agents in infancy. (In preparation.)

Leekam, S., Baron-Cohen, S., Perret, D., Milders, M. and Brown, S. (1997). Eye-direction detection: a dissociation between geometric and joint attention skills in autism. *Br. J. Devl Psychol.* **15**, 77–95.

Legerstee, M. (1991). The role of person and object in eliciting early imitation. *J. Exp. Child Psychol.* **51**, 423–33.

Legerstee, M. (1992). A review of the animate-inanimate distinction in infancy: implications for models of social and cognitive knowing. *Early Dev. Parenting* **1**, 59–67.

Legerstee, M. (1994). Patterns of 4-month-old infant responses to hidden silent and sounding people and objects. *Early Dev. Parenting* **3**, 71–80.

Legerstee, M. (1997). Contingency effects of people and objects on subsequent cognitive functioning in 3-month-old infants. *Social Dev.* **6**, 307–21.

Legerstee, M., Pomerleau, A., Malcuit, G. and Feider, H. (1987). The development of infants' responses to people and a doll: implications for research in communication. *Infant Behav. Dev.* **10**, 81–95.

Lempers, J. D. (1979). Young children's production and comprehension of nonverbal deictic behaviors. *J. Genet. Psychol.* **135**, 93–102.

Leslie, A. M. (1994). ToMM, ToBy, and agency: core architecture and domain specificity. In *Mapping the mind: domain specificity in cognition and culture* (ed. L. A. Hirschfeld and S. A. Gelman), pp. 119–48. New York: Cambridge University Press.

Leslie, A. M. (1995). A theory of Agency. In *Causal cognition: a multidisciplinary debate* (ed. D. Sperber, D. Premack and A. J. Premack), pp. 121–41. Oxford: Clarendon Press.

Leung, E. H. L. and Rheingold, H. L. (1981). Development of pointing as a social gesture. *Dev. Psychol.* **17**, 215–20.

Lycan, W. (1999). Intentionality. In *MIT Encyclopedia of Cognitive Science* (ed. R. Wilson and F. Keil), pp. 413–15. Cambridge, MA: MIT Press.

McDonough, L. and Mandler, J. M. (1998). Inductive generalization in 9- and 11-month-olds. *Devl Sci.* **1**, 227–32.

Meltzoff, A. N. (1995). Understanding the intention of others: re-enactment of intended acts by 18-month-old children. *Devl Psychol.* **31**, 838–50.

Meltzoff, A. N. and Moore, M. (1983). Newborn infants imitate adult facial gestures. *Child Dev.* **54**, 702–9.

Meltzoff, A. N. and Moore, M. K. (1977). Imitation of facial and manual gestures by human neonates. *Science* **198**, 75–8.

Moore, C. and Corkum, V. (1994). Social understanding at the end of the first year of life. *Devl Rev.* **14**, 349–72.

Morton, J. and Johnson, M. M. (1991). CONSPEC and CONLERN: a two-process theory of infant face recognition. *Psychol. Rev.* **98**, 164–81.

Moses, L. J., Baldwin, D. A., Rosicky, J. G. and Tidball, G. (2001). Evidence for referential understanding in the emotions domain at twelve and eighteen months. *Child Dev.* **72**, 718–35.

Perner, J. (1991). *Understanding the representational mind.* Cambridge, MA: MIT Press.

Poulin-Dubois, D. (1999). Infants' distinction between animate and inanimate objects: the origins of naive psychology. In *Early social cognition* (ed. P. Rochat), pp. 257–80. Hillsdale, NJ: Lawrence Erlbaum Associates.

Poulin-Dubois, D., Lepage, A. and Ferland, D. (1996). Infants' concept of animacy. *Cogn. Dev.* **11**, 19–36.

Premack, D. (1990). The infant's theory of self-propelled objects. *Cognition* **36**, 1–16.

Premack, D. (1991). The infant's theory of self-propelled objects. In *Children's theories of mind: mental states and social understanding* (ed. D. Frye and C. Moore), pp. 39–48. Hillsdale, NJ: Lawrence Erlbaum Associates.

Repacholi, B. M. and Gopnik, A. (1997). Early reasoning of desires: evidence from 14- to 18-month-olds. *Devl Psychol.* **33**, 12–21.

Ricard, M. and Allard, L. (1993). The reaction of 9- to 10-monthold infants to an unfamiliar animal. *J. Genet. Psychol.* **154**, 5–16.

Rock, I. (1983). *The logic of perception.* Cambridge, MA: MIT Press.

Rovee-Collier, C. K., Earley, L. and Stafford, S. (1989). Ontogeny of early event memory: III. Attentional determinants of retrieval at 2 and 3 months. *Infant Behav. Dev.* **12**, 147–61.

Scaife, J. F. and Bruner, J. S. (1975). The capacity for joint visual attention in the infant. *Nature* **253**, 265–6.

Scholl, B. J. and Tremoulet, P. D. (2000). Perceptual causality and animacy. *Trends Cogn. Sci.* **4**, 299–309.

Shimizu, Y. A. and Johnson, S. C. (2003). The attribution of goals to morphologically novel agents by twelve-month-olds. (In preparation.)

Slater, A. and Quinn, P. C. (2001). Face recognition in the newborn infant. *Infant Child Dev.* (Special Issue: Face Processing in Infancy and Early Childhood) **10**, 21–4.

Slater, A., Bremner, G., Johnson, S. P., Sherwood, P., Hayes, R. and Brown, E. (2000). Newborn infants' preference for attractive faces: the role of internal and external facial features. *Infancy* **1**, 265–74.

Spelke, E., Phillips, A. and Woodward, A. (1995). Infants' knowledge of object motion and human action. In *Causal cognition: a multidisciplinary debate* (ed. D. Sperber, D. Premack and A. Premack), pp. 44–78. Oxford: Clarendon Press.

Watson, J. S. (1972). Smiling, cooing, and 'the game'. *Merrill-Palmer Q.* **118**, 323–40.

Watson, J. S. (1979). Perception of contingency as a determinant of social responsiveness. In *Origins of the infant's social responsiveness: the Johnson and Johnson baby products company pediatric round table*, II (ed. E. G. Thoman), pp. 33–64. Hillsdale, NJ: Lawrence Erlbaum.

Wellman, H. M. (1993). Early understanding of mind: the normal case. In *Understanding other minds: perspectives from autism* (ed. S. Baron-Cohen, H. Tager-Flusberg and D. J. Cohen), pp. 10–39. Oxford: Oxford University Press.

Woodward, A. (1998). Infants selectively encode the goal object of an actor's reach. *Cognition* **69**, 1–34.

Glossary

STS: superior temporal sulcus

11

Facial expressions, their communicatory functions and neuro-cognitive substrates

R. J. R. Blair

Human emotional expressions serve a crucial communicatory role allowing the rapid transmission of valence information from one individual to another. This paper will review the literature on the neural mechanisms necessary for this communication: both the mechanisms involved in the production of emotional expressions and those involved in the interpretation of the emotional expressions of others. Finally, reference to the neuro-psychiatric disorders of autism, psychopathy and acquired sociopathy will be made. In these conditions, the appropriate processing of emotional expressions is impaired. In autism, it is argued that the basic response to emotional expressions remains intact but that there is impaired ability to represent the referent of the individual displaying the emotion. In psychopathy, the response to fearful and sad expressions is attenuated and this interferes with socialization resulting in an individual who fails to learn to avoid actions that result in harm to others. In acquired sociopathy, the response to angry expressions in particular is attenuated resulting in reduced regulation of social behaviour.

Keywords: facial expressions; amygdala; communication; psychopath; autism

11.1 Introduction

Facial expressions are a crucial component of human emotional and social behaviour and are believed to represent innate and automatic behaviour patterns (Darwin 1872). The purpose of this paper is to consider facial expressions: the stimuli that elicit their presentation, the neuro-cognitive systems necessary for their production, the neuro-cognitive systems that interpret the expressions produced by others and the conditions under which the interpreter may respond to the emoter thus closing the communicatory loop. To do this, I will make one fundamental assumption: that facial expressions of emotion do indeed have a communicatory function, and that they impart specific information to the observer. Thus, the suggestion will be that expressions of fearfulness, sadness and happiness are reinforcers that modulate the probability that a particular behaviour will be performed in the future. Indeed, fearful faces have been seen as aversive unconditioned stimuli that rapidly convey information to others that a novel stimulus is aversive and should be avoided

(Mineka and Cook 1993). Similarly, it has been suggested that sad facial expressions also act as aversive unconditioned stimuli discouraging actions that caused the display of sadness in another individual and motivating reparatory behaviours (Blair 1995). Happy expressions, in contrast, are appetitive unconditioned stimuli which increase the probability of actions to which they appear causally related (Matthews and Wells 1999). Disgusted expressions are also reinforcers but are used most frequently to provide information about foods (Rozin *et al*. 1993). Displays of anger or embarrassment, it is argued, do not act as unconditioned stimuli for aversive conditioning or instrumental learning. Instead, they are important signals to modulate current behavioural responding, particularly in situations involving hierarchy interactions (Blair and Cipolotti 2000; Keltner and Anderson 2000).

In contrast to the communicatory function assumption, there have been suggestions that emotional expressions are automatic displays that occur as a function of the emotional experience of the individual (Darwin 1872; Buck 1984; Izard and Malatesta 1987; Ekman 1997). According to these authors, although the expression may impart information to observers, the transmission of information is not their function. Instead, the expression is an automatic consequence of the individual's experience (Ekman 1997). However, the empirical literature does not indicate that individuals display emotional expressions automatically as a function of the degree to which they feel a particular emotion (Fridlund 1991; Camras 1994). Instead social context predicts probability of emotional expression in humans as it does probability of non-verbal displays in non-human species (Cheney and Seyfarth 1980; Hinde 1985). Thus, participants smile more at a humourous video or show greater distress to the sound of an individual in distress if they are together with another rather than if they are alone (Chovil 1991; Fridlund 1991). Similarly, infant smiling from the age of 10 months is almost entirely dependent on visual contact with the caregiver: without such contact the infant is very unlikely to smile (Jones and Raag 1989; Jones *et al*. 1991).

Importantly, the argument here is not that the display of an emotional expression implies intent to convey a specific message to the observer. The argument is simply that emotional expressions serve a communicatory function that they have evolved so that information on the valence of objects/ situations can be transmitted rapidly between conspecifics. Thus, important triggers for an emotional display include both an emotional event and also a potential observer. If there is no observer, the emotional display will either not occur or be considerably muted.

A particularly clear illustration of the communicatory function of emotional expressions can be seen after an infant's discovery of a novel object. The infant will look towards the primary caregiver and their behaviour will be determined by the caregiver's emotional display. If the caregiver displays an expression of fear or disgust, the child will avoid the novel object. If the caregiver displays a happy expression, the child will approach the novel object. This process is known as social referencing and is seen in children from the age of eight to ten months (Klinnert *et al*. 1983, 1987; Walker-Andrews 1998). Interestingly, comparable social referencing is seen in chimpanzees (Russell *et al*. 1997) and a very similar process has been shown in other monkeys and labelled observational fear (Mineka and Cook 1993).

Mineka characterizes the process of observational fear within an aversive conditioning framework (Mineka and Cook 1993). The US is the mother macaque's expression of fear, which she shows to the CS, the novel object. This maternal fearful expression, the US, elicits an unconditioned response, a fearful reaction, in the infant monkey. Pairing of the US with the CS, the novel object, allows the CS to elicit a conditioned response; the infant monkey comes to show a fearful reaction to the novel object.

A simple conditioning approach is, however, unlikely to be appropriate in humans. In humans, the representation of the emoter's intent has been shown to be crucial. Indeed, the learning of valences for novel objects can be thought of similarly to the learning of names for novel objects. When hearing a new word, children do not automatically associate this word with whatever novel object is in their immediate field of view. Instead, they turn towards the speaker, calculate the object that they are attending to, and associate the new word with this novel object (Baldwin *et al*. 1996; Bloom 2002). Similarly, during social referencing, if the child is attending to one object when the caregiver displays an emotional response to another, the child will look at the caregiver to determine the direction of their attention. The child will then form the appropriate association between the information communicated by the caregiver's expression and the object to which the caregiver had been attending (Moses *et al*. 2001). Thus, the communication of valence to objects, like the communication of names to objects, involves association of the affective information with a CS that corresponds to the communicator's referent.

11.2 The production of emotional expressions

The suggestion developed above is that emotional expressions are communicatory signals that function to convey valence information rapidly to conspecifics. Specifically, they are particularly likely to be elicited under conditions when there is an emotional stimulus in the environment and there is an audience to perceive the expression. But emotional expressions are not automatically elicited under these conditions. Individuals are capable of intentionally manipulating their emotional displays, they may follow 'display rules', societal proscriptions as to what emotion should be displayed in given circumstances and how intensely it should be displayed (Ekman and Friesen 1969). Indeed, one major task faced by the child in middle childhood is to learn the culture's display rules governing the conditions that are appropriate for the display of specific emotions. In a classic study of the development of display rules and control over emotional expressions, age-related changes were demonstrated in the ability of children to cover their disappointment at the discovery that their gift for helping out an adult was much less interesting than the gift they had been expecting; the disappointment of the younger children was far easier to detect (Saarni 1984).

There is thus a suggestion of spontaneous or over-learned emotional expressions to emotional stimuli in the presence of observers as well as controlled or posed emotional expressions as a function of display rules. It has been argued that the neuropsychological data about the production of emotional expressions echo this dichotomy (Rinn 1984; Hopf *et al.* 1992). Thus, it has been claimed that sub-cortical regions are necessary for spontaneous emotional displays but not controlled ones, whereas cortical regions are necessary for controlled emotional displays but not automatic emotional displays (Rinn 1984). However, this strict dichotomy overstates the empirical picture. Thus, investigations of patients with Parkinson's disease and other patients with damage to the basal ganglia report marked reductions in the production of spontaneous emotional expressions; such patients show reduced displays of emotional expressions when watching emotionally arousing videos relative to comparison individuals (Borod *et al.* 1990; Pitcairn *et al.* 1990; Weddell 1994; Smith *et al.* 1996). However, such patients also show some impairment in the production of posed emotional displays, though to a lesser degree (Borod *et al.* 1990; Weddell 1994; Smith *et al.* 1996). Similarly, there have been reports that lesions of frontal cortex impair the ability of the patient to pose emotional expressions but spare the production of spontaneous emotional expressions (Hopf *et al.* 1992). However, other studies find significant impairment in the production of both posed and spontaneous emotional expressions in patients with frontal cortex lesions (Weddell *et al.* 1988, 1990; Weddell 1994).

The data therefore suggest that sub-cortical regions, in particular basal ganglia, and cortical regions, particularly frontal cortex, are involved in both the production of spontaneous and controlled emotional displays. A schematic of regions known to be involved is presented in Fig. 11.1. Basal ganglia and frontal cortex are represented as reciprocally interconnected such that damage to either structure impairs the production of emotional expressions. The greater output from the frontal cortex represents the fact that while frontal cortical lesions cause significant impairment to both the production of spontaneous and controlled expressions (Weddell *et al.* 1988, 1990; Weddell 1994), lesions to the basal ganglia disproportionately affect the production of spontaneous expressions (Borod *et al.* 1990; Weddell 1994; Smith *et al.* 1996). Frontal cortex is likely to be crucial for representing goals to either show or suppress an emotional expression. The basal ganglia receives inputs from both the amygdala and other structures processing emotional information. Although amygdala lesions do reduce the display of spontaneous fearful

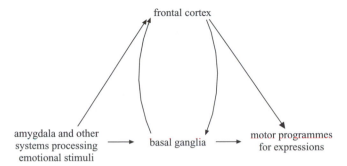

Fig. 11.1 A schematic of regions known to be involved in the production of emotional expressions.

displays to novel objects (Prather *et al.* 2001), they do not affect the production of controlled fearful or other emotional displays (Anderson and Phelps 2000).

11.3 Responding to the emotional expressions of others

Two dissociable routes have been shown to be involved in processing fear conditioning (Armony *et al.* 1997; LeDoux 2000). Thus, information on conditioned stimuli during auditory fear conditioning can be mediated by projections to the amygdala from either the auditory thalamus or auditory cortex (LeDoux *et al.* 1984; Romanski and LeDoux 1992*a,b*; Campeau and Davis 1995). Analogously, there have been suggestions that information on the emotional expressions of others can be conveyed either by a sub-cortical pathway (retinocollicular–pulvinar–amygdalar) or by a cortical pathway (retinogeniculostriate–extrastriate–fusiform) (de Gelder *et al.* 1999; Morris *et al.* 1999; Adolphs 2002).

The suggestion is that the sub-cortical pathway is fast and allows immediate automatic access of information on emotional expressions to the amygdala that can then modulate the processing of information through the cortical pathway (Pizzagalli *et al.* 1999; Adolphs 2002). In support of a sub-cortical pathway, positive covariations of cerebral blood flow (as measured by positron emission tomography imaging) have been demonstrated in the pulvinar, superior colliculus and amygdala in response to masked facial expressions of anger that had been previously associated with an aversive stimulus (Morris *et al.* 1999). Visual masking is assumed to be a result of interference between the induction of neural activity by the stimulus and the mask, which occurs within the relatively slow response time of primary visual cortex neurons (Macknik and Livingstone 1998). Neurons in the superior colliculus are capable of responding to much more rapid changes in visual input and hence produce quite distinct responses to the facial expression and neutral mask. However,

such responses fail to elicit conscious experience. Additional support for the
suggestion of a sub-cortical pathway has been provided by work with G.Y., a
patient with a long-standing right-sided hemianopia after occipital lobe damage at the age of 8 years (de Gelder *et al.* 1999). This 'blindsight' patient
showed some ability to discriminate (by guessing) between different facial
expressions in his blind hemifield. Later neuro-imaging work with G.Y.
demonstrated differential amygdala responses to fearful versus happy expressions when these were presented to both the blind and seeing hemifields.
However, striate and fusiform activity only occurred in response to stimuli
presented to the seeing hemifield. In addition, amygdala responses to fear conditioned faces exhibit condition-specific covariations with neural activity in
the posterior thalamus and superior colliculus (Morris *et al.* 2001).

The cortical route involves regions of occipital and posterior temporal
visual cortex (Haxby *et al.* 2000, 2002). In particular, neuro-imaging studies
have indicated that three specific areas are involved in face processing: the
lateral occipital gyri, bilateral regions in the lateral fusiform gyrus and the
posterior superior temporal sulcus (Kanwisher *et al.* 1997, 2000; Haxby *et al.*
1999). Moreover, there are strong suggestions of a dissociation in function
between the fusiform gyrus and superior temporal sulcus (Hasselmo *et al.*
1989; Hoffman and Haxby 2000). The suggestion is that the fusiform gyrus is
more involved in the processing of facial identity whereas the superior
temporal sulcus is more involved in the processing of social communication
(Haxby *et al.* 2002).

Recent event-related potential and magnetoencephalography studies have
allowed considerable specification of the time-course for the processing of
emotional expressions (Pizzagalli *et al.* 1999, 2002; Streit *et al.* 1999; Halgren
et al. 2000). The earliest activity that discriminates between emotional facial
expressions is seen in midline occipital cortex from between 80 to 110 ms
post-stimulus (Pizzagalli *et al.* 1999; Halgren *et al.* 2000). From around 160
ms, activity is seen in the fusiform gyrus and superior temporal sulcus (Streit
et al. 1999; Halgren *et al.* 2000; Pizzagalli *et al.* 2002). This literature has yet
to find evidence of early amygdala activity that the sub-cortical route should
predict. Indeed, the earliest activity seen is at around 220 ms in the right
amygdala (Streit *et al.* 1999). However, there has been a report of neuronal
discrimination, as single unit responses, between the emotions of fear and
happiness after only 120 ms in the orbital frontal cortex of a patient (Kawasaki
et al. 2001). This would suggest a sub-cortical route to orbital frontal cortex.

There appear to be further activations of superior temporal cortex after
the amygdala activation (Streit *et al.* 1999), perhaps as a consequence of the
amygdala activity. Indeed, a recent study examining single unit activity in the
temporal visual cortex in monkeys found that information sufficient to distinguish different emotional expressions occurred around 50 ms after information
sufficient to distinguish faces from other objects was available (Sugase *et al.*
1999). This again suggests the possibility that response to emotional stimuli

in the temporal cortex is modulated by feedback from structures such as the amygdala (Adolphs 2002). Moreover, many imaging studies investigating the neural response to emotional expressions have reported greater superior temporal sulcus and fusiform gyrus activity to emotional expressions relative to neutral expressions (Phillips *et al.* 1998; Critchley *et al.* 2000; Iidaka *et al.* 2001). In addition, task conditions that increase attention to emotional expressions result in increased superior temporal sulcus and fusiform gyrus activity (Narumoto *et al.* 2001; Vuilleumier *et al.* 2001; Pessoa *et al.* 2002).

Two additional cortical areas that have been linked to the processing of emotional expressions are bilateral regions of inferior frontal cortex and inferior parietal cortex. Three neuro-imaging studies have observed inferior frontal cortex activity to emotional expressions (George *et al.* 1993; Nakamura *et al.* 1999; Gorno-Tempini *et al.* 2001) although, it should be noted, many other studies have not. Activity in the inferior parietal cortex, or at least the proximal region of superior temporal sulcus, is frequently implicated in the processing of face stimuli (Haxby *et al.* 2000) and expression processing (Phillips *et al.* 1997; Streit *et al.* 1999; Halgren *et al.* 2000; Kesler-West *et al.* 2001; Pizzagalli *et al.* 2002). Moreover, two studies investigating which cortical regions, when damaged, most effected expression recognition stressed the importance of the inferior parietal cortex (Adolphs *et al.* 1996, 2000). These areas are of potential interest as proximal areas are activated when either an individual is initiating a movement or when they are observing another initiate the same movement (Iacoboni *et al.* 1999). This has prompted suggestions that responding to another individual's expression relies on the activation of motor programmes that the individual uses for the production of expressions (Preston and de Waal 2003).

As stated in the beginning of this chapter a fundamental assumption of this paper is that emotional expressions are communicatory signals that serve specific purposes. The claim is that this perspective allows an understanding into specific patterns of activation seen for specific emotions. Importantly, fearful, sad and happy expressions can all be viewed as reinforcers that modulate the probability that a particular behaviour will be performed in the future. The amygdala has been implicated in aversive and appetitive conditioning including instrumental learning (Killcross *et al.* 1997; Everitt *et al.* 2000; LeDoux 2000). It is thus unsurprising, given the suggested role of fearful, sad and happy expressions as reinforcers, that neuro-imaging studies, with a few exceptions (Kesler-West *et al.* 2001), have generally found that fearful, sad and happy expressions all modulate amygdala activity (Schneider *et al.* 1994; Breiter *et al.* 1996; Morris *et al.* 1996; Phillips *et al.* 1997, 1998; Baird *et al.* 1999; Blair *et al.* 1999; Drevets *et al.* 2000), though it should be noted that happy expressions have been reported to both increase and decrease amygdala activity (Breiter *et al.* 1996; Morris *et al.* 1996). The neuropsychological literature supports the neuro-imaging literature about the importance of the amygdala in the processing of fearful expressions. There have been occasional suggestions that amygdala damage leads to general expression recognition impairment but these reports are typically from patients whose lesions extend considerably beyond the amygdala (Rapcsak *et al.* 2000). Instead, amygdala lesions have been consistently associated with impairment in the recognition of fearful expressions (Adolphs *et al.* 1994, 1999; Calder *et al.* 1996; Schmolck and Squire 2001). Impairment in the processing of sad expressions is not uncommonly found in patients with amygdala lesions (Adolphs *et al.* 1999; Schmolck and Squire 2001). Indeed, a recent review of patient performance across studies, reported that around 50% of patients with amygdala damage present with impairment for the recognition of sad expressions (Fine and Blair 2000). Amygdala lesions rarely result in impairment in the recognition of happy expressions (Adolphs *et al.* 1999; Fine and Blair 2000). However, this may reflect the ease with which happy expressions are recognized (Ekman and Friesen 1976).

Disgusted expressions are also reinforcers but are used most frequently to provide information about foods (Rozin *et al.* 1993). In particular, they allow the rapid transmission of taste aversions; the observer is warned not to approach the food that the emoter is displaying the disgust reaction to. Functional imaging studies have consistently shown that disgusted expressions engage the insula and putamen (Phillips *et al.* 1997, 1998; Sprengelmeyer *et al.* 1998) and patients with damage to the insula present with selective impairment for the recognition of disgusted expressions (Sprengelmeyer *et al.* 1996; Calder *et al.* 2000). Experimental investigations in macaques have shown that there is a primary taste cortical region in the anterior insula (Rolls 1997) and neuro-imaging studies in humans have also shown the insula to be involved in the representation of taste (O'Doherty *et al.* 2001*b*; Small *et al.* 2001). Crucially, insula lesions have been found to block the acquisition and expression of taste aversion learning (Cubero *et al.* 1999). Thus, the suggestion is that the disgusted expressions of others activate in particular the insula allowing taste aversion (disgust expression US–novel food CS associations) to occur.

In contrast to the expressions considered above, it is far less clear that the angry expression is a basic reinforcer. Angry expressions are known to curtail the behaviour of others in situations where social rules or expectations have been violated (Averill 1982). They appear to serve to inform the observer to stop the current behavioural action rather than to convey any information as to whether that action should be initiated in the future. In other words, angry expressions can be seen as triggers for response reversal (Blair *et al.* 1999; Blair and Cipolotti 2000). Orbital frontal cortex is crucially implicated in response reversal (Dias *et al.* 1996; O'Doherty *et al.* 2001*a*; Cools *et al.* 2002). Interestingly, similar areas of lateral orbital frontal cortex are activated by angry expressions and response reversal as a function of contingency change (Sprengelmeyer *et al.* 1998; Blair *et al.* 1999; Kesler-West *et al.* 2001). In addition, most neuro-imaging studies do not observe amygdala activation to angry expressions (Sprengelmeyer *et al.* 1998; Blair *et al.* 1999;

Kesler-West *et al.* 2001). The only study, to my knowledge, that did observe amygdala activation by angry expressions found very weak activation that was significantly less than that seen to fearful expressions (Whalen *et al.* 2001).

11.4 Neurotransmitter involvement in responding to the expressions of others

There is a growing body of data indicating a degree of differential neurotransmitter involvement in systems responsible for the processing of emotional expressions. Thus, pharmacological interventions can alter the communicatory salience of emotional expressions. For example, serotonergic manipulations have been found to differentially affect the processing of fearful and happy expressions (Harmer *et al.* 2001*a*), noradrenergic manipulations to differentially affect the processing of sad expressions (Harmer *et al.* 2001*b*) whereas dopaminergic and GABAergic manipulations differentially affect the processing of angry expressions (Borrill *et al.* 1987; Blair and Curran 1999; Zangara *et al.* 2002). Given these differential effects one might predict that the serotonergic and noradrenergic manipulations are differentially affecting the amygdala's role in responding to fearful, sad and happy expressions as unconditioned stimuli for aversive and appetitive conditioning and instrumental learning, whereas GABAergic manipulations impact the role of orbital frontal cortex in modulating the response to interpersonal signals of conflict such as anger. Certainly, it is known that there is considerable serotonergic and noradrenergic innervation of the amygdala (Amaral *et al.* 1992) and the impact of noradrenergic manipulations of the amygdala's role in the augmentation of episodic memory is well known (Cahill and McGaugh 1998; Cahill 2000). There are high concentrations of benzodiazepine receptor sites in both amygdala and the frontal cortex (Dennis *et al.* 1988; Bremner *et al.* 2000). However, although the central nucleus of the amygdala which projects to autonomic centres in the brain stem is densely innervated by GABA neurons, the basolateral nucleus of the amygdala, projecting to cortical regions, contains only scattered GABA neurons (Swanson and Petrovich 1998). It is plausible that the basolateral nucleus, as a function of its interconnections with cortical regions, is more involved in responding to fearful expressions and thus relatively unaffected by GABAergic manipulations.

At present only one study, to my knowledge, has examined the neural underpinnings of the effects of these pharmacological agents (Blair *et al.* 2003). This investigated the impact of diazepam on the neural response to morphed angry and fearful expressions. Interestingly, while diazepam abolished the increase in lateral orbital frontal cortex activity as a function of increased angry expression intensity, the increase in amygdala activity as a function of increased fearful expression intensity was not affected by diazepam. This study thus adds support to the suggestion that GABAergic manipulations impact the role of orbital frontal cortex in modulating the response to interpersonal signals of conflict such as anger.

11.5 Acknowledging other individuals' expressions: closing the communicatory loop

In this paper the communicatory function of emotional expressions has been stressed. Reference was made to a crucial determinant of whether an expression will be elicited: the presence of others (Jones and Raag 1989; Chovil 1991; Fridlund 1991; Jones *et al.* 1991). Individuals typically display expressions when there is an audience to witness these expressions. This might suggest that individuals should stop displaying emotional expressions when the audience has demonstrated that they have registered the display of the emoter. Thus, for example, in the social referencing example provided above, the caregiver should stop to display fear when the infant demonstrates that they will now not approach the aversive novel object. However, although this would intuitively appear to be the case, I know of no empirical literature demonstrating it to be so.

One particular case where there are clear indications that the audience demonstrates that they have registered the display of the emoter is seen during embarrassment displays. Embarrassment is associated with gaze aversion, shifting eye positions, speech disturbances, face touches, a nervous smile and a rigid, slouched posture (Goffman 1967; Asendorpf 1990; Lewis *et al.* 1991). More recent work has demonstrated that embarrassment display unfolds in the following reliable sequence. This involves gaze aversion; a smile control, which is a lower facial action that potentially inhibits the smile; a non-Duchenne smile, which only involves the zygomatic major muscle action that pulls the corners of the lips upwards; a second smile control; head movements down; and then face touching, which occurred around 25% of the time (Keltner 1995).

Leary and Meadows (1991), Leary *et al.* (1996) and others (Keltner 1995; Miller 1996; Gilbert 1997; Keltner and Buswell 1997) have suggested that embarrassment serves an important social function by signalling appeasement to others. When a person's untoward behaviour threatens his/her standing in an important social group, visible signs of embarrassment function as a non-verbal acknowledgement of shared social standards. Leary argues that embarrassment displays diffuse negative social evaluations and the likelihood of retaliation. The basic idea is that embarrassment serves to aid the restoration of relationships following social transgressions (Keltner and Buswell 1997). In other words, embarrassment displays may be initiated by an individual following an emoter's display of anger: if the individual's behaviour was unintentional or the angry observer is of high status.

There is a good deal of empirical evidence to support this 'appeasement' or remedial function of embarrassment from studies of both humans and non-human primates (Leary and Meadows 1991; Gilbert 1997; Keltner and Buswell 1997; Keltner and Anderson 2000). For example, Semin and Manstead (1982) found that people reacted more positively to others after a social transgression if the transgressors were visibly embarrassed. In addition, Leary *et al.* (1996) presented evidence that people are actually motivated to convey embarrassment to others as a way of repairing their social image.

11.6 Pathological expression processing: the cases of autism, developmental psychopathy and acquired sociopathy

If emotional expressions serve a communicatory function, as I have been arguing, we might expect that atypical responding to the emotional expressions of others would adversely affect development. Three ways in which development can be affected will be discussed below with reference to the neuro-psychiatric conditions of autism, developmental psychopathy and acquired sociopathy.

Autism is a severe developmental disorder described by the American Psychiatric Association's diagnostic and statistical manual (DSM-IV) as 'the presence of markedly abnormal or impaired development in social interaction and communication and a markedly restricted repertoire of activities and interests' (American Psychiatric Association 1994, p. 66). The main criteria for the diagnosis in DSM-IV can be summarized as qualitative impairment in social communication and restricted and repetitive patterns of behaviour and interests. These criteria must be evident before 3 years of age.

As long as autism has been recognized, the idea has existed that the main difficulty for people with autism is an inability to enter into emotional relationships. Thus, Kanner, the psychiatrist who originally described the disorder in 1943, wrote 'these children have come into the world with an innate inability to form the usual, biologically provided affective contact with other people, just as other children come into the world with innate physical or intellectual handicaps' (Kanner 1943, p. 250). More recently, it has been suggested that autism is due to an innate impairment in the ability to perceive and respond to the affective expressions of others, and that this deficit leads to their profound difficulties in social interaction (Hobson 1993).

Many studies have investigated the ability of individuals with autism to recognize the emotional expressions of others. Many have reported that children with autism have difficulty recognizing the emotional expressions of others (Hobson 1986; Bormann-Kischkel *et al.* 1995; Howard *et al.* 2000) with a recent claim suggesting that this is specific for fearful expressions (Howard *et al.* 2000). However, the above only applies to studies where the groups have not been matched on mental age. When they are, children with autism have usually been found to be unimpaired in facial affect recognition (Ozonoff *et al.* 1990; Prior *et al.* 1990; Baron-Cohen *et al.* 1997*b*; Adolphs *et al.* 2001). In addition, several studies have found the emotion processing impairment to be pronounced only when the emotion is a complex 'cognitive' emotion such as surprise or embarrassment (Capps *et al.* 1992; Baron-Cohen *et al.* 1993; Bormann-Kischkel *et al.* 1995).

I would therefore argue that autism does not represent a disorder where there is atypical recognition of emotional expressions. However, autism is interesting because of the well-documented impairment in theory of mind shown by patients with this disorder (Frith 2001). Theory of mind refers to the ability to represent the mental states of others, i.e. their thoughts, desires, beliefs, intentions and knowledge (Premack and Woodruff 1978; Leslie 1987; Frith 1989). Impairment in theory of mind is interesting for the communicatory role of emotional expressions. Thus, a healthy individual, when witnessing the emotional display of another individual, will attempt to represent the intended cue that elicited the emoter's expression. So, for example, during social referencing, if the child is attending to one object when the caregiver displays an emotional response to another, the child will look at the caregiver to determine the direction of their attention (Moses *et al.* 2001). Theory of mind should be involved in the representation of the emoter's intention. If it is, we might predict anomalous behavioural reactions to the emotional displays of other individuals in children with autism given their theory-of-mind impairment. In particular, we should see a reduction in the usual orientation response to the emoter to calculate the eliciting stimulus. Indeed, this is exactly what is seen in children with autism. A series of studies has examined the behavioural reactions of individuals with autism when the child has been playing with the experimenter and the experimenter has feigned an emotional reaction, usually distress (Sigman *et al.* 1992; Dissanayake *et al.* 1996; Bacon *et al.* 1998; Corona *et al.* 1998). All four of these studies have reported reduced orientation to the caregiver by the children with autism although this was only in the lower ability sample in the Bacon *et al.* (1998) study. However, this does not reflect a lack of responsiveness to other individuals' emotion. A child with autism presented with another individual in distress will show aversive autonomic arousal to the other's distress (Blair 1999) and, as has been argued above, children with autism present with no impairment in expression recognition (Ozonoff *et al.* 1990; Prior *et al.* 1990; Baron-Cohen *et al.* 1997*b*; Adolphs *et al.* 2001).

The above argument generates further predictions about emotion in autism. Social referencing, the learning of emotional valence for novel objects, should be impaired in children with autism. The child with autism should fail to use the emoter's gaze direction to calculate the correct object to associate the valence elicited by the emoter's display in the same way that they fail to use a speaker's gaze direction during novel word use to calculate the speaker's referent (Baron-Cohen *et al.* 1997*a*). This, in turn, predicts that children with autism may present with very unusual emotional reactions to objects. That is, without representing the emoter's referent they may associate valence to novel objects inappropriately or not at all.

Psychopathy is a developmental disorder characterized in part by callousness, a diminished capacity for remorse, impulsivity and poor behavioural control (Hare 1991). It is identified in children with the antisocial process screening device (Frick and Hare 2001) and in adults with the revised psychopathy checklist (Hare 1991). Importantly, this disorder is not equivalent to the psychiatric diagnoses of conduct disorder or antisocial personality disorder (American Psychiatric Association 1994). These psychiatric diagnoses are relatively poorly specified and concentrate almost entirely on the antisocial behaviour shown by the individual rather than any form of functional impairment. Because of this lack of specification, rates of diagnosis of conduct disorder reach up to 16% of boys in mainstream education (American Psychiatric Association 1994) and rates of diagnosis of antisocial personality disorder are over 80% in forensic institutions (Hart and Hare 1996). Because of these high rates of diagnosis, populations identified with these diagnostic tools are highly heterogeneous and also include many individuals with other disorders. Psychopathy, in contrast, is shown by less than 1% of individuals in mainstream education (Blair and Coles 2000) and less than 30% of individuals incarcerated in forensic institutions (Hart and Hare 1996).

One account of psychopathy has linked the disorder to early amygdala dysfunction and consequent impairment in processing fearful and sad expressions (Blair 1995, 2001; Blair *et al.* 1999). The basic suggestion is that psychopathic individuals represent the developmental case where sad and fearful expressions are not aversive unconditioned stimuli. As a consequence of this, the individual does not learn to avoid committing behaviours that cause harm to others and will commit them if, by doing them, he receives reward (Blair 1995). In line with this theory, psychopathic individuals have been found to present with reduced amygdaloid volume relative to comparison individuals (Tiihonen *et al.* 2000) and reduced amygdala activation, relative to comparison individuals, during an emotional memory task (Kiehl *et al.* 2001) and aversive conditioning tasks (Veit *et al.* 2002). Moreover, in functions that recruit the amygdala such as aversive conditioning and instrumental learning, the augmentation of startle reflex by visual threat primes or arousal to the anticipation of punishment are all impaired in psychopathic individuals (Blair 2001). Also in line with the theory, psychopathic individuals show pronounced impairment in processing sad and fearful expressions. They show reduced autonomic responses to these expressions (Aniskiewicz 1979; Blair *et al.* 1997) and, particularly in childhood, impaired ability to recognize these expressions (Blair *et al.* 2001). Finally, their socialization is markedly impaired. Thus, although it has been repeatedly shown that the use of empathy inducing positive parenting strategies by caregivers decreases the probability of antisocial behaviour in healthy developing children, it does not decrease the probability of antisocial behaviour in children who present with the emotional dysfunction of psychopathy (Wootton *et al.* 1997).

Acquired sociopathy represents an interesting counterpoint to developmental psychopathy. 'Acquired sociopathy' was a term introduced by Damasio *et al.* (1990) to characterize individuals who, following acquired lesions of the orbitofrontal cortex, fulfil the DSM-III diagnostic criteria for 'sociopathic disorder' (American Psychiatric Association 1980). Previously, Blumer and Benson (1975) had used the term 'pseudo-psychopathy' to refer to patients with frontal lobe lesions presenting in this manner. Although there have been suggestions that developmental psychopathy and acquired sociopathy might be different forms of the same disorder (Damasio 1994), this now appears unlikely (Blair 2001). Indeed, developmental psychopathy and acquired sociopathy present very differently. Psychopathic individuals present with pronounced levels of goal-directed instrumental aggression and antisocial behaviour, reflecting an impairment that interferes with their ability to be socialized (Cornell *et al.* 1996). In contrast, patients with acquired sociopathy present with frustration- or threat-induced reactive aggression whether their acquired lesion of the orbital frontal cortex occurs in childhood (Pennington and Bennetto 1993; Anderson *et al.* 1999) or adulthood (Grafman *et al.* 1996; Blair and Cipolotti 2000).

I have argued for the communicatory role of angry and embarrassment expressions in regulating social hierarchical interactions, in particular, the role of angry expressions in stopping the current behavioural action and the role of embarrassment displays in communicating a lack of intent to commit the action that has resulted in social disapproval. We might expect therefore that an individual whose response to angry/embarrassment expressions is dysfunctional should present with impaired modulation of their social behaviour. The orbital frontal cortex is implicated in the response to angry expressions (Sprengelmeyer *et al.* 1998; Blair *et al.* 1999; Kesler-West *et al.* 2001). Interestingly, then, patients with acquired sociopathy following lesions of the orbital frontal cortex present with generally impaired expression recognition but this impairment is particularly marked for angry expressions (Hornak *et al.* 1996; Blair and Cipolotti 2000). The strong suggestion is therefore that this impairment underlies their socially inappropriate behaviour.

11.7 Conclusions

In this chapter I have stressed the communicatory function of emotional expressions. Importantly, the argument is not that the display of expressions implies that the emoter intended to convey a specific message to the observer, it is simply that emotional expressions serve a communicatory function. Crucially, the emoter's emotional displays are a function of the presence of observers and the observer will attempt to determine the referent of the emoter's display.

Assuming the observer accomplishes this, appropriate information will have been transferred from the emoter to the observer.

Although emotional expressions are not intentional communications, their display can be intentionally manipulated. Children learn display rules; social rules that stipulate when it is, and when it is not, appropriate to display emotional expressions. Thus we can learn to intentionally mask or alter our expressions as a function of these display rules. Presumably, the emoter's intent modulates the frontal lobe–basal ganglia circuitry that has been implicated in the production of emotional expressions.

Although systems generally involved in processing facial stimuli, such as the occipital cortex, fusiform and the superior temporal sulcus process expressions, the communicatory function of emotional expressions is reflected in the partly dissociable neural systems that are additionally involved in processing emotional expressions. Thus, expressions that serve as positive or negative reinforcers preferentially activate the amygdala (fearfulness, sadness and happiness). Although disgusted expressions are also reinforcers, they are used most frequently to provide information about foods. As such they engage the insula, a region involved in taste aversion. Angry expressions initiate response reversal and activate regions of orbital frontal cortex that are involved in the modulation of behavioural responding.

If we assume that emotional expressions serve a communicatory function, we must predict that they will be more likely to be displayed when a potential observer is present. This is indeed the case. In addition, we must predict that the display of the expression will be terminated when the observer has shown clear indication that they have received the communication. This remains to be investigated.

The consequences of impairment in being able to adequately process the emotional displays of others can be severe. I have argued that although individuals with autism may be able to recognize the expressions of others, it is highly likely that they fail to adequately process the emoter's referent and that they therefore process the display incorrectly because of their impairment in theory of mind. In contrast, individuals with the developmental disorder of psychopathy and individuals with acquired sociopathy following lesions of the orbital frontal cortex fail to respond appropriately to specific expressions. In psychopathic individuals, the processing of other individuals' sadness and fear is particularly affected. This leads to a failure in socialization. The psychopathic individual does not learn to avoid actions that cause harm to others. In acquired sociopathy, the processing of others' anger and probably embarrassment is particularly affected. This leads to a failure to adequately modulate behaviour according to the social context.

In short, emotional expressions allow the rapid communication of valence information between individuals. They allow the observer to rapidly learn which behaviours and objects (including foods) to approach or avoid, as well as information allowing rapid modification of behaviour according to the social environment and hierarchy. Impairment in systems that respond to the emotional expressions of others can have devastating effects.

References

Adolphs, R. (2002). Neural systems for recognizing emotion. *Curr. Opin. Neurobiol.* **12**, 169–77.

Adolphs, R., Tranel, D., Damasio, H. and Damasio, A. (1994). Impaired recognition of emotion in facial expressions following bilateral damage to the human amygdala. *Nature* **372**, 669–72.

Adolphs, R., Damasio, H., Tranel, D. and Damasio, A. R. (1996). Cortical systems for the recognition of emotion in facial expressions. *J. Neurosci.* **16**, 7678–87.

Adolphs, R., Tranel, D., Young, A. W., Calder, A. J., Phelps, E. A., Anderson, A. K., *et al.* (1999). Recognition of facial emotion in nine individuals with bilateral amygdala damage. *Neuropsycholgia* **37**, 1111–17.

Adolphs, R., Damasio, H., Cooper, G. and Damasio, A. R. (2000). A role of somatosensory cortices in the visual recognition of emotion as revealed by three-dimensional lesion mapping. *J. Neurosci.* **20**, 2683–90.

Adolphs, R., Sears, L. and Piven, J. (2001). Abnormal processing of social information from faces in autism. *J. Cogn. Neurosci.* **13**, 232–40.

Amaral, D. G., Price, J. L., Pitkanen, A. and Carmichael, S. T. (1992). Anatomical organization of the primate amygdaloid complex. In *The amygdala: neurobiological aspects of emotion, memory, and mental dysfunction* (ed. J. P. Aggleton), pp. 1–66. New York: John Wiley.

American Psychiatric Association (1980). *Diagnostic and statistical manual of mental disorders* (*DSM-III*), 3rd edn. Washington, DC: American Psychiatric Association.

American Psychiatric Association (1994). *Diagnostic and statistical manual of mental disorders*, 4th edn. Washington, DC: American Psychiatric Association.

Anderson, A. K. and Phelps, E. A. (2000). Expression without recognition: contributions of the human amygdala to emotional communication. *Psychol. Sci.* **11**, 106–11.

Anderson, S. W., Bechara, A., Damasio, H., Tranel, D. and Damasio, A. R. (1999). Impairment of social and moral behaviour related to early damage in human prefrontal cortex. *Nature Neurosci.* **2**, 1032–7.

Aniskiewicz, A. S. (1979). Autonomic components of vicarious conditioning and psychopathy. *J. Clin. Psychol.* **35**, 60–7.

Armony, J. L., Servan-Schreiber, D., Romanski, L. M., Cohen, J. D. and LeDoux, J. E. (1997). Stimulus generalization of fear responses: effects of auditory cortex lesions in a computational model and in rats. *Cerebr. Cortex* **7**, 157–65.

Asendorpf, J. B. (1990). The expression of shyness and embarrassment. In *Shyness and embarrassment: perspectives from social psychology* (ed. W. R. Crozier), pp. 87–118. Cambridge: Cambridge University Press.

Averill, J. R. (1982). *Anger and aggression: an essay on emotion.* New York: Springer-Verlag.

Bacon, A. L., Fein, D., Morris, R., Waterhouse, L. and Allen, D. (1998). The responses of autistic children to the distress of others. *J. Autism Devl Disord.* **28**, 129–42.

Baird, A. A., Gruber, S. A., Fein, D. A., Maas, L. C., Steingard, R. J., Renshaw, P. F., *et al.* (1999). Functional magnetic resonance imaging of facial affect recognition in children and adolescents. *J. Am. Acad. Child Adolescent Psychiat.* **38**, 195–9.

Baldwin, D. A., Markman, E. M., Bill, B., Desjardins, R. N., Irwin, J. M. and Tidball, G. (1996). Infants' reliance on a social criterion for establishing word–object relations. *Child Dev.* **67**, 3135–53.

Baron-Cohen, S., Spitz, A. and Cross, P. (1993). Do children with autism recognize surprise? A research note. *Cogn. Emotion* **7**, 507–16.

Baron-Cohen, S., Baldwin, D. A. and Crowson, M. (1997*a*). Do children with autism use the speaker's direction of gaze strategy to crack the code of language? *Child Dev.* **68**, 48–57.

Baron-Cohen, S., Wheelwright, S. and Joliffe, T. (1997*b*). Is there a 'language of the eyes'? Evidence from normal adults, and adults with autism or Asperger syndrome. *Vis. Cogn* **4**, 311–31.

Blair, R. J. R. (1995). A cognitive developmental approach to morality: investigating the psychopath. *Cognition* **57**, 1–29.

Blair, R. J. R. (1999). Psycho–physiological responsiveness to the distress of others in children with autism. *Personal. Indiv. Diff.* **26**, 477–85.

Blair, R. J. R. (2001). Neuro–cognitive models of aggression, the antisocial personality disorders and psychopathy. *J. Neurol. Neurosurg. Psychiat.* **71**, 727–31.

Blair, R. J. R. and Cipolotti, L. (2000). Impaired social response reversal: a case of 'acquired sociopathy'. *Brain* **123**, 1122–41.

Blair, R. J. R. and Coles, M. (2000). Expression recognition and behavioural problems in early adolescence. *Cogn. Dev.* **15**, 421–34.

Blair, R. J. R. and Curran, H. V. (1999). Selective impairment in the recognition of anger induced by diazepam. *Psychopharmacology* **147**, 335–8.

Blair, R. J. R., Jones, L., Clark, F. and Smith, M. (1997). The psychopathic individual: a lack of responsiveness to distress cues? *Psychophysiology* **34**, 192–8.

Blair, R. J. R., Morris, J. S., Frith, C. D., Perrett, D. I. and Dolan, R. (1999). Dissociable neural responses to facial expressions of sadness and anger. *Brain* **122**, 883–93.

Blair, R. J., Colledge, E., Murray, L. and Mitchell, D. G. (2001). A selective impairment in the processing of sad and fearful expressions in children with psychopathic tendencies. *J. Abnormal Child Psychol.* **29**, 491–8.

Blair, R. J. R., Maratos, E. J., Berthoz, S., Glaser, D. and Dolan, R. (2003). Impact of diazpem on the neural response to angry and fearful facial expressions. (Submitted.)

Bloom, P. (2002). Mindreading, communication and the learning of names for things. *Mind Lang.* **17**, 37–54.

Blumer, D. and Benson, D. F. (1975). Personality changes with frontal and temporal lobe lesions. In *Psychiatric aspects of neurological disease* (ed. D. F. Benson and D. Blumer), pp. 151–70. New York: Grune and Stratton.

Bormann-Kischkel, C., Vilsmeier, M. and Baude, B. (1995). The development of emotional concepts in autism. *J. Child Psychol. Psychiat.* **36**, 1243–59.

Borod, J. C., Welkowitz, J., Alpert, M., Brozgold, A. Z., Martin, C., Peselow, E., *et al.* (1990). Parameters of emotional processing in neuropsychiatric disorders: conceptual issues and a battery of tests. *J. Commun. Disord.* **23**, 247–71.

Borrill, J. A., Rosen, B. K. and Summerfield, A. B. (1987). The influence of alcohol on judgment of facial expressions of emotion. *Br. J. Med. Psychol.* **60**, 71–7.

Breiter, H. C., Etcoff, N. L., Whalen, P. J., Kennedy, W. A., Rauch, S. L., Buckner, R. L., *et al.* (1996). Response and habituation of the human amygdala during visual processing of facial expression. *Neuron* **17**, 875–87.

Bremner, J. D., Innis, R. B., Southwick, S. M., Staib, L., Zoghbi, S. and Charney, D. S. (2000). Decreased benzodiazepine receptor binding in prefrontal cortex in combat-related post-traumatic stress disorder. *Am. J. Psychiat.* **157**, 1120–6.

Buck, R. (1984). *The communication of emotion*. New York: Guilford Press.

Cahill, L. (2000). Neurobiological mechanisms of emotionally influenced, long-term memory. *Prog. Brain Res.* **126**, 29–37.

Cahill, L. and McGaugh, J. L. (1998). Mechanisms of emotional arousal and lasting declarative memory. *Trends Neurosci.* **21**, 294–9.

Calder, A. J., Young, A. W., Rowland, D. and Perrett, D. I. (1996). Facial emotion recognition after bilateral amygdala damage: differentially severe impairment of fear. *Cogn. Neuropsychol.* **13**, 699–745.

Calder, A. J., Keane, J., Manes, F., Antoun, N. and Young, A. W. (2000). Impaired recognition and experience of disgust following brain injury. *Nature Neurosci.* **3**, 1077–8.

Campeau, S. and Davis, M. (1995). Involvement of the central nucleus and basolateral complex of the amygdala in fear conditioning measured with fear-potentiated startle in rats trained concurrently with auditory and visual conditioned stimuli. *J. Neurosci.* **15**, 2301–11.

Camras, L. A. (1994). Two aspects of emotional development: expression and elicitation. In *The nature of emotion: fundamental questions* (ed. P. Ekman and R. J. Davidson), pp. 347–51. New York: Oxford University Press.

Capps, L., Yirmiya, N. and Sigman, M. (1992). Understanding of simple and complex emotions in non-retarded children with autism. *J. Child Psychol. Psychiat.* **33**, 1169–82.

Cheney, D. L. and Seyfarth, R. M. (1980). Vocal recognition in free-ranging vervet monkeys. *Anim. Behav.* **28**, 362–7.

Chovil, N. (1991). Social determinants of facial displays. *J. Non-verbal Behav.* **15**, 141–54.

Cools, R., Clark, L., Owen, A. M. and Robbins, T. W. (2002). Defining the neural mechanisms of probabilistic reversal learning using event-related functional magnetic resonance imaging. *J. Neurosci.* **22**, 4563–7.

Cornell, D. G., Warren, J., Hawk, G., Stafford, E., Oram, G. and Pine, D. (1996). Psychopathy in instrumental and reactive violent offenders. *J. Consulting Clin. Psychol.* **64**, 783–90.

Corona, C., Dissanayake, C., Arbelle, A., Wellington, P. and Sigman, M. (1998). Is affect aversive to young children with autism? Behavioural and cardiac responses to experimenter distress. *Child Dev.* **69**, 1494–502.

Critchley, H., Daly, E., Phillips, M., Brammer, M., Bullmore, E., Williams, S., *et al.* (2000). Explicit and implicit neural mechanisms for processing of social information from facial expressions: a functional magnetic resonance imaging study. *Hum. Brain Mapping* **9**, 93–105.

Cubero, I., Thiele, T. E. and Bernstein, I. L. (1999). Insular cortex lesions and taste aversion learning: effects of conditioning method and timing of lesion. *Brain Res.* **839**, 323–30.

Damasio, A. R. (1994). *Descartes' error: emotion, rationality and the human brain*. New York: Putnam (Grosset Books).

Damasio, A. R., Tranel, D. and Damasio, H. (1990). Individuals with sociopathic behaviour caused by frontal damage fail to respond autonomically to social stimuli. *Behav. Brain Res.* **41**, 81–94.

Darwin, C. (1872). *The expression of the emotions in man and animals*. London: Albemarle.

de Gelder, B., Vroomen, J., Pourtois, G. and Weiskrantz, L. (1999). Non-conscious recognition of affect in the absence of striate cortex. *NeuroReport* **10**, 3759–63.

Dennis, T., Dubois, A., Benavides, J. and Scatton, B. (1988). Distribution of central omega 1 (benzodiazepine1) and omega 2 (benzodiazepine2) receptor subtypes in the monkey and human brain. An autoradiographic study with [3H]flunitrazepam and the omega 1 selective ligand [3H]zolpidem. *J. Pharmacol. Exp. Theor.* **247**, 309–22.

Dias, R., Robbins, T. W. and Roberts, A. C. (1996). Dissociation in prefrontal cortex of affective and attentional shifts. *Nature* **380**, 69–72.

Dissanayake, C., Sigman, M. and Kasari, C. (1996). Long-term stability of individual differences in the emotional responsiveness of children with autism. *J. Child Psychol. Psychiat.* **37**, 461–7.

Drevets, W. C., Lowry, T., Gautier, C., Perrett, D. I. and Kupfer, D. J. (2000). Amygdalar blood flow responses to facially expressed sadness. *Biol. Psychiatry* **47**(Suppl. 8), 160S.

Ekman, P. (1997). Should we call it expression or communication? *Innovations Social Sci. Res.* **10**, 333–44.

Ekman, P. and Friesen, W. V. (1969). The repertoire of non-verbal behavior: categories, origins, usage, and coding. *Semiotica* **1**, 49–98.

Ekman, P. and Friesen, W. V. (1976). *Pictures of facial affect*. Palo Alto, CA: Consulting Psychologists Press.

Everitt, B. J., Cardinal, R. N., Hall, J., Parkinson, J. A. and Robbins, T. W. (2000). Differential involvement of amygdala sub-systems in appetitive conditioning and drug addiction. In *The amygdala: a functional analysis* (ed. J. P. Aggleton), pp. 289–310. Oxford: Oxford University Press.

Fine, C. and Blair, R. J. R. (2000). Mini review: the cognitive and emotional effects of amygdala damage. *Neurocase* **6**, 435–50.

Frick, P. J. and Hare, R. D. (2001). *The antisocial process screening device*. Toronto, Ontario: Multi-Health Systems.

Fridlund, A. J. (1991). Sociality of solitary smiling: potentiation by an implicit audience. *J. Personality Social Psychol.* **60**, 229–46.

Frith, U. (1989). *Autism: explaining the enigma*. Oxford: Blackwell.

Frith, U. (2001). Mind blindness and the brain in autism. *Neuron* **32**, 969–79.

George, M. S., Ketter, T. A., Gill, D. S., Haxby, J. V., Ungerleider, L. G., Herscovitch, P., *et al.* (1993). Brain regions involved in recognizing facial emotion or identity: an oxygen-15 PET study. *J. Neuropsychiatry* **5**, 384–93.

Gilbert, P. (1997). The evolution of social attractiveness and its role in shame, humiliation, guilt and therapy. *Br. J. Med. Psychol.* **70**, 113–47.

Goffman, E. (1967). *Interaction ritual: essays on face-to-face behavior*. Garden City, NY: Anchor.

Gorno-Tempini, M. L., Pradelli, S., Serafini, M., Pagnoni, G., Baraldi, P., Porro, C., *et al.* (2001). Explicit and incidental facial expression processing: an fMRI study. *Neuroimage* **14**, 465–73.

Grafman, J., Schwab, K., Warden, D., Pridgen, B. S. and Brown, H. R. (1996). Frontal lobe injuries, violence, and aggression: a report of the Vietnam head injury study. *Neurology* **46**, 1231–8.

Halgren, E., Raij, T., Marinkovic, K., Jousmaki, V. and Hari, R. (2000). Cognitive response profile of the human fusiform face area as determined by MEG. *Cerebr. Cortex* **10**, 69–81.

Hare, R. D. (1991). *The Hare psychopathy checklist: revised.* Toronto, Ontario: Multi-Health Systems.

Harmer, C. J., Bhagwagar, Z., Cowen, P. J. and Goodwin, G. W. (2001*a*). Acute adimin-stration of citalopram in healthy volunteers facilitates recognition of happiness and fear. *J. Psychopharmacol.* **15**(Suppl.), A16.

Harmer, C. J., Perrett, D. I., Cowen, P. J. and Goodwin, G. M. (2001*b*). Administration of the beta-adrenoceptor blocker propranolol impairs the processing of facial expressions of sadness. *Psychopharmacol. Berl.* **154**, 383–9.

Hart, S. D. and Hare, R. D. (1996). Psychopathy and antisocial personality disorder. *Curr. Opin. Psychiat.* **9**, 129–32.

Hasselmo, M. E., Rolls, E. T. and Baylis, G. C. (1989). The role of expression and iden-tity in the face-selective responses of neurons in the temporal visual cortex of the monkey. *Behav. Brain Res.* **32**, 203–18.

Haxby, J. V., Ungerleider, L. G., Clark, V. P., Schouten, J. L., Hoffman, E. A. and Martin, A. (1999). The effect of face inversion on activity in human neural systems for face and object perception. *Neuron* **22**, 189–99.

Haxby, J. V., Hoffman, E. A. and Gobbini, M. I. (2000). The distributed human neural system for face perception. *J. Cogn. Neurosci.* **4**, 223–33.

Haxby, J. V., Hoffman, E. A. and Gobbini, M. I. (2002). Human neural systems for face recognition and social communication. *Biol. Psychiatry* **51**, 59–67.

Hinde, R. A. (1985). Was 'the expression of the emotions' a misleading phrase? *Anim. Behav.* **33**, 985–92.

Hobson, P. (1986). The autistic child's appraisal of expressions of emotion. *J. Child Psychol. Psychiat.* **27**, 321–42.

Hobson, R. P. (1993). *Autism and the development of mind.* Hove, East Sussex: Lawrence Erlbaum.

Hoffman, E. A. and Haxby, J. V. (2000). Distinct representations of eye gaze and identity in the distributed human neural system for face perception. *Nature Neurosci.* **3**, 80–4.

Hopf, H. C., Muller-Forell, W. and Hopf, N. J. (1992). Localization of emotional and volitional facial paresis. *Neurology* **42**, 1918–23.

Hornak, J., Rolls, E. T. and Wade, D. (1996). Face and voice expression identification in patients with emotional and behavioural changes following ventral frontal dam-age. *Neuropsychologia* **34**, 247–61.

Howard, M. A., Cowell, P. E., Boucher, J., Broks, P., Mayes, A., Farrant, A., *et al.* (2000). Convergent neuroanatomical and behavioural evidence of an amygdala hypothesis of autism. *NeuroReport* **11**, 1931–5.

Iacoboni, M., Woods, R. P., Brass, M., Bekkering, H., Mazziotta, J. C. and Rizzolatti, G. (1999). Cortical mechanisms of human imitation. *Science* **286**, 2526–8.

Iidaka, T., Omori, M., Murata, T., Kosaka, H., Yonekura, Y., Okada, T., *et al.* (2001). Neural interaction of the amygdala with the prefrontal and temporal cortices in the processing of facial expressions as revealed by fMRI. *J. Cogn. Neurosci.* **13**, 1035–47.

Izard, C. E. and Malatesta, C. (1987). Perspectives on emotional development I: differential emotions theory of early emotional development. In *Handbook of infant development* (ed. J. D. Osofsky), pp. 494–554. New York: John Wiley.

Jones, S. S. and Raag, T. (1989). Smile production in older infants: the importance of a social recipient for the facial signal. *Child Dev.* **60**, 811–18.

Jones, S. S., Collins, K. and Hong, H. W. (1991). An audience effect on smile production in 10-month-old infants. *Psychol. Sci.* **2**, 45–9.

Kanner, L. (1943). Autistic disturbances of affective contact. *Nervous Child* **2**, 217–50.

Kanwisher, N., McDermott, J. and Chun, M. M. (1997). The fusiform face area: a module in human extrastriate cortex specialized for face perception. *J. Neurosci.* **17**, 4302–11.

Kanwisher, N., Stanley, D. and Harris, A. (2000). The fusiform face area is selective for faces not animals. *NeuroReport* **18**, 183–7.

Kawasaki, H., Kaufman, O., Damasio, H., Damasio, A. R., Granner, M., Bakken, H., *et al.* (2001). Single-neuron responses to emotional visual stimuli recorded in human ventral prefrontal cortex. *Nature Neurosci.* **4**, 15–16.

Keltner, D. (1995). Signs of appeasement: evidence for the distinct displays of embarrassment, amusement, and shame. *J. Personality Social Psychol.* **68**, 441–54.

Keltner, D. and Anderson, C. (2000). Saving face for Darwin: the functions and uses of embarrassment. *Curr. Directions Psychol. Sci.* **9**, 187–92.

Keltner, D. and Buswell, B. N. (1997). Embarrassment: its distinct form and appeasement functions. *Psychol. Bull.* **122**, 250–70.

Kesler-West, M. L., Andersen, A. H., Smith, C. D., Avison, M. J., Davis, C. E., Kryscio, R. J., *et al.* (2001). Neural substrates of facial emotion processing using fMRI. *Cogn. Brain Res.* **11**, 213–26.

Kiehl, K. A., Smith, A. M., Hare, R. D., Mendrek, A., Forster, B. B., Brink, J., *et al.* (2001). Limbic abnormalities in affective processing by criminal psychopaths as revealed by functional magnetic resonance imaging. *Biol. Psychiat.* **50**, 677–84.

Killcross, S., Robbins, T. W. and Everitt, B. J. (1997). Different types of fear-conditioned behaviour mediated by separate nuclei within amygdala. *Nature* **388**, 377–80.

Klinnert, M. D., Campos, J. J. and Source, J. (1983). Emotions as behavior regulators: social referencing in infancy. In *Emotions in early development* (ed. R. Plutchik and H. Kellerman), pp. 57–86. New York, NY: Academic.

Klinnert, M. D., Emde, R. N., Butterfield, P. and Campos, J. J. (1987). Social referencing: the infant's use of emotional signals from a friendly adult with mother present. *A. Prog. Child Psychiatry Child Dev.* **22**, 427–32.

Leary, M. R. and Meadows, S. (1991). Predictors, elicitors, and concomitants of social blushing. *J. Personal. Social Psychol.* **60**, 254–62.

Leary, M. R., Landel, J. L. and Patton, K. M. (1996). The motivated expression of embarrassment following a self-presentational predicament. *J. Personality* **64**, 619–37.

LeDoux, J. E. (2000). Emotion circuits in the brain. *A. Rev. Neurosci.* **23**, 155–84.

LeDoux, J. E., Sakaguchi, A. and Reis, D. J. (1984). Sub-cortical efferent projections of the medial geniculate nucleus mediate emotional responses conditioned to acoustic stimuli. *J. Neurosci.* **4**, 683–98.

Leslie, A. M. (1987). Pretense and representation: the origins of 'theory of mind'. *Psychol. Rev.* **94**, 412–26.

Lewis, M., Stanger, C., Sullivan, M. W. and Barone, P. (1991). Changes in embarrassment as a function of age, sex, and situation. *Br. J. Devl Psychol.* **9**, 485–92.

Macknik, S. L. and Livingstone, M. S. (1998). Neuronal correlates of visibility and invisibility in the primate visual system. *Nature Neurosci.* **1**, 144–9.

Matthews, G. and Wells, A. (1999). The cognitive science of attention and emotion. In *Handbook of cognition and emotion* (ed. T. Dalgleish and M. J. Power), pp. 171–92. New York: Wiley.

Miller, R. S. (1996). *Embarrassment: poise and peril in everyday life.* New York: Guilford Press.

Mineka, S. and Cook, M. (1993). Mechanisms involved in the observational conditioning of fear. *J. Exp. Psychol. Gen.* **122**, 23–38.

Morris, J. S., Frith, C. D., Perrett, D. I., Rowland, D., Young, A. W., Calder, A. J., *et al.* (1996). A differential response in the human amygdala to fearful and happy facial expressions. *Nature* **383**, 812–15.

Morris, J. S., Ohman, A. and Dolan, R. (1999). A sub-cortical pathway to the right amygdala mediating 'unseen' fear. *Proc. Natl Acad. Sci. USA* **96**, 1680–5.

Morris, J. S., DeGelder, B., Weiskrantz, L. and Dolan, R. J. (2001). Differential extrageniculostriate and amygdala responses to presentation of emotional faces in a cortically blind field. *Brain* **124**, 1241–52.

Moses, L. J., Baldwin, D. A., Rosicky, J. G. and Tidball, G. (2001). Evidence for referential understanding in the emotions domain at twelve and eighteen months. *Child Dev.* **72**, 718–35.

Nakamura, K., Kawashima, R., Ho, K., Sugiura, M., Kato, T., Nakamura, A., *et al.* (1999). Activation of the right inferior frontal cortex during assessment of facial emotion. *J. Neurophysiol.* **82**, 1610–14.

Narumoto, J., Okada, T., Sadato, N., Fukui, K. and Yonekura, Y. (2001). Attention to emotion modulates fMRI activity in human right superior temporal sulcus. *Brain Res. Cogn. Brain Res.* **12**, 225–31.

O'Doherty, J., Kringelbach, M. L., Rolls, E. T., Hornak, J. and Andrews, C. (2001*a*). Abstract reward and punishment representations in the human orbitofrontal cortex. *Nature Neurosci.* **4**, 95–102.

O'Doherty, J., Rolls, E. T., Francis, S., Bowtell, R. and McGlone, F. (2001*b*). Representation of pleasant and aversive taste in the human brain. *J. Neurophysiol.* **85**, 1315–21.

Ozonoff, S., Pennington, B. and Rogers, S. (1990). Are there emotion perception deficits in young autistic children? *J. Child Psychol. Psychiat.* **31**, 343–63.

Pennington, B. F. and Bennetto, L. (1993). Main effects or transaction in the neuropsychology of conduct disorder? Commentary on 'the neuropsychology of conduct disorder'. *Dev. Psychopathol.* **5**, 153–64.

Pessoa, L., McKenna, M., Gutierrez, E. and Ungerleider, L. G. (2002). Neural processing of emotional faces requires attention. *Proc. Natl Acad. Sci. USA* **99**, 11 458–63.

Phillips, M. L., Young, A. W., Senior, C., Brammer, M., Andrew, C., Calder, A. J., *et al.* (1997). A specified neural substrate for perceiving facial expressions of disgust. *Nature* **389**, 495–8.

Phillips, M. L., Young, A. W., Scott, S. K., Calder, A. J., Andrew, C., Giampietro, V., *et al.* (1998). Neural responses to facial and vocal expressions of fear and disgust. *Proc. R. Soc. Lond.* B **265**, 1809–17. (DOI 10.1098/rspb.1998. 0506.)

Pitcairn, T. K., Clemie, S., Gray, J. M. and Pentland, B. (1990). Non-verbal cues in the self-presentation of parkinsonian patients. *Br. J. Clin. Psychol.* **29**, 177–84.

Pizzagalli, D., Regard, M. and Lehmann, D. (1999). Rapid emotional face processing in the human right and left brain hemispheres: an ERP study. *NeuroReport* **10**, 2691–8.

Pizzagalli, D., Lehmann, D., Hendrick, A., Regard, M., Pascual-Marqui, R. and Davidson, R. (2002). Affective judgments of faces modulate early activity (approximately 160 ms) within the fusiform gyri. *Neuroimage* **16**, 663–77.

Prather, M. D., Lavenex, P., Mauldin-Jourdain, M. L., Mason, W. A., Capitanio, J. P., Mendoza, S. P., *et al.* (2001). Increased social fear and decreased fear of objects in monkeys with neonatal amygdala lesions. *Neuroscience* **106**, 653–8.

Premack, D. and Woodruff, G. (1978). Does the chimpanzee have a theory of mind? *Behav. Brain Sci.* **1**, 515–26.

Preston, S. D. and de Waal, F. B. (2003). Empathy: its ultimate and proximate bases. *Behav. Brain Sci.*, in press.

Prior, M., Dahlstrom, B. and Squires, T. (1990). Autistic children's knowledge of thinking and feeling states in other people. *J. Autism Devl Disord.* **31**, 587–602.

Rapcsak, S. Z., Galper, S. R., Comer, J. F., Reminger, S. L., Nielsen, L., Kaszniak, A. W., *et al.* (2000). Fear recognition deficits after focal brain damage: a cautionary note. *Neurology* **54**, 575–81.

Rinn, W. E. (1984). The neuropsychology of facial expression: a review of the neurological and psychological mechanisms for producing facial expressions. *Psychol. Bull.* **95**, 52–77.

Rolls, E. T. (1997). Taste and olfactory processing in the brain and its relation to the control of eating. *Crit. Rev. Neurobiol.* **11**, 263–87.

Romanski, L. M. and LeDoux, J. E. (1992). Bilateral destruction of neocortical and perirhinal projection targets of the acoustic thalamus does not disrupt auditory fear conditioning. *Neurosci. Lett.* **142**, 228–32.

Romanski, L. M. and LeDoux, J. E. (1992). Equipotentiality of thalamoamygdala and thalamocorticoamygdala circuits in auditory fear conditioning. *J. Neurosci.* **12**, 4501–9.

Rozin, P., Haidt, J. and McCauley, C. R. (1993). Disgust. In *Handbook of emotions* (ed. M. Lewis and J. M. Haviland), pp. 575–94. New York: Guilford Press.

Russell, C. L., Bard, K. A. and Adamson, L. B. (1997). Social referencing by young chimpanzees (*Pan troglodytes*). *J. Comp. Psychol.* **111**, 185–93.

Saarni, C. (1984). An observational study of children's attempts to monitor their expressive behavior. *Child Dev.* **55**, 1504–13.

Schmolck, H. and Squire, L. R. (2001). Impaired perception of facial emotions following bilateral damage to the anterior temporal lobe. *Neuropsychology* **15**, 30–8.

Schneider, F., Gur, R. C., Gur, R. E. and Muenz, L. R. (1994). Standardized mood induction with happy and sad facial expression. *Psychiat. Res.* **51**, 19–31.

Semin, G. R. and Manstead, A. S. (1982). The social implications of embarrassment displays and restitution behaviour. *Eur. J. Social Psychol.* **12**, 367–77.

Sigman, M. D., Kasari, C., Kwon, J. and Yirmiya, N. (1992). Responses to the negative emotions of others by autistic, mentally retarded, and normal children. *Child Dev.* **63**, 796–807.

Small, D. M., Zatorre, R. J., Dagher, A., Evans, A. C. and Jones-Gotman, M. (2001). Changes in brain activity related to eating chocolate: from pleasure to aversion. *Brain* **124**, 1720–33.

Smith, M. C., Smith, M. K. and Ellgring, H. (1996). Spontaneous and posed facial expression in Parkinson's disease. *J. Int. Neuropsychol. Soc.* **2**, 383–91.

Sprengelmeyer, R., Young, A. W., Calder, A. J., Karnat, A., Lange, H. W. and Homberg, V. (1996). Loss of disgust: perception of faces and emotions in Huntington's disease. *Brain* **119**, 1647–65.

Sprengelmeyer, R., Rausch, M., Eysel, U. T. and Przuntek, H. (1998). Neural structures associated with the recognition of facial basic emotions. *Proc. R. Soc. Lond.* B **265**, 1927–31. (DOI 10.1098/rspb.1998.0522.)

Streit, M., Ioannides, A. A., Liu, L., Wolwer, W., Dammers, J., Gross, J., *et al.* (1999). Neurophysiological correlates of the recognition of facial expressions of emotion as revealed by magnetoencephalography. *Brain Res. Cogn. Brain Res.* **7**, 481–91.

Sugase, Y., Yamane, S., Ueno, S. and Kawano, K. (1999). Global and fine information coded by single neurons in the temporal visual cortex. *Nature* **400**, 869–73.

Swanson, L. W. and Petrovich, G. D. (1998). What is the amygdala? *Trends Neurosci.* **21**, 323–31.

Tiihonen, J., Hodgins, S., Vaurio, O., Laakso, M., Repo, E., Soininen, H., *et al.* (2000). Amygdaloid volume loss in psychopathy. *Soc. Neurosci. Abstr.* **15**, 2017.

Veit, R., Flor, H., Erb, M., Hermann, C., Lotze, M., Grodd, W., *et al.* (2002). Brain circuits involved in emotional learning in antisocial behavior and social phobia in humans. *Neurosci. Lett.* **328**, 233–6.

Vuilleumier, P., Armony, J. L., Driver, J. and Dolan, R. J. (2001). Effects of attention and emotion on face processing in the human brain: an event-related fMRI study. *Neuron* **30**, 829–41.

Walker-Andrews, A. S. (1998). Emotions and social development: infants' recognition of emotions in others. *Pediatrics* **102**(Suppl. E), 1268–71.

Weddell, R. A. (1994). Effects of sub-cortical lesion site on human emotional behavior. *Brain Cogn* **25**, 161–93.

Weddell, R. A., Trevarthen, C. and Miller, J. D. (1988). Reactions of patients with focal cerebral lesions to success or failure. *Neuropsychologia* **28**, 49–60.

Weddell, R. A., Miller, J. D. and Trevarthen, C. (1990). Voluntary emotional facial expressions in patients with focal cerebral lesions. *Neuropsychologia* **28**, 49–60.

Whalen, P. J., Shin, L. M., McInerney, S. C., Fischer, H., Wright, C. L. and Rauch, S. L. (2001). A functional MRI study of human amygdala responses to facial expressions of fear versus anger. *Emotion* **1**, 70–84.

Wootton, J. M., Frick, P. J., Shelton, K. K. and Silverthorn, P. (1997). Ineffective parenting and childhood conduct problems: the moderating role of callous-unemotional traits. *J. Consult. Clin. Psychol.* **65**, 292–300.

Zangara, A., Blair, R. J. and Curran, H. V. (2002). A comparison of the effects of a beta-adrenergic blocker and a benzodiazepine upon the recognition of human facial expressions. *Psychopharmacol. Berl.* **163**, 36–41.

Glossary

CS: conditioned stimulus
US: unconditioned stimulus

12

Models of dyadic social interaction

Dale Griffin and Richard Gonzalez

We discuss the logic of research designs for dyadic interaction and present statistical models with parameters that are tied to psychologically relevant constructs. Building on Karl Pearson's classic nineteenth-century statistical analysis of within-organism similarity, we describe several approaches to indexing dyadic interdependence and provide graphical methods for visualizing dyadic data. We also describe several statistical and conceptual solutions to the 'levels of analysis' problem in analysing dyadic data. These analytic strategies allow the researcher to examine and measure psychological questions of interdependence and social influence. We provide illustrative data from casually interacting and romantic dyads.

Keywords: dyads; statistical analysis; interdependence; research design

12.1 Introduction

Social interaction is a fundamental aspect of psychological life for humans, chimpanzees, dolphins and other 'social animals'. In humans, social interaction, especially dyadic social interaction, can have profound effects, promoting both happiness and depression, and possibly even physical well-being and longevity. Ethology, the study of animals in their natural environments, is dominated by the naturalistic observation of social interaction. Social psychology, often defined—at least in the classic American tradition—as the study of the individual in the social context, is finally turning back to the study of natural social interaction. We begin with the story of how and why social psychology turned its back on the study of social interaction, and then describe models of dyadic social interaction that are guiding the field back to studying this central issue.

The most well-known and influential social psychology studies are controlled experiments that demonstrate the power of the social situation to change behaviour in surprising and profound ways. Probably the best-known series of such studies is that conducted by Solomon Asch (1952), which demonstrated that a unanimous group could impose such conformity pressure on an individual as to make the individual report that a long line was relatively short (and vice versa). Second in prominence is the series of studies by Stanley Milgram (1974) which demonstrated that an insistent 'expert' experimenter with the trappings of authority (e.g. a white laboratory coat) could impose such compliance pressure on an individual that the volunteer 'teacher' would give apparently fatal electric shocks to a 'learner' subject. These and a long list of similarly profound experiments illustrate the power of social interaction *without* ever creating any natural contact between the 'interacting' individuals. Whether it is the unyielding and unanimously mistaken majority of the conformity studies of Asch (1952), the magisterial and unshakeable experimenter of the compliance studies of Milgram (1974), the forbidding and frightening scientist of the fear and affiliation studies of Schachter (1959), or the unconcerned and distracted onlookers of the bystander intervention studies of Darley and Latane (1968), the social contexts—that is, the other people—are constrained to uniformity to provide a controlled experience for the 'real' participants in the studies. There are good reasons for the individualistic approach of classic experiments on the influence of 'social' context. The experimental method itself, the manipulation and control of factors that allows the experimenter to draw the cherished causal inference, brings with it some basic ground rules: individuals within conditions should be treated identically to eliminate confounding and to reduce within-cell error variance.

There is no doubt that these and similar experiments have taught us much about the nature of social influence (most importantly, that an individual's thoughts, feelings and behaviour are powerfully determined by the presence and behaviour of others), and each of these scholars clearly acknowledged the interplay between individual and group in real life. However, the experimental methodology of the individual subject faced with pre-programmed confederates has stifled the study of actual group or dyadic processes. From the perspective of the classic experimental tradition, actual interaction brings with it two undesirable consequences. First, extraneous or uncontrolled variation and covariation are introduced, whereas the goal of the controlled experiment is to maximize the systematic effect relative to the uncontrolled variation. Second, the interaction brings with it the threat of a statistical 'nuisance', the statistical dependence of data across individuals. As the methodologist David Kenny (1994) has noted, this nuisance is actually the 'very stuff' of social interaction, because it indicates that interacting individuals actually affect each other. However, to the social psychology experimenter, this statistical dependence across subjects within conditions was devastating because it required moving the level of statistical analysis from the individual to that of the group, and this dramatically reduced the number of units analysed and hence the power of that analysis. Thus, a study of 16 interacting groups, each with five individuals, would not have 80 units or total degrees of freedom to analyse, but only 16.

These methodological challenges helped deter experimentalists from studying actual social interaction. However, a few brave souls were committed to studying relationships such as those between romantic partners, between siblings or between parents and children. Although it was clear that such relationships could not simply be studied by controlled experiments, the individual level of analysis still reigned supreme because of a third problem with conceptualizing and analysing dyadic and group interaction. That is, from disciplines more at home with data from aggregates (in particular, sociology and political science) came warnings of the dangers of making cross-level inferences. Robinson (1950) illustrated the 'ecological fallacy' with the following example: across the 48 US states represented in the 1930 census the correlation between percentage foreign born (i.e. immigrants) and percentage literate was +0.58; however, within the states the average correlation between the two dichotomous variables was −0.11. As Freedman (2001) summarizes, 'The ecological correlation suggests a positive correlation between foreign birth and literacy: the foreign-born are more likely to be literate . . . than the nativeborn . . . . The ecological correlation gives the wrong inference. The sign of the correlation [at the aggregate between-state level] is positive because the foreign-born tend to live in states where the native-born are relatively literate' (p. 4027). Freedman also demonstrates that the same patterns of correlation are found today between measures of income and immigration: large and positive between-state correlation and small and negative within-state correlation— primarily because immigrants are attracted to large cities in wealthy areas.

As Robinson (1950) recognized, the difference between the ecological and individual correlations combines two biases: an aggregation bias whereby the individual-level effect is amplifed by the combination process, and a level-specific confounding whereby the relation at each level is determined by a different set of causal factors. If only the first bias is operating, then the aggregate correlation will be of the same sign as the individual-level correlation, only larger. However, a confounding bias (as in the census examples) can result in the sign of the correlation switching.

The message of Robinson (1950) was that researchers should restrict their inferences to the level at which they collected their data and that they should be sensitive to different causal influences at each level, across and within units. However, in psychology, this warning had the effect of reinforcing the bias towards studying individual behaviour and avoiding the effects of actual social context. Thus, relationship researchers routinely measured only one member of a couple, or if they collected data on both members, they would analyse the data for each sex separately. Why was this so wrong, other than making it impossible to find evidence of social interaction or social influence effects? Consider the cross-state example again. What level of analysis is represented by examining a national census and correlating foreign-born status and literacy *ignoring states*? This 'total' correlation combines the individual (within-state) and ecological (between-state) relationship and tells us nothing about each level of analysis separately. Note that a proper individual-level correlation in the census example was always computed *within-state*. In a dyadic design, the individual-level correlation is not the total correlation across all individuals, but is instead the within-dyad correlation. Thus, whenever effects may operate at both the individual and the dyadic level, no problems are solved by analysing only one individual per dyad. The results will represent a conglomeration of individual and dyadic effects.

In the dyadic case, this can be described by the following identity:

$$r_{xy} = \sqrt{r_{xx'}} r_\mathrm{d} \sqrt{r_{yy'}} + \sqrt{(1 - r_{xx'})} r_\mathrm{i} \sqrt{(1 - r_{yy'})},$$

where r_{xy} represents the total correlation across individuals, r_d represents the corrected dyad-level correlation, r_i represents the corrected individual-level correlation, and $r_{xx'}$ and $r_{yy'}$ represent the ICCs, or proportion of shared variance on each variable. The 'pieces' of this equation are the building blocks of interdependence theory and are thrown away by the kind of designs that throw away statistical dependence. The ICCs represent the similarity within dyad members, and are the fundamental building blocks for measuring interpersonal influence. We begin with this and build up models for dyadic social interaction.

We consider the problems and opportunities of dyadic data analysis in light of a specific example. Stinson and Ickes (1992) observed pairs of male students interacting in an unstructured 'waiting room' situation. These interactions, some between friends and some between strangers, were videotaped and coded on a number of dimensions including the frequency of verbalizations, gestures and gazes. Note that this is a special situation because the researchers randomly assigned the pairs of strangers. This provides a rare opportunity to examine how interdependence *emerges*. That is, any similarity between individuals within these dyads can be seen as an emergent property of the social interaction. Owing to the random assignment, we can assume that individuals start off no more similar to their partners than they are to any other person in the sample. However, if interaction leads to interdependence—so that the dyads are no longer simply the 'sum of their individual parts'—then interaction might lead individuals to become more (a positive ICC) or less (a negative ICC) similar to their partners than to the other people in the sample. When dyadic sorting is non-random, as in the case of heterosexual romantic relationships or male friends as in the Stinson and Ickes (1992) study, this inference is not so straightforward. Similarity within dyads may indicate interdependence arising through interaction, but it may also be an artefact of sorting owing to common interests, common abilities or common status.

A second aspect of the study of Stinson and Ickes (1992) is noteworthy. Dyads made up of male friends or male strangers have members that are (in statistical terms) *exchangeable* because they are not readily distinguished on the basis of sex or any other non-arbitrary variable. When the dyad members are distinguishable it is possible for the scores of the members within each 'type' or category to have different means, different variances and different covariances. For example, if the dyads were made up of a teacher and a learner, the two types of individuals might behave very differently. When the dyad members are exchangeable, however, their scores have the same mean, the same variance and the same distribution because there is no meaningful way to divide them into distinct categories. We do not dwell on this categorization but simply note that the analytic methods are generally more complex in the exchangeable case (Gonzalez and Griffin 2000).

12.2 Assessing interdependence on a single variable: the intraclass correlation

In the case of dyadic and group designs, the ICC has a special meaning because it assesses the degree of agreement within group members. For example, if we assess how often two strangers speak, the ICC provides a measure of agreement within dyads, and so it provides a natural measure of interdependence. If each individual vocalizes at a rate that is equal to his dyadic partner's, but different dyads have different mean levels of vocalization, then the ICC will be a perfect 1 because pairs are maximally similar (i.e. all the variance is between couples). If ratings vary within dyads just as much as they vary between dyads, then the ICC will equal 0 because there is no evidence of similarity or dissimilarity across coupled individuals. If ratings vary more within dyads than they do between dyads, the ICC will be negative, indicating that individuals within groups are more dissimilar than expected by chance, that is, individuals within a dyad are behaving in a *complementary* fashion.

The ICC can be used to index non-independence or interdependence across a wide range of applications, from diary studies where individuals are measured a number of times (time is embedded within individuals and an individual's scores may be similar across those times) to educational studies where students within classes share a common environment (students are nested within schools and the students within a school may be similar) to studies of close relationships where individuals mutually influence each other. In each of these designs and many others, the presence of non-independence or interdependence provides a challenge and an opportunity. The challenge is to deal with the level-of-analysis problem (e.g. individuals versus classes versus schools), both statistically and conceptually. The opportunity is to go beyond merely acknowledging the degree of non-independence and unpack the meaning of the shared effects. Clearly, if a researcher is examining the impact of social interaction, then the degree of interdependence might be a central phenomenon of interest, and should be modelled directly rather than treated as a statistical nuisance that needs to be corrected.

The ICC is one of the oldest, as well as one of the most versatile, statistics. The original computational method for the ICC was proposed by Karl Pearson

(1901). He was searching for an index of similarity in plants for use in genetic research. For example, early genetics researchers could have studied whether the pea blossoms on a particular plant tended to be of a similar size. Pearson (1901) proposed a method for listing all the measurements of interest across all plants and tagging those that came from 'within' the same plant. He focused on the similarity of all possible pairwise combinations of the blossoms within a plant. Imagine there are three blossoms on the first plant: 1 is compared to 2, 1 is compared to 3 and 2 is compared to 3. If they are all the same size—but different from the overall mean across all plants—that adds up to evidence for within-plant similarity.

Originally, this pairwise ICC was computed using a special way of coding data, although other methods of computation have been developed for this maximum-likelihood estimate of the ICC. Consider a simple example of the frequency of vocalization in the members of five male dyads. Let us say that the scores on this dependent variable were (1,2), (3,4), (4,4), (5,4) and (2,3). Each member of the same couple is denoted within parentheses. We could enter these ten data points in one long column, 1, 2, 3, 4, 4, 4, 5, 4, 2, 3, along with an associated column of codes that tell us of which dyad the individual was a member. The pairwise approach involves re-entering the same data but in a different order, an order that switches the two individuals within the same dyad. So, for these data the second column would be 2, 1, 4, 3, 4, 4, 5, 4, 3 and 2. To understand how this coding actually codes the level of agreement within dyads, it is helpful to plot these data, calling the first column X and the second column of reordered data X' (see Fig. 12.1).

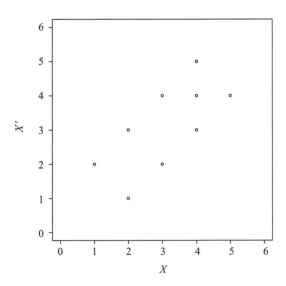

Fig. 12.1   Demonstration of pairwise coding—points only.

This plot appears to show a positive correlation between the two columns regardless of dyadic membership, but actually it shows more. If we connect the two points from the same dyad with a line segment, we see some structure around the identity line. It is this very structure that is the experimental 'nuisance', the violation of statistical independence: these data are not randomly scattered on the plane, instead points are coupled according to dyadic structure. Fig. 12.2 displays the additional structure.

This second plot shows that the two members of each dyad tended to share a tendency to vocalize, as the behaviour of the two members in four of the five couples differed by only one point. Note that perfect agreement corresponds to a point on the identity line, as seen in the dyad scoring (4,4). Importantly, not only do pairs within dyads tend to be similar but there is quite a bit of variation across dyads. It turns out that the traditional Pearson product-moment correlation between these two variables (i.e. variables that have been 'pairwise' or double coded, X and X' in our nomenclature) provides the pairwise or Pearson ICC. In this example, the intraclass is relatively high at 0.706, suggesting a high level of within-dyad agreement.

Consider the data plotted in Fig. 12.3, demonstrating a lack of similarity within dyads. This plots the data (1,5), (2,5), (3,1), (4,1) and (5,3). Again, string these data into one long column, create a second column that contains the re-coded pairwise data, examine the plot and compute the Pearson correlation between the two columns. As one would expect with these data, there is relatively little agreement within dyads but instead there is marked dissimilarity in

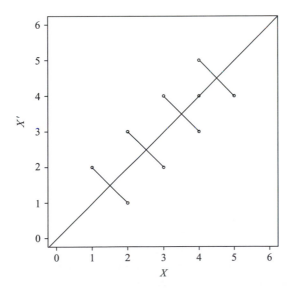

Fig. 12.2 Demonstration of pairwise coding—points and dyad indicator.

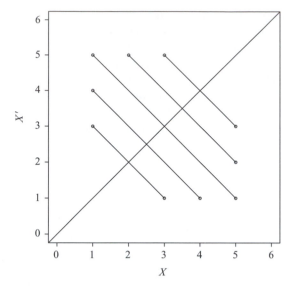

Fig. 12.3   Demonstration of pairwise coding—relatively low agreement.

that when one member of the couple scored relatively high (i.e. above the mean) the other member scored relatively low, indicating some sort of process of complementarity. Indeed, the plots show that the pairs of points are not close to the identity line (which would have signified agreement) and the Pearson correlation between X and X' is -0.615.

From the data of Stinson and Ickes (1992), we selected three variables on which to measure dyadic interdependence: gazes, verbalizations and gestures. Our example focuses on the 24 dyads of same-sex strangers. Each variable was coded in the pairwise fashion, creating a total of six columns of data for the three variables (e.g. the $2N$ gaze scores in column 1, and the $2N$ gaze scores in reversed order in column 2, and so on). The corresponding value of $r_{xx'}$ for the frequency of gazes was 0.57; for the frequency of verbalizations, 0.84; and for the frequency of gestures, 0.23 (i.e. 57%, 84% and 23% of the variance in each variable, respectively, was shared between dyad members). These values of $r_{xx'}$ suggest that dyad members were quite similar on the frequency of their gazes and the frequency of their verbalizations, but it appears that the similarity between dyad members in the frequency of their gestures was low. Recall our argument about the role of random assignment in allowing inferences about emergent properties in dyads. Clearly, individuals allocated to dyads started out with varying norms of how much to gaze at their partner. There was no reason for individuals within groups to show such concordance in amount of gazing unless something like a group norm emerged spontaneously in these waiting-room interactions. When dyads are sorted more naturalistically, then sorting may occur based on the similarity of

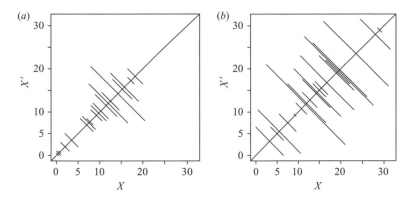

Fig. 12.4 Comparing two types of dyads: the laughter of (a) strangers ($r_{xx'} = 0.72$) and (b) friends ($r_{xx'} = 0.4$).

any number of variables. Then, the standard of proof for identifying emergent norms is much higher, and such inferences may require a multivariate form of dyadic similarity as captured in the dyad-level correlation described in the next section.

Fig. 12.4 presents two intraclass plots displaying actual data from another variable collected by Stinson and Ickes (1992): frequency of smiles and laughter. This variable shows an interesting difference in interdependence between dyads made up of strangers and dyads made up of friends. Strangers share 72% of the variance in smiles and laughter (intuitively, if one member of the dyad smiles, so does the other). However, the data from 24 dyads of best friends reveal the percentage of shared variance is lower (intuitively, there was less matching of smiles in laughter in the dyads of best friends than in the dyads of strangers). This difference in agreement complements the more traditional analysis of the mean, which shows that the best friends smiled and laughed more on average than did the strangers. The agreement analysis provides additional information about the degree of (in)dependence between the two individuals on this variable.

12.3 Three statistical models

Building on the ICC as the fundamental building block of measures of interpersonal influence, we develop models for conceptualizing different types of dyadic processes. We describe three prototypical designs for modelling dyad-level data: the latent dyadic model, the actor–partner model, and the slopes-as-outcomes (HLM) model. Although each model is built upon a common building block, the ICC, each solves the levels of analysis or multilevel problem in a different way, with very different implications for theory building and theory testing.

Consider each model in relation to the study of dyads of Stinson and Ickes (1992). The latent dyadic model (Fig. 12.5) places the main causal forces giving rise to shared behaviour or attitudes at the level of latent or underlying dyadic effects. This model is consistent with such notions as a 'group mind' or a 'dyadic personality'. This model requires substantial dyadic similarity on both variables as a given behaviour is modelled as the combination of an underlying emergent dyadic effect that is shared by the dyadic members and an individual effect that is unique to one of the members. The emergent effects on each variable are then related to yield an estimate of the dyad-level correlation: an example of a research question that can be tackled by the latent dyadic model is 'What is the dyad-level correlation between a dyad's tendency to gaze and a dyad's tendency to talk?' We return to this example and explore it more thoroughly in the following paragraphs.

The actor–partner model (Fig. 12.6) models the causal forces entirely at the level of individuals: in particular, is an actor's behaviour primarily a function of his own qualities or the qualities of his partner? Here, interdependence as assessed by the ICCs is not an indicator of some underlying shared force or emergent dyadic property but is simply a statistical artefact to be corrected. This model does not require dyadic similarity on either variable, but can accommodate any degree of similarity or dissimilarity. An example of a research question that can be addressed by the actor–partner model is 'is an actor's tendency to gaze at his partner primarily determined by his own level of vocalization or his partner's level of vocalization?' A phenomenon that is significantly affected by partner effects demonstrates social influence.

The slopes-as-outcomes (also known as HLM) model emphasizes causal forces acting between levels. Like the actor–partner model, the HLM model corrects for interdependence but does not require it or model it directly. The key assumption is that structure within groups, or individuals across time, can be captured in a within-unit regression model described by an intercept

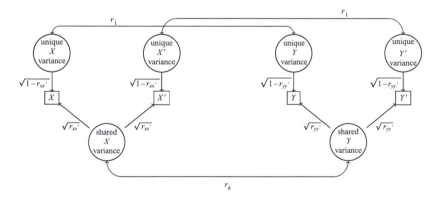

Fig. 12.5 The latent variable model.

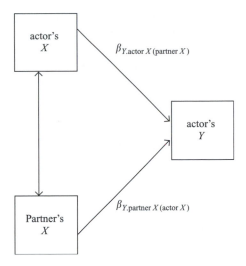

Fig. 12.6   The actor–partner model.

(representing the elevation of the set of outcome points) and a set of slopes
(representing the within-group relation between predictors and the outcome).
These within-unit intercepts and slopes are then described in terms of a 'fixed'
component that is common to all units, and a 'random' component that
consists of the variability among the units. When significant 'random' variation
exists among the within-unit parameter values, the analyst searches for 'cross-
level interactions', higher-level group factors that predict variations in the
within-unit parameter of interest. Note that this model is not appropriate for
the data of Stinson and Ickes (1992) because the dyad members were randomly assigned (thus there are no higher-level variables associated with
dyads) and because there are not enough observations to permit within-dyad
regressions to be estimated.

Let us consider an HLM model that builds on the actor–partner model of
figure 6 and is based on the actual model of Murray *et al.* (2002). They examined how individuals (nested in married couples) responded to daily conflicts
with their partners. Reports of conflict from each partner on day t were used
to predict reported feelings of intimacy on day $t + 1$. Each individual within
each couple filled out a set of daily diaries for 21 days. Thus, it was possible
to model each actor's intimacy as a function of an average level (an intercept)
and slope coefficients for the actor's prior report of conflict and the partner's
prior report of conflict. These within-dyad processes (the relative magnitude
and direction of the actor and partner coefficients) were then related to higher-
level variables, such as the duration and quality of the relationship.

Before we delve more deeply into our three focal models, we mention a
hybrid model that combines a classic experimental approach with actual social

interaction. The 'social relations model' of Kenny (1994) brings the logic of factorial composition to interpersonal interaction by systematically pairing different interaction partners (a round-robin design) and measuring the outcome. This approach, which can be seen as a rare marriage of social and personality psychology, is not reviewed here because it solves the non-independence problem by design (the experimenter's control over the sequence of interaction partners) rather than by analysis *per se*. In fact, in a full round-robin or factorial design, the experimenter can reduce the ICC to zero.

The notion of a dyad-level correlation or even of emergent behaviour is not easy to communicate. We build up these intuitions with graphical examples. Let us make up a simple example with five all-male dyads such as those studied by Stinson and Ickes (1992), i.e. five exchangeable dyads. The scores for the five dyads on level of vocalization are as before with the example showing high agreement: (1,2), (3,4), (4,4), (5,4) and (2,3). The scores for gazing also show high agreement (pairwise ICC = 0.834): (5,5), (2,1), (3,3), (3,2) and (4,5). Let us call these two variables X and Y, respectively, and we will also create the pairwise coded version of these variables X' and Y'. The two pairwise plots for vocalization and gaze frequency are presented in Fig. 12.7. Next to each line segment depicting a dyad, we place a number corresponding to which dyad it is, for example, on vocalization frequency the point (4,4) corresponds to dyad 3 in our hypothetical dataset.

Both of these plots show a relatively high level of dyad agreement (positive correlation within variables, meaning the lines perpendicular to the identity line are relatively 'short' compared with the variation along the identity line); it is also instructive to compare the dyad numbers listed in the vocalization plot with the dyad numbers listed in the gaze plot. At the dyadic level of analysis, there appears to be a negative correlation between the placement of these

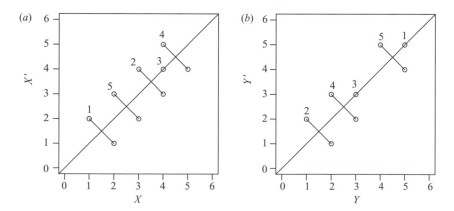

Fig. 12.7   Pairwise plots for two variables: (*a*) vocalization and (*b*) gazing. Numbers in the figure refer to couple identification numbers.

dyad numbers across variables: when both dyad members are low on vocalization such as dyad 1, both dyad members tend to be high on gazes. This dyad-level relationship between joint standing on one variable and joint standing on a second variable is the dyadic or dyad-level correlation. Another way to visualize this is to plot what Pearson (1901) called the cross-ICC or $r_{xy'}$, in this case the relation between standing on vocalization frequency (variable X) and standing on gaze frequency (variable Y'), as shown in Fig. 12.8.

In Fig. 12.8, the Pearson correlation between an individual's vocalization and the partner's gaze, the cross-ICC, is -0.656. The negative correlation can be seen by looking at the 10 points in the plot (ignoring the line segments connecting dyad members). To see the negative correlation note that the scatterplot of points moves from the northwest corner to the southeast corner of the scatterplot. The line segments provide further information because they identify the pairs of points that belong to the same dyad—again giving a visual measure of the considerable within-dyad similarity on each variable. The key conclusions from this plot are:

(i)   that when individual-level relations are stripped out of the data (by examining across-partner relations) there is a strong negative correlation; and

(ii) the dyads appear to be similar on both vocalization and gaze.

These two conclusions are jointly modelled in the dyad-level correlation that captures the relation between the two variables at the level of dyadic latent variables. Such a latent variable correlation also can be interpreted as the correlation between the 'true' dyad-level scores on each variable—scores that have been purged of the unique individual-level effect of each dyad member. This is one possible solution to the levels of the analysis problem: shared variance

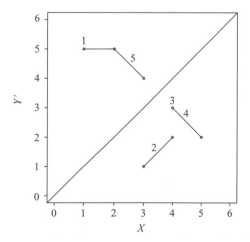

Fig. 12.8   Cross variable pairwise plot. Numbers in the figure refer to couple identification numbers.

within a dyad is treated as a dyadic effect and related across variables to create a dyad-level correlation or regression; unshared variance is treated as an individual effect and related across variables to create an individual-level correlation or regression (as we describe in the following paragraphs). Note, however, that such a model is first and foremost a theoretical choice that implies that there is some underlying and unobserved group-level construct (Dyadic personality? Shared environment? Group mind?) that gives rise to the observed similarity. Alternatively, this model also helps define and give substance to fuzzy concepts such as dyadic personality: it is a coherent network of dyad-level relationships among variables.

We continue using the Stinson and Ickes (1992) data to illustrate the exchangeable case. Having determined that there was dyad-level variance—as indexed by the pairwise ICC—in at least two of the three variables of interest, we calculate and test r_d and r_i. In the case of verbalizations and gazes, $r_d =$ 0.680. The observed Z and p values for r_d were $Z = 2.56$, $p < 0.01$. The latent dyad-level correlation (r_d) between gaze frequency and gesture frequency was 0.906, $Z = 1.94$, $p = 0.052$. The dyad-level correlation (r_d) between verbalization frequency and gesture frequency was 1.10, which is 'out of bounds'. Such out-of-bounds values are most likely to occur when the ICC for one or both of the variables is marginal or non-significant (as in the case of gestures). In sum, the significant, positive values of r_d (and $r_{xy'}$) indicate that dyads in which both members gaze frequently are also dyads in which both members speak to each other frequently and gesture to each other frequently.

Were the three variables related at the level of *individuals* within dyads? The computation of the individual-level correlation, r_i, between verbalizations and gazes is -0.325. In contrast to the positive dyad-level correlation between verbalization and gaze (0.680), the individual-level correlation is negative. That is, the dyad member who speaks *more* often tends to be the dyad member who looks at the other *less* often. This negative individual-level correlation emerges despite the fact that dyads in which there is frequent speaking also tend to be dyads in which there is frequent gazing. However, the individual-level correlation is also only marginally significant. The individual-level correlations for the other pairs of variables were relatively small and non-significant. For verbalizations and gestures $r_i = -0.086$, and for gestures and gazes $r_i = 0.258$. All three values of r_i were markedly discrepant from the corresponding values of r_d and r_{xy}, underlining the importance of separating the dyad-level and individual-level relationships.

Note that all three overall correlations (across all individuals ignoring dyadic membership) were moderate and positive. However, the overall correlation represents a combination of underlying dyadic and individual-level correlations. A more detailed picture of the social interactions that occurred in this study emerges when the two levels are decomposed. Verbalizations and gazes were negatively correlated at the individual level, but positively correlated at the dyad level. Verbalizations and gestures were unrelated at the individual level, but positively correlated at the dyad level. Finally, gazes and gestures were positively correlated at both the individual and dyadic levels.

The latent variable model of dyadic influence implies that dyadic influence flows from a shared dyadic construct to each individual's behaviour. However, the same data can be analysed under the assumption that the influence flows from individual to individual (without latent variable constructs), and that an individual's outcome is created by his or her own qualities (the 'actor effect') plus the qualities of the partner (the 'partner effect'). In the actor–partner model, there is no underlying dyadic effect giving rise to observed similarity; similarity on X is simply an unexplained correlation (the ICC) to be modelled but not explained by multiple regression methods.

For the data of Stinson and Ickes (1992) that we have been using throughout this chapter, the actor correlation r_{xy} between gaze and verbalization was 0.386. In the context of the model shown in figure 6, the standardized regression coefficient was 0.173 ($Z = 0.97$)—thus, stripping this coefficient of its shared variance (by partialling out the ICC) substantially reduced its predictive power. This standardized regression coefficient is interpreted as the influence on an actor's frequency of verbalization given one standard deviation change on the actor's frequency of gaze, holding constant the partner's frequency of gaze. In this case, the actor effect was not statistically significant. Similarly, the partner correlation r_{xy} between gaze and verbalization was 0.471. The standardized regression coefficient was 0.372 ($Z = 2.09$). In other words, the influence on the actor's frequency of verbalization given one standard deviation change on the partner's frequency of gaze, holding constant the actor's frequency of gaze, was statistically significant. The partner's gaze frequency was a more powerful predictor of the actor's verbalization frequency than the actor's own gaze frequency. For one possible theoretical analysis of these results see Duncan and Fiske (1977). Note again how the purpose of this model is to apportion relative predictive power between characteristics of the actor and of the partner.

To illustrate the slopes-as-outcomes approach, data from five dyads are plotted in Fig. 12.9. We look only at the actor effects. Each dotted line represents a best-fitting line for the 20 daily points where today's feeling of intimacy is predicted by the amount of conflict experienced yesterday (Murray et al. 2002). The X variable (amount of conflict yesterday) has been centred so that the 0 point corresponds to the mean level for that individual. In such a transformed model, the level 1 or within-individual across-time intercept reflects how intimate one partner feels the day after an average amount of conflict. The level 1 slope reflects reactivity: how much one's level of intimacy today depends on the amount of conflict experienced yesterday. The solid line defines the best-fitting line (defined by the slope and intercept) across all individuals—this is the fixed effect. There is a small but non-significant negative slope between conflict and intimacy for men and women. The average level of intimacy, the elevation of the famed line, is virtually identical for men and

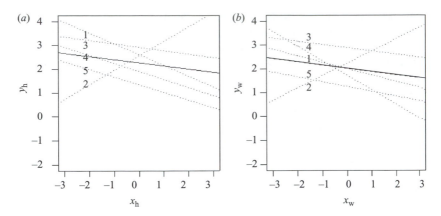

Fig. 12.9 Example from the slopes-as-outcomes model. (*a*) Husbands and (*b*) wives.
Numbers in the figure refer to couple identification numbers.

women. But the focus of the slopes-as-outcomes model is on explaining
the variability of the individual lines around the fixed line, not the degree of
similarity across partners.

Consider the partners from marriage 2 (the number next to each regression
line refers to couple number). In this small sub-sample of men and women,
they are the only ones who show a positive slope between yesterday's conflict
and today's feelings of intimacy. This illustrates both the covariation between
partners (essentially the ICC between partner's level 1 coefficients) and the so-
far unexplained variability of the slopes and intercepts. This variability is then
explained in terms of higher-level factors (e.g. individual or couple-level
factors) that cause some individuals or couples to be more reactive than
others, or for some to react positively and others to react negatively. In accord
with the hypothesis of Murray *et al.* (2002), individuals with high levels of felt
security responded to higher levels of conflict than average by drawing closer
to their partners, whereas those with low levels of felt security responded to
higher than average conflict days by drawing away from their partners. In this
model, romantic partners are treated as parallel multivariate measures so
that interdependence is modelled (i.e. accounted for in the model) but is not
the focus. The focus, instead, is on explaining or predicting the level 1 slopes
and intercepts by higher-level factors.

12.4 Future directions

We have briefly sketched some methods and models for capturing the social
part of social interaction. Some of these methods are rather simple, even
simplistic, but they still serve to direct attention to some key measures of

similarity and influence that have been too long ignored in social psychology. The same basic issues can be modelled at any level of complexity, as demonstrated by Gottman *et al.* (2003) who use general systems theory to model the behaviour of married couples. But simple or complex, it is high time that social psychological models begin to focus on—and not hide from—the statistics of interdependence.

The authors thank W. Ickes for kindly allowing them to use his data for purposes of illustration.

References

Asch, S. E. (1952). *Social psychology*. New York: Prentice-Hall.

Darley, J. M. and Latane, B. (1968). Bystander intervention in emergencies: diffusion of responsibility. *J. Personality Soc. Psychol.* **8**, 377–83.

Duncan, S. and Fiske, D. W. (1977). *Face-to-face interaction: research, methods, and theory*. Hillsdale, NJ: Lawrence Erlbaum Associates.

Freedman, D. A. (2001). Ecological inference and the ecological fallacy. In *International encyclopedia for the social and behavioral sciences*, vol. 6, pp. 4027–30. Amsterdam: Elsevier Science.

Gonzalez, R. and Griffin, D. (2000). The statistics of interdependence: treating dyadic data with respect. In *The social psychology of personal relationships* (ed. W. Ickes and S. W. Duck), pp. 181–213. Chichester, UK: Wiley.

Gottman, J., Murray, J., Swanson, C., Tyson, R. and Swanson, K. (2003). *The mathematics of marriage: nonlinear dynamic models*. Cambridge, MA: MIT Press.

Kenny, D. A. (1994). *Interpersonal perception: a social relations analysis*. New York: Guilford Press.

Milgram, S. (1974). *Obedience to authority*. New York: Harper and Row.

Murray, S. L., Bellavia, G. M., Rose, P. and Griffin, D. W. (2002). Once hurt, twice hurtful: how perceived regard regulates daily marital interactions. *J. Personality Soc. Psychol.* **84**, 126–47.

Pearson, K. (1901). Mathematical contributions to the theory of evolution IX. On the principle of homotyposis and its relation to heredity, to the variability of the individual, and to that of the race. *Phil. Trans. R. Soc. Lond.* A **197**, 285–379.

Robinson, W. S. (1950). Ecological correlations and the behavior of individuals. *Am. Sociol. Rev.* **15**, 351–7.

Schachter, S. (1959). *The psychology of affiliation*. Stanford, CA: Stanford University Press.

Stinson, L. and Ickes, W. (1992). Empathic accuracy in the interactions of male friends versus male strangers. *J. Personality Soc. Psychol.* **62**, 787–97.

Glossary

HLM: hierarchical linear model
ICC: intraclass correlation

13

Dressing the mind properly for the game
David Sally

Game theory as a theoretical and empirical approach to interaction has spread from economics to psychology, political science, sociology and biology. Numerous social interactions—foraging, talking, trusting, coordinating, competing—can be formally represented in a game with specific rules and strategies. These same interactions seem to rely on an interweaving of mental selves, but an effective strategy need not depend on explicit strategizing and higher mental capabilities, as less sentient creatures or even lines of software can play similar games. Human players are distinct because we are less consistent and our choices respond to elements of the setting that appear to be strategically insignificant. Recent analyses of this variable response have yielded a number of insights into the mental approach of human players: we often mentalize, but not always; we are endowed with social preferences; we distinguish among various types of opponents; we manifest different personalities; we are often guided by security concerns; and our strategic sophistication is usually modest.

Keywords: game theory; theory of mind; rationality; social preferences; risk dominance; strategic sophistication

13.1 Introduction

Society is an interweaving and interworking of mental selves. I imagine your mind, and especially what your mind thinks about my mind, and what your mind thinks about what my mind thinks about your mind. I dress my mind before yours and expect that you will dress yours before mine. Whoever cannot or will not perform these feats is not properly in the game.

(Cooley 1927, pp. 200–201)

If society is an interweaving of mental selves, then games are a particularly useful way to look more closely at the quality and hang of the fabric. To play a game is to engage in a certain kind of interaction, and the general claim of the research has been that the way players dress their minds here is indicative of their mental attire in other social situations. Games have become a critical theoretical and empirical tool in the social and biological sciences. A game is a formal representation of an interaction among strategies and 'strategy-carriers'. Examples of such carriers in the game theory literature range from automata, lines of software, viruses, hungry vampire bats, protective fishes, colluding corporations and warring countries, to individual human beings. An explosion of experimental work in the past 20 years has shown that this last category of strategy-carriers, despite their advantages in the areas of reasoning, rationality and mentalizing, can be the most befuddling and the least consistent game-players. These assays have shown humans to be at various times cooperative, altruistic, competitive, selfish, generous, equitable, spiteful, communicative, distant, similar, mindreading or mindblind as small elements in the game structure or social setting are altered.

There is no possible way to do justice to the wealth of work, the thousands of studies and the manifold models that comprise modern game theory in this chapter. Rather, I will focus on recent results from behavioural economics and social and cognitive psychology that detail some of the mental apparel donned by human players under various social conditions. Just as we might dress unthinkingly and automatically in the early morning hours and knowingly grab a light jacket on a windy afternoon, just as we might wear socks every day and a suit on only special occasions, there are similar, discernible patterns in the mental garments we display while playing different games. Human players are not the buttoned-up, conservative, uniform dressers that early game theory expected them to be. Rather, our mental dress is much more casual, simple and flexible. The key findings of our mental fashion review are the following:

(i) Mentalizing is employed in many, but not all, games, as are rules and norms.
(ii) The way the game is displayed significantly affects strategies.
(iii) Players bring strong social preferences to a game.
(iv) Games can be used to diagnose individual differences and personality consistencies.
(v) Concerns about risk and security can determine player choices.
(vi) In general, most players are not very strategically sophisticated.

13.2 Formal wear: morning suits and dinner jackets

As the inventors of game theory stated, formally a game 'is simply the totality of the rules which describe it' (Von Neumann and Morgenstern 1944). The key rules are those that govern the number of players, their possible moves, the flow of information and the outcomes resulting from terminal combinations of moves. A strategy is an action plan developed by a player that uses all the information available and that prescribes a move at each stage of the game. Outcomes are usually represented by simple payoff functions. In the standard theory, these are utility functions of the form

$$v_i = u_i(\pi_i(a_i, a_{-i})), \tag{2.1}$$

where $\pi_i(a_i, a_{-i})$ is the payoff to player i resulting from his/her own action and those of all other players (a_{-i}). The standard restrictions placed on the function, $u_i(\cdot)$, allow analysis to be based on a direct identification of utility, v_i, with the payoff.

We can distinguish some important categories of games. Zero-sum games are those in which any gain for a single player is offset by an equivalent loss spread across all other players; all other games present players with the opportunity to create or destroy common value. Games can be repeated or single-shot. Finally, they can be normal form or extensive, that is, drawn as a matrix or a tree. The simple zero-sum children's game of rock, paper, scissors is displayed in both normal and extensive forms in Fig. 13.1. The payoffs here are normalized so that the winner and loser receive 1 and -1, respectively, and a draw gives each player 0. The dotted line, an information set, connecting the second-stage nodes in Fig. 13.1*b* indicates that player 2 is uncertain which of the branches he/she is on as he/she chooses. Information sets allow any game to be displayed as either a box or a tree, a cross-dressing that proves theoretically that player strategies should be independent of the game form.

One solution concept that is both prescriptive and descriptive is the Nash equilibrium. An equilibrium is a combination of player strategies that is stable. Stability in a Nash equilibrium arises because each player's strategy is a best response to the strategies of all of the other players (Nash 1950). To see this, imagine that, before a single move was made, each player announced honestly to all of the other players what he or she was tentatively planning to do. These tentative plans form a Nash equilibrium if each player answers 'no' to the following question: 'Given what everyone else just said, is there a strategy that would make me better off than my tentative plan does?' Here, suppose that our children announced 'rock' and 'scissors'. This is not a Nash equilibrium because the scissors player wants to change to 'paper'. There are, in fact, no pairs of strategies that would be confirmed; the only truthful dialogue that would cause no subsequent change is if each says: 'I have no idea what I'm going to do' or 'I could choose anything'. Hence, the only Nash equilibrium

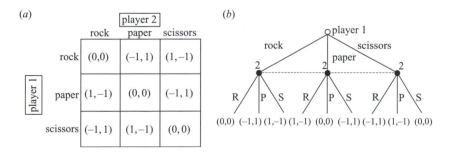

Fig. 13.1   The rock, paper, scissors game. (*a*) Normal form, (*b*) extensive form.

has each child randomizing uniformly among her three moves. If the game were repeated, this equilibrium would result in each player winning, losing and drawing one-third of the games. These were exactly the proportions found in an imaging study of this game conducted by Gallagher *et al.* (2002).

The Nash equilibrium can involve a back-and-forth mentalizing process that was most vividly dramatized in an encounter in the film, *The Princess Bride*. The game here involves a duel over two goblets of wine, one of which has seemingly been poisoned by the mysterious Man in Black. Vizzini must choose one of the goblets and attempts to read the cloaked knowledge and masked intentions of the Man in Black as follows.

> But it's so simple. All I have to do is divine from what I know of you. Are you the sort of man who would put the poison into his own goblet, or his enemy's? ... Now, a clever man would put the poison into his own goblet, because he would know that only a great fool would reach for what he was given. I'm not a great fool, so I can clearly not choose the wine in front of you. But you must have known I was not a great fool; you would have counted on it, so I can clearly not choose the wine in front of me ... You've beaten my giant, which means you're exceptionally strong. So, you could have put the poison in your own goblet, trusting on your strength to save you. So I can clearly not choose the wine in front of you. But, you've also bested my Spaniard which means you must have studied. And in studying, you must have learned that man is mortal so you would have put the poison as far from yourself as possible, so I can clearly not choose the wine in front of me.
>
> (Goldman 2003, p. 2)

Vizzini finally brings his mentalizing to a close, drinks and dies, not realizing that both goblets were poisoned, the Man in Black having built an immunity to the toxin.

The plight of this sophisticated rationalizer was due to his ignorance of the other's resistance. In general, however, Aumann and Brandenburger (1995) showed that if two players' actions are based on mutual knowledge of their payoff functions, of their rationality and of their strategic conjectures, then these actions will constitute a Nash equilibrium. Knowledge of another's conjectures can be derived through the application of theory of mind—our awareness, as vividly portrayed by Vizzini, that others have mental states that differ from our own and that this unique cerebral dress explains their behaviours (Frith and Frith 1999). Hence, the formal result above means that for a two-person game a first-order theory of mind is sufficient to support a Nash equilibrium: a player does not have to interpret what the other's conjectures of his/her conjectures are.

Demands on mentalizing increase when there are more than two players. It can be proved formally that with three or more players in a game, common knowledge of the others' strategic conjectures is now required to support a rational, premeditated Nash equilibrium (Aumann and Brandenburger 1995). Common knowledge of intentions requires higher orders of theory of mind to perceive levels of conjectures about conjectures. Also, many of the most frequently studied games become much more difficult in practice as the roster of players increases. For those researchers exploring the relationship between mentalizing and games, these facts indicate that experiments involving more than two players may be worth pursuing for they can sometimes be an even more acute test of theory of mind.

Cooley might call Vizzini and any player who hews to the Nash equilibrium in every game, who is supremely logical and self-interested, a rational dandy, one whose mind is clothed in the most sophisticated morning coat or evening wear. Such a person might find himself in a finitely repeated Prisoner's Dilemma as shown in Fig. 13.2. The Prisoner's Dilemma has been used in hundreds of experiments and models to portray the conflict between doing what is best for the individual (defection) and helping maximize the group's outcome (cooperation) (for comprehensive reviews see Sally (1995) and Allison *et al.* (1996)). The only Nash equilibrium is to defect in each of the n rounds, as any thoughts of cooperation are banished by the inevitability of defection. For example, the popinjay might hypothesize a completely cooperative relationship up through the last round, but then he/she would see that there is an incentive to defect in the nth trial. Since the rational counterpart knows this as well, mutual defection is assured, making the cooperative relationship last for $n - 1$ rounds. With another cycle of theory of mind, he/she realizes that both he/she and the other will recognize the $n - 1$ round as the new 'last' round and will defect here as well, cutting mutual cooperation down to $n - 2$ rounds. This inevitable logic, usually called backward induction, unzips the cooperative relationship completely.

There is only one problem with this story: backward induction is rarely, if ever, seen among real players (Johnson *et al.* 2002). Most players will cooperate for many of the rounds, not defecting until the last or second to last trial, if they defect at all (data: Sally 1995; theory: Kreps *et al.* 1982). This is but one example of a general finding: most players are not rational dandies and most games do not encourage or reward such naive and calculating behaviour.

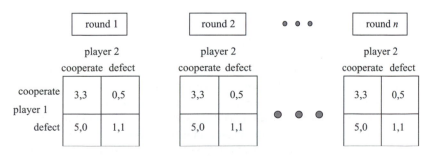

Fig. 13.2   A finitely repeated Prisoner's Dilemma.

In fact, the formal definition of a game given above misstates its reality: 'The game, one would like to say, has not only rules but also a *point*' (Wittgenstein 1958, Section 564). Much of the recent research on game theory has been directed towards determining what these points might be and in what ways people will regularly vary from the Nash equilibrium.

13.3 Emperor's new clothes?

The emperor was convinced as he marched through court to his throne that his robes were luxurious, his breeches well fitted and his blouses radiant. Of course, well suited, or dressed at all, he was not. In the same way, *contra* Cooley, perhaps we believe that our minds are dressed when we participate in society, but really they are quite naked. Perhaps mentalizing is a grand illusion.

We have learned from studies of those with autistic spectrum disorder that mental attire is not incidental to the interweaving of larger society. Many researchers agree that one of the core deficits of autism is a damaged theory of mind (Baron-Cohen *et al*. 1985, 1993; Frith *et al*. 1991). An autistic individual manifests this deficit in the laboratory in an inability to interpret stories involving false knowledge, bluffs and deceptions (Happe 1994) and to automatically ascribe motivations, intentions and emotions to moving and interacting abstract figures (Castelli *et al*. 2002; by contrast, see Heider and Simmel 1944). Largely due to their malfunctioning theory of mind, those with autism, in keeping with Cooley's statement, are not properly dressed in many critical social games (Sally 2001). For example, they infrequently engage in spontaneous pretend play (Carruthers 1996); their language tends to be overly literal and devoid of metaphor, irony, implication and indirectness (Mitchell *et al*. 1997; Tager-Flusberg 2000); they find fictional drama to be unrewarding or frustrating (Sacks 1995); their friendship and acquaintance networks are sparsely peopled (Frith *et al*. 1994); and their gifts are inclined to be incongruous (Park 1998).

Autism is an organic brain disorder with multiple (known and unidentified) causes that injure the innate theory of mind and hamper its full development. Scanning studies of those with autism and those with focal brain lesions indicate that the theory of mind is found in a distributed neural system incorporating the medial prefrontal cortex, which includes areas activated in monitoring the self 's inner states, and the superior temporal sulcus, which is associated with the detection of the movement of animate objects, especially eyes, hands and mouth (Sabbagh and Taylor 2000; Frith and Frith 2000; Chapters 1 and 3 of this volume). So, this neural system may be the physical loom upon which the interworking of mental selves occurs and the social games of friendship, language, gift-giving, etc., are woven. The activity of specific neurons indicates that mentalizing is not a majestic illusion in these games.

Still, it could be true that in the formal games of concern here, as the social trappings are removed to reveal the bare bones of the underlying matrix or branching tree, the minds of players also are unclothed despite their sensations of strategic finery. It is possible that it is not the game itself but its social setting that promotes mentalizing, and in the starkness of the laboratory our minds are simple and unadorned. There are two very recent sources of evidence relevant here as follows:

(i) imaging studies that examine the brains of active participants in games; and

(ii) a study comparing the decisions of autistic and control subjects.

Gallagher *et al.* (2002) had normal subjects play the rock, paper, scissors game of Fig. 13.1 while positron emission tomography was employed to document their neural activity. In two conditions subjects were told that they were playing either another person or a rule-following, pre-programmed computer. In addition, those facing the first type of opponent were explicitly encouraged to outwit and outguess him/her, while half of those facing the computer were told to just randomize each round across the moves. The one region of significant difference in the brain activity of these experimental groups appeared in the most anterior portion of the paracingulate cortex bilaterally—a region solidly within the hypothesized theory-of-mind neural system (see Chapter 3, this volume). There is an another implication of this study: there are approaches to games in which full mentalizing does not occur. Facing a computer and just generating random moves does not engage the medial prefrontal cortex in the same way that outsmarting a human counterpart does.

A similar comparison, but a different game, was used by Rilling *et al.* (2002). These researchers scanned the brains of players matched with another person or a computer in a finitely repeated Prisoner's Dilemma (Fig. 13.2). The scanning took place both when the players were deciding on a move and after an outcome was revealed. Relative to the other three outcomes, mutual cooperation with a human partner elicited more activity in a variety of areas of the brain associated with reward processing—the medial prefrontal cortex (Brodmann's area 11) and rostral anterior cingulate gyrus (BA 32). By contrast to the previous study, there was overlap in activation between human and machine: the ventromedial/orbitofrontal cortex also responded to mutual cooperation with the computer. As there were no special instructions regarding the computer opponent, these experimental participants may have anthropomorphically and quite naturally mentalized. Finally, the decision to reciprocate the human counterpart's cooperative move in the prior round also evoked BA 32, whose role may be to bring an emotional tone to the theory-of-mind system (Bush *et al.* 2000; Chapter 3 of this volume).

The extensive-form game shown in Fig. 13.3a is representative of those used by a number of researchers. In this 'trust game,' player 1 must decide whether to end the game right away with matching payoffs of 45 for each player, or to pass the decision-making power to player 2 who must then choose to move left or right, resulting in outcome pairs of (180, 225) or (0, 405), respectively.

A decision to continue the game implies that the first player trusts the second to not be overly greedy and choose the fairer outcome. Rigdon (2002) compared choices made in trust games that were presented in the theoretically equivalent normal and extensive forms, and found that the tree form increased the frequency of the most cooperative outcome from 15% to 50%. In an imaging study (McCabe *et al.* 2001), participants played extensive-form trust games against human and computer opponents, and they were told all the details of the latter's probabilistic strategy. A human–computer comparison of brain activation in those subjects who cooperated at least one-third of the time overall showed heightened responses in a number of areas including the medial prefrontal cortex.

These imaging studies indicate that whether a game evokes mentalizing can depend on the identity of the opponent, the form of the game, and whether the strategic approach is one of problem solving in the form of rule detection and rule application. E. Hill and D. Sally (unpublished data) reported somewhat similar findings from their research on autism and games. Among children who played a finitely repeated Prisoner's Dilemma (Fig. 13.2), the degree of development of theory of mind was correlated with greater levels of cooperation. However, among adults, those with autism and those normal adults with less sophisticated and accurate mentalizing skills were less reactive to changes in the settings of the games. Theory of mind seemed to be used by the control adults to compete more vigorously and cooperate more thoroughly, in accordance with the altered rules of the game.

Autistic and control subjects also played the ultimatum game in Fig. 13.3*b*. This game represents the essence of many bargaining situations. The first player is given 10 points and must make an offer, *x*, of some portion of the total to the second player. The latter can say 'yes' or 'no', resulting in payoffs of $(10 - x, x)$ and $(0,0)$, respectively. In other words, the second player can scotch the whole deal if *x* is too small or unfair. There were the many interesting comparisons and contrasts among the participants, adults and children,

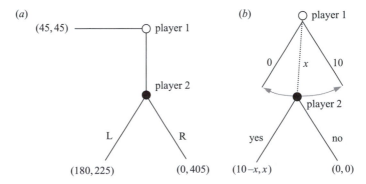

Fig. 13.3   Two extensive-form bargaining games. (*a*) Trust game, (*b*) ultimatum game.

controls and autistics, including the following: if a child failed a second-order false belief test (which was much more probable among the autistics), then he/she was significantly more prone to offer nothing or only one point to the second player. Alternatively, most of the children who passed this test initially offered an even split of the total points. Most autistic adults proposed offers of either zero or 50%, while adults without autism tendered bids that were strategically shaded a notch or two below half.

These and other distinctions between the autistics and the controls, though significant, were outnumbered by the similarities. Hill and Sally (2002) claimed that this was a surprising finding since the literatures of behavioural economics, developmental psychology and cognitive neuroscience predicted gross differences. The decisions of autistic participants were not founded on a well-developed, innate theory of mind but, rather, on a rule-based, awkward, compensatory mechanism (Happé 1994), and yet, they were often reasonable approximations of those of the mentalizers. This type of norm-based behaviour has been witnessed in other games (Henrich et al. 2001), and it raises a question for future researchers—what is the relationship between theory of mind and norms? Is one a necessary input to the other? In what social games are they complementary or discordant?

Taken as a group, these studies provide compelling testimony that mentalizing does occur in formal games: the emperor is at least partially clad some of the time. It may be that the extensive form encourages theory of mind, but we do not know why. Does the tree illustrate movement and progress; does it reduce uncertainty; does it underscore intentions, and if so, how? Mentalizing does not always occur naturally. Gallagher et al. (2002) felt they had to advocate for it in their game, and Hoffman et al. (2000) raised the average offer in their ultimatum game by recommending that subjects consider the other's expectations. To the questions about norms raised above, one might ask, what is the relationship between learning within a repeated game and mentalizing? Lastly, what elements of the identity of the counterpart make the neurally based theory of mind wax and wane?

13.4 Mao jackets and pinstriped suits

One reason that strategy with a machine can be quite distinct is that it is difficult for a player to identify with his/her silicon-based counterpart. Clothing, whether it is donned for a party rally in the Forbidden City or a meeting in the board room, is often used to express solidarity, and it should come as no surprise that mental dress frequently fulfils the same function. Researchers have determined that most players bring social preferences to a game, preferences that place some weight on the intentions and outcomes of other players.

A variety of functional forms have been proposed to represent these social preferences (Edgeworth 1881; Sawyer 1966; Loewenstein et al. 1989;

Rabin 1993; Montgomery 1994; Levine 1998; Fehr and Schmidt 1999; Sethi and Somanathan 2001; Charness and Rabin 2002). These proposals place a non-zero weight on the other players' payoffs (unlike the asocial utility of equation (2.1)), and most include factors representing pure altruism and reciprocity. Sally (2000) reviewed the history of thought on social preferences within a variety of disciplines and developed a modern theory of sympathy. This model of sympathy is a recasting of the original theory developed by Hume (1740), Smith (1790) and Darwin (1936), and it is a variant of these recent approaches—the balance theory of Heider (1958), the simulation theory of Goldman (1989), the notion of identification of Coleman (1990) and the concept of empathy of Gallese (Chapter 7). Following the tradition of functional forms listed here and borrowing the mathematics of kinship altruism as developed by Hamilton (1964) and Hirshleifer (1978), one version of sympathetic preferences (for a two-person game) is the following:

$$v_i = \pi_i + (1 - \alpha_i) \exp(-\alpha_i \varphi_{ij} \psi_{ij}) \pi_j. \tag{4.1}$$

The pure altruism of player i is α_i, and φ_{ij} and ψ_{ij} are player i's perceived physical and psychological distances from player j. Simply, the closer another is to us, the more readily we have fellow-feeling, identification, sympathy for them.

Personal consistency (α_i) across a variety of games is the focus of the burgeoning literature on social values orientation. Individuals are categorized as one of three types—prosocial, individualistic, competitive—corresponding to $\alpha_i < 1$, $\alpha_i = 1$, $\alpha_i > 1$, respectively. A panel of decomposed games, i.e. sets of paired payoffs without any moves, is used to screen and identify a person's orientation (Messick and McClintock 1968). Arithmetically, a smaller α_i means a heavier weight on the other's payoff and a greater return from an other-oriented strategy in a particular game. Hence, a prosocial orientation fosters cooperation in the Prisoner's Dilemma (McClintock and Liebrand 1988), helping behaviour (McClintock and Allison 1989) and more productive negotiations (DeDreu *et al.* 2000). In a very interesting study on the developmental aspects of social value orientation, Van Lange *et al.* (1997) discovered that individuals with a prosocial orientation had more siblings and more sisters than did the other two types. Also, across the lifespan the proportion of individualists and competitors decreases from 45% in the 15–29 age group to 18% in the over 60 group. As yet, there is no research addressing the neural foundations of α_i or how it might be related to theory of mind.

Equation (4.1) predicts that physical and psychological closeness will also motivate prosocial individuals to employ an other-oriented strategy in a given game. Indeed, physical proximity will promote cooperation in the repeated Prisoner's Dilemma and generosity in bargaining games (Wichman 1970; Michelini 1971; Bohnet and Frey 1999). In addition, psychological similarity and familiarity will support prosocial behaviour in these same games (McNeel and Reid 1975; Hoffman *et al.* 1996). Finally, in a protocol that allowed participants to meet each other, identify commonalities, and then play a 'trust' game, participants were significantly more likely to trust than were the anonymous, distant subjects in previous experiments (Glaeser *et al*. 2000).

The cognitive assessment of distance is inextricably bound with the emotions (Hume 1740; Zajonc 1998), in particular with how much we like another person and how good we believe another to be (Heider 1958). So, perceptions of distance interact with evaluation and attraction in such social phenomena as clustered friendship networks in schools and workplaces (Newcomb 1956; Segal 1974), an instinctive approach towards the good and avoidance of the bad (Solarz 1960; Bargh 1997), a positive evaluation of something solely because it is near to us (Cacioppo *et al*. 1993) and affection for someone who mimics our gestures (Chartrand and Bargh 1998). (For a comprehensive review of this evidence on sympathy, see Sally (2000).)

It is a simple and yet profound point that most social interaction involves physical closeness. The result, as Goffman (1983) points out, is that 'emotion, mood, cognition, bodily orientation, and muscular effort are intrinsically involved, introducing an inevitable psychobiological element' (p. 5). There is no doubt that this psychobiological element has a real impact on the strategies players employ in a variety of games. Emerging work on the innateness, pervasiveness and mechanisms of imitation (see Chapter 5, this volume), mirror neurons, simulation, and sympathy (see Chapter 7), and the perception of motion, intentions and goals (see Chapters 2 and 10) promises to generate insight into player strategizing and social preferences. This research might find game theory an attractive arena in which to rigorously test hypotheses about interaction.

13.5 Chain mail and macs

The primary purpose of some habiliments is to protect the body beneath: for armour, from an aggressive opponent; for raincoats, from the elements. When they invented game theory, Von Neumann and Morgenstern (1944) analysed many games from a 'maximin' perspective. This solution focuses on what move in a game would maximize the player's worst, or minimum, payoff. A conservative, risk-averse player might play maximin in order to preclude large losses and boost the guaranteed outcome.

Similar security concerns lie behind the solution concept of risk dominance. To explore this principle, we need to examine another category of interaction—coordination games. Two examples are shown in Fig. 13.4. The first (Fig. 13.4*a*) is a problem of pure coordination: players need to pick the same move and mismatching is costly to both; however, no equilibrium is better than another. This game can represent an encounter between two people moving in opposite directions who will pass successfully only if they both move either to their left or their right (Schelling 1960), or the semantics shared

David Sally

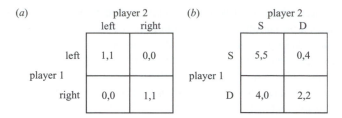

Fig. 13.4 Two coordination games. (*a*) Pure coordination, (*b*) impure coordination.

by a speaker and a listener, i.e. 'left' and 'right' meaning left and right instead of one of the other infinite possibilities (Lewis 1969). Convention is often used to solve these problems: on the roadways, depending on the country, all drivers use the left or the right lane. Difficulties arise in less defined spaces such as rectangular mall parking lots where the drivers slow down dramatically, reducing simultaneity of decision, transforming the game into its extensive form equivalent, and allowing them to pass each other on the 'wrong' side if necessary. (The same extensive, sequential, unconventional solution can happen on the sidewalk as pedestrians are able to identify a potential miscoordination and take unilateral action to prevent it.) In the semantic game, convention is essential and is documented in the dictionary. Finally, players able to solve the semantic game will be able to communicate and untangle other coordination problems more easily, especially if only one person can speak (e.g. 'you go left') or they can talk sequentially (Cooper *et al.* 1992).

The 'impure' coordination game shown in Fig. 13.4 has two Nash equilibria—(S, S) and (D, D). The first equilibrium is payoff dominant relative to the second as both players have a higher return. However, the second is risk dominant as it arises from a move that is psychologically more secure and is confirmed by a wider range of beliefs about the other's move (it also, in this case, happens to be maximin as well). More generally, with two Nash equilibria, (a'_1, a'_2) and (a^*_1, a^*_2), the first is strictly payoff dominant if

$$\pi_1(a'_1, a'_2) > \pi_1(a^*_1, a^*_2), \quad \pi_2(a'_1, a'_2) > \pi_2(a^*_1, a^*_2) \tag{5.1}$$

and the second is risk dominant if

$$(\pi_1(a^*_1, a^*_2) - \pi_1(a'_1, a^*_2))(\pi_2(a^*_1, a^*_2) - \pi_2(a^*_1, a'_2))$$
$$> (\pi_1(a'_1, a'_2) - \pi_1(a^*_1, a'_2))(\pi_2(a'_1, a'_2) - \pi_2(a'_1, a^*_2)). \tag{5.2}$$

Although it seems obvious that payoff dominance should trump risk dominance (and does so when one equilibrium's return is far greater than the rest), game theorists have discovered that many evolutionary models and experimental participants are guided by risk dominance. In a simulated ecology of matrix games, reproductive success accrued to players who favoured the risk-dominant action (Kandori *et al.* 1993; Young 1993). Subjects in numerous tests of matrices like the one in Fig. 13.4*b* were very likely to coordinate on the risk-dominant (D, D) cell (Cooper *et al.* 1992; Straub 1995; Battalio *et al.* 2001; Schmidt *et al.* 2003).

So, risk dominance is a central principle of choice, but are there any essential impure coordination games? One example is that of the stag hunt in which the success of a group of hunters closing in on their prey depends on the absence of any gaps in the narrowing circle. If a single hunter falters, the stag will escape (Battalio *et al.* 2001). Such a weakest-link structure can be found in many team or group production situations, whether on the factory floor, the executive suite or the game-show stage.

Another instance may be the utterance game studied by pragmatics (Sally 2002, 2003). The game in Fig. 13.4*b* is created by the first player saying to the second, 'you are such a moron'. This utterance has a multiplicity of meanings and possible implications: the speaker could be intending to denigrate or praise the listener's intelligence. This particular array of payoffs can be shown to arise from a combination of distinctive cognitive effects (e.g. emphasis, surprise, negative politeness), altered processing costs and the efficiency loss of miscoordination (see Sally (2002) for details). The literal interpretation (Dumb, Dumb) risk dominates the ironic interpretation (Smart, Smart), while the latter is payoff dominant.

A number of authors have asserted that meaning coordination is determined by maximizing the difference between the benefits and costs of interpretation (Prieto 1966; Bourdieu 1977; Parikh 1991). The most important of these efforts is the principle of optimal relevance (Sperber and Wilson 1995).

(i) The utterance is relevant enough for it to be worth the addressee's effort to process it.
(ii) The utterance is the most relevant one compatible with the communicator's abilities and preferences.

The first part of the principle guarantees the addressee a positive payoff, and the second part that the outcome will be payoff dominant. However, as the research concludes, payoff dominance is no guarantee of selection. The addressee has security concerns as well and his/her mind may be draped with protective garb.

There can be situations, then, in which optimal relevance is trumped by risk dominance. Empirically, the interpretation of 'you are such a moron' depends on the relationship between the speaker and listener, not just their individual abilities and efforts: friends will coordinate on (S, S) while acquaintances or strangers will settle on (D, D). In experimental settings, subjects were more likely to interpret insult or sarcasm non-literally and to view it as appropriate verbal behaviour if the phrase was spoken between friends (Slugoski and Turnbull 1988; Jorgensen 1996; Kreuz *et al.* 1999). Technically, this arises when the social preferences of equation (4.1) are inserted into the calculation of risk dominance in equation (5.2) and, if the players are physically and psychologically close enough, the payoff-dominant cell becomes also risk dominant (Sally 2002). There is, then, a connection between sympathy, mind-reading and identification and perceptions of risk dominance.

The impure coordination game of utterance meaning may be neurally represented in the right hemisphere of the brain. Individuals who have sustained damage to this hemisphere, as well as those with autism, have problems picking out punch lines to jokes, revising initial interpretations, understanding metaphors and comprehending discourse (Van Lancker 1997). The summary by Brownell *et al.* (2000) of the neurological evidence incorporates the model of a deciding player and an uncertain matrix.

> The right hemisphere is more likely than the left to process weak or diffuse associations and low frequency alternative meanings, and the right hemisphere maintains activation over longer prime-target intervals. The left hemisphere actively dampens or inhibits activation of alternatives and focuses on the contextually most dominant reading.
>
> (Brownell *et al.* 2000, p. 320)

For those researchers studying connections between the mind and brain, coordination games offer the chance to examine more closely a number of elements of social interaction: norm- and rule-based behaviours, risk dominance and the effect of uncertainty, the role of the language coordination game in other social games.

13.6 Fashion on the cutting edge

View the plight of the one who would be a fashion leader: this person has to be able to predict the taste of the 'hoi polloi' and then stay just one step ahead. It is a cutting edge: half a step ahead and the leader is undistinguished, two steps ahead and the leader is bizarre. The quandary of the stylish dresser is the same as that of the equities and bonds trader: ideally, you are one step ahead of the average dealer—half a step and transaction costs eat up your gains; two steps and either the rest of the world never makes it out to you or holding costs erode profits while you wait. Keynes (1936) originally drew this comparison between investment in stock and the selection of something (or someone) stylish or beautiful.

> It is not a case of choosing those which, to the best of one's judgment, are really the prettiest, not even those which average opinion genuinely thinks the prettiest. We have reached the third degree where we devote our intelligences to anticipating what average opinion expects the average opinion to be.
>
> (Keynes 1936, p. 156)

A new set of experiments has emerged recently in game theory to test what degree of intelligence people really employ when trying to guess what the majority will do. These games and protocols may be of interest to those studying cognition from a developmental or neural perspective.

Nagel (1995) staged a version of the beauty contest of Keynes (1936). Instead of a stylish outfit, 15–18 (N) participants had to choose an integer, x_i, between 0 and 100. The choices would be averaged and then the average would be multiplied by a factor, p. In one condition, for example, $p = 0.5$. A prize was offered to the individual whose guess was closest to the target, $p(\Sigma x_i / N)$. The only Nash equilibrium, in the example, has every player guessing zero. To see the logic of this, suppose the mean guess is greater than zero. Then at least one player is above the mean and that player, holding everyone else's choice fixed, can be made better off by reducing his/her number. As this is true for every player, the guesses should unravel all the way down the number line to zero.

As with the other games we have considered, the Nash equilibrium is a very unlikely outcome in this game unless players are experienced. Rather, one can distinguish the degrees of strategic intelligence proposed by Keynes. Zero-step players decide randomly; one-step players make the best response to opponents who are all zero step; two-step players make the best response to opponents who are all one step; etc. If the zero-step players randomize across the entire number range of 100, then the expected mean of their choices is 50. Accordingly, one-step players will target 25 (shaded by a little to account for their own impact on the overall mean), and two-step players will point towards 12. Nagel (1995) discovered that most of her subjects were either one- or two-step players; a finding replicated by Ho et al. (1995) in a greater variety of 'beauty contest' games.

A single or double layer of strategic sophistication was also the dress chosen by most of the participants in a study by Costa-Gomes et al. (2001). A wide range of two-person, normal-form games confronted each subject. The twist in the protocol was that all the payoffs displayed on a computer screen were masked. To learn what their own or the other's payoff was in a given cell, the subject had to move the cursor over the appropriate region in the matrix. The subject's information search could be recorded and analysed. (MOUSELAB, the name of this laboratory technology, is the equivalent of a mind's-eye-movement tracking device. It was developed by Payne et al. (1993) and has been applied in decision-making experiments by Camerer et al. (1993), X. Gabaix and D. Laibson (unpublished data), and others.)

A one-step player in a normal-form game just has to determine their own payoffs as they are assuming that their counterpart is randomizing across the available moves. A two-step player has to search across all the outcomes for both participants and needs to make certain paired comparisons. By combining search information with actual choices, Costa-Gomes et al. (2001) estimated that 45% of their subjects were one-step and 44% were two-step players.

There is clearly a great deal of overlap between the concepts of mentalizing and strategic sophistication. One might be cut from the whole cloth of the other. If they are not identical, the latter process may be more manifest in the anonymous, multi-player setting epitomized by the beauty contest, and the other may be more important in the more intimate repeated dyadic game. There may also be differences with respect to the search for information and the effects of uncertainty. Those scientists researching theory of mind may be able to help the game theorists get a better feel for the texture and grain of strategic sophistication.

13.7 Headwear: caps and hats

For a number of decades, the formal models and empirical tests of game theory developed in parallel with relatively little contact. The tweed jacket of the theorist and the laboratory coat of the experimenter were rarely observed together. Recent developments in the field, only some of which have been reviewed here, have attempted to knit the models and observed decisions into a single fabric. New games have been invented; old games have been modified; new technologies, such as imaging and MOUSELAB, have been applied; game forms, trees and boxes, have been distinguished; risk dominance and social preferences have been appreciated; new pools of players, autistics and members of small-scale societies, have been analysed. In all, the varied mental garments of players have been more completely identified.

Cognitive psychologists, neuroscientists and animal behaviourists can contribute mightily to a greater understanding of decisions and actions within games. In turn, the uniting of theory and data in modern game theory may make its models and procedures more valuable for these scientists. The time is ripe for cross-disciplinary collaboration. Here are some ideas:

(i) Can we adapt the protocols discussed above to diagnose the strategic sophistication of chimpanzees or children? What is its developmental path? Similar questions could be asked with respect to risk dominance.

(ii) Imaging studies have isolated the neural system that controls the value of a perceived object (Tremblay and Schultz 1999). Scanning and MOUSELAB could be used together as people play a masked game. Would the value-related neural system be activated by the revelation of a large own payoff? What areas of the brain are stimulated when the payoffs of the counterpart are unmasked?

(iii) How are a prosocial or competitive orientation and, more generally, sympathy and theory of mind connected? Also, how are rule-based behaviour and mentalizing distinguished?

(iv) The extensive form may promote the use of theory of mind in a game. What other changes in the game structure or environment would produce the level of mentalizing we believe exists in a casual conversation? Or, contrary to our current belief, are many social games, including conversation, conducted with undressed minds?

Lastly, even the essay is an example of the interweaving of mental selves that Cooley postulated. As occurs in all social interactions, such as a sales call, the essayist dresses his mind for the reader as he writes. With a nod to Tversky (1977) one might ask, how is the essayist like a well-dressed salesperson? He dons his best suit, starts with a greeting and a little small talk, makes his pitch, remains ever polite, crafts his offer, asks for an agreement and ends with a tip of his cap.

References

Allison, S. T., Beggan, J. K. and Midgley, E. H. (1996). The quest for 'similar instances' and 'simultaneous possibilities': metaphors in social dilemma research. *J. Personality Social Psychol.* **71**, 479–97.

Aumann, R. and Brandenburger, A. (1995). Epistemic conditions for Nash equilibrium. *Econometrica* **63**, 1161–80.

Bargh, J. A. (1997). The automaticity of everyday life. *Adv. Social Cogn* **10**, 1–61.

Baron-Cohen, S., Leslie, A. and Frith, U. (1985). Does the autistic child have a 'theory of mind'? *Cognition* **21**, 37–46.

Baron-Cohen, S., Tager-Flusberg, H. and Cohen, D. J. (1993). *Understanding other minds: perspectives from autism.* Oxford: Oxford University Press.

Battalio, R., Samuelson, L. and Van Huyck, J. (2001). Optimization incentives and coordination failure in laboratory stag hunt games. *Econometrica* **69**, 749–64.

Bohnet, I. and Frey, B. S. (1999). The sound of silence in prisoners' dilemma and dictator games. *J. Econ. Behav. Org.* **38**, 43–57.

Bourdieu, P. (1977). The economics of linguistic exchanges. *Social Sci. Inform.* **16**, 645–68.

Brownell, H., Griffin, R., Winner, E., Friedman, O. and Happé, F. (2000). Cerebral lateralization and theory of mind. In *Understanding other minds: perspectives from developmental cognitive neuroscience*, 2nd edn (ed. S. Baron-Cohen, H. Tager-Flusberg and D. J. Cohen), pp. 306–33. Oxford: Oxford University Press.

Bush, G., Luu, P. and Posner, M. I. (2000). Cognition and emotional infuences in anterior cingulate cortex. *Trends Cogn. Sci.* **4**, 215–22.

Cacioppo, J. T., Priester, J. R. and Berntson, G. G. (1993). Rudimentary determinants of attitudes. II. Arm flexion and extension have differential effects on attitudes. *J. Personality Social Psychol.* **65**, 5–17.

Camerer, C., Johnson, E., Rymon, T. and Sen, S. (1993). Cognition and framing in sequential bargaining for gains and losses. In *Frontiers of game theory* (ed. K. Binmore, A. Kirman and P. Tani), pp. 27–47. Cambridge, MA: MIT Press.

Carruthers, P. (1996). Autism as mind-blindness: an elaboration and partial defence. In *Theories of theories of mind* (ed. P. Carruthers and P. K. Smith), pp. 257–74. Cambridge: Cambridge University Press.

Castelli, F., Frith, C., Happé, F. and Frith, U. (2002). Autism, Asperger syndrome and brain mechanisms for the attribution of mental states to animated shapes. *Brain* **125**, 1839–49.

Charness, G. and Rabin, M. (2002). Understanding social preferences with simple tests. *Q. J. Econ.* **117**, 817–69.

Chartrand, T. L. and Bargh, J. A. (1998). The chameleon effect: the perception-behavior link and social interaction. *J. Personality Social Psychol.* **76**, 893–910.

Coleman, J. S. (1990). *Foundations of social theory*. Cambridge, MA: Belknap.

Cooley, C. H. (1927). *Life and the student*. New York: Knopf.

Cooper, R., DeJong, D. V., Forsythe, R. and Ross, T. W. (1992). Communication in coordination games. *Q. J. Econ.* **107**, 739–71.

Costa-Gomes, M., Crawford, V. P. and Broseta, B. (2001). Cognition and behavior in normal-form games: an experimental study. *Econometrica* **69**, 1193–235.

Darwin, C. (1936). *The origin of the species and the descent of man*. New York: The Modern Library.

De Dreu, K. W., Weingart, L. R. and Kwon, S. (2000). Influence of social motives on integrative negotiations: a meta-analytic review and test of two theories. *J. Personality Social Psychol.* **78**, 889–905.

Edgeworth, F. Y. (1881). *Mathematical psychics*. New York: Augustus M. Kelley (reprinted 1967).

Fehr, E. and Schmidt, K. M. (1999). A theory of fairness, competition, and cooperation. *Q. J. Econ.* **114**, 817–68.

Frith, C. D. and Frith, U. (1999). Interacting minds—a biological basis. *Science* **286**, 1692–5.

Frith, C. D. and Frith, U. (2000). The physiological basis of theory of mind: functional neuroimaging studies. In *Understanding other minds: perspectives from developmental cognitive neuroscience*, 2nd edn (ed. S. Baron-Cohen, H. Tager-Flusberg and D. J. Cohen), pp. 334–56. Oxford: Oxford University Press.

Frith, U., Morton, J. and Leslie, A. M. (1991). The cognitive basis of a biological disorder: autism. *Trends Neurosci.* **14**, 433–8.

Frith, U., Happé, F. and Siddons, F. (1994). Autism and theory of mind in everyday life. *Social Dev.* **3**, 108–24.

Gallagher, H. L., Jack, A. I., Roepstorff, A. and Frith, C. D. (2002). Imaging the intentional stance in a competitive game. *NeuroImage* **16**, 814–21.

Glaeser, E. L., Laibson, D. I., Scheinkman, J. A. and Soutter, C. L. (2000). Measuring trust. *Q. J. Econ.* **115**, 811–46.

Goffman, E. (1983). The interaction order. *Am. Sociol. Rev.* **48**, 1–17.

Goldman, A. I. (1989). Interpretation psychologized. *Mind Lang.* **4**, 161–85.

Goldman, W. (2003). *The princess bride*. See http://www.heatherbryson.com/princess/pbscript.htm

Hamilton, W. D. (1964). The genetical evolution of social behavior: I and II. *J. Theor. Biol.* **7**, 1–52.

Happé, F. G. E. (1994). An advanced test of theory of mind: understanding of story characters' thoughts and feelings by able autistic, mentally handicapped and normal children and adults. *J. Autism Dev. Disorders* **24**, 129–54.

Heider, F. (1958). *The psychology of interpersonal relationships*. Hillsdale, HJ: Lawrence Erlbaum Associates.

Heider, F. and Simmel, M. (1944). An experimental study of apparent behavior. *Am. J. Psychol.* **57**, 243–59.

Henrich, J., Boyd, R., Bowles, S., Camerer, C., Fehr, E., Gintis, H., *et al.* (2001). In search of homo economicus: behavioral experiments in 15 small-scale societies. *Am. Econ. Rev.* **91**, 73–8.

Hill, E. and Sally, D. (2002). *Dilemmas and bargains: theory-of-mind, cooperation and fairness.* Institute for Cognitive Neuroscience, University College of London.

Hirshleifer, J. (1978). Competition, cooperation, and conflict in economics and biology. *Am. Econ. Rev. Proc.* **68**, 238–43.

Ho, T. H., Camerer, C. and Weigelt, K. (1995). Iterated dominance and iterated best response in experimental 'p-beauty contests'. *Am. Econ. Rev.* **88**, 947–69.

Hoffman, E., McCabe, K. and Smith, V. L. (1996). Social distance and other-regarding behavior in dictator games. *Am. Econ. Rev.* **86**, 653–60.

Hoffman, E., McCabe, K. and Smith, V. L. (2000). The impact of exchange context on the activation of equity in ultimatum games. *Exp. Econ.* **3**, 5–9.

Hume, D. (1740). *A treatise of human nature.* Oxford: Oxford University Press (reprinted 1978).

Johnson, E. J., Camerer, C., Sen, S. and Rymon, T. (2002). Detecting failures of backward induction: monitoring information search in sequential bargaining. *J. Econ. Theory* **104**, 16–47.

Jorgensen, J. (1996). The functions of sarcastic irony in speech. *J. Pragmatics* **26**, 613–34.

Kandori, M., Mailath, G. J. and Rob, R. (1993). Learning, mutation, and long run equilibria in games. *Econometrica* **61**, 29–56.

Keynes, J. M. (1936). *The genera theory of employment, interest and money.* New York: Harcourt Brace (reprinted 1964).

Kreps, D. M., Milgrom, P., Roberts, J. and Wilson, R. (1982). Rational cooperation in the finitely repeated prisoners' dilemma. *J. Econ. Theory* **27**, 245–52.

Kreuz, R. J., Kassler, M. A., Coppenrath, L. and Allen, B. M. (1999). Tag questions and common ground effects in the perception of verbal irony. *J. Pragmatics* **31**, 1685–700.

Levine, D. K. (1998). Modeling altruism and spitefulness in experiments. *Rev. Econ. Dynam.* **1**, 593–622.

Lewis, D. K. (1969). *Convention.* Cambridge, MA: Harvard University Press.

Loewenstein, G. F., Thompson, L. and Bazerman, M. H. (1989). Social utility and decision making in interpersonal contexts. *J. Personality Social Psychol.* **57**, 426–41.

McCabe, K., Houser, D., Ryan, L., Smith, V. and Trouard, T. (2001). A functional imaging study of cooperation in two-person reciprocal exchange. *Proc. Natl Acad. Sci. USA* **98**, 11 832–11 835.

McClintock, C. G. and Allison, S. (1989). Social value orientation and helping behavior. *J. Appl. Social Psychol.* **19**, 353–62.

McClintock, C. G. and Liebrand, W. B. G. (1988). Role of interdependence structure, individual value orientation, and another's strategy in social decision making: a transformational analysis. *J. Personality Social Psychol.* **55**, 396–409.

McNeel, S. P. and Reid, E. C. (1975). Attitude similarity, social goals, and cooperation. *J. Conflict Resolution* **19**, 665–81.

Messick, D. M. and McClintock, C. G. (1968). Motivational basis of choice in exper-
    imental games. *J. Exp. Social Psychol.* **4**, 1–25.
Michelini, R. L. (1971). Effects of prior interaction, contact, strategy, and expectation
    of meeting on game behavior and sentiment. *J. Conflict Resolution* **15**, 97–103.
Mitchell, P., Saltmarsh, R. and Russell, H. (1997). Overly literal interpretations of
    speech in autism: understanding that messages arise from minds. *J. Child Psychol.
    Psychiat.* **38**, 685–91.
Montgomery, J. (1994). Revisiting Tally's Corner: mainstream norms, cognitive disso-
    nance, and underclass behavior. *Rationality Soc.* **6**, 462–88.
Nagel, R. (1995). Unraveling in guessing games: an experimental study. *Am. Econ.
    Rev.* **85**, 1313–26.
Nash, J. (1950). Equilibrium points in n-person games. *Proc. Natl Acad. Sci. USA* **36**,
    48–9.
Newcomb, T. M. (1956). The prediction of interpersonal attraction. *Am. Psychol.* **11**,
    575–86.
Parikh, P. (1991). Communication and strategic inference. *Linguistics Phil.* **14**, 473–514.
Park, C. C. (1998). Exiting nirvana. *Am. Scholar* **67**(Spring), 28–42.
Payne, J., Bettman, J. and Johnson, E. (1993). *The adaptive decision maker*. Cambridge
    University Press.
Prieto, L. J. (1966). *Messages et signaux*. Paris: P.U.F.
Rabin, M. (1993). Incorporating fairness into game theory and economics. *Am. Econ.
    Rev.* **83**, 1281–302.
Rigdon, M. L. (2002). Theory of mind in two-person experiments. In *Encyclopedia of
    cognitive science* (ed. L. Nadel). London: Macmillan.
Rilling, J. K., Gutman, D. A., Zeh, T. R., Pagnoni, G., Berns, G. S. and Kilts, C. D.
    (2002). A neural basis for social cooperation. *Neuron* **35**, 395–405.
Sabbagh, M. A. and Taylor, M. (2000). Neural correlates of theory-of-mind reasoning:
    an event-related potential study. *Psychol. Sci.* **11**, 46–50.
Sacks, O. (1995). *An anthropologist on Mars*. New York: Knopf.
Sally, D. (1995). Conversation and cooperation in social dilemmas: a meta-analysis of
    experiments from 1958 to 1992. *Rationality Soc.* **7**, 58–92.
Sally, D. (2000). A general theory of sympathy, mind-reading, and social interaction,
    with an application to the prisoners' dilemma. *Social Sci. Inform.* **39**, 567–634.
Sally, D. (2001). Into the looking glass: discerning the social mind through the mind-
    blind. *Adv. Group Processes* **18**, 99–128.
Sally, D. (2002). 'What an ugly baby!' Risk dominance, sympathy, and the coordina-
    tion of meaning. *Rationality Soc.* **14**, 78–108.
Sally, D. (2003). Risky speech: behavioral game theory and pragmatics. *J. Pragmatics*
    (Submitted.)
Sawyer, J. (1966). The altruism scale: a measure of co-operative, individualistic, and
    competitive interpersonal orientation. *Am. J. Sociol.* **71**, 407–16.
Schelling, T. (1960). *The strategy of conflict*. Cambridge, MA: Harvard University Press.
Schmidt, D., Shupp, R., Walker, J. M. and Ostrom, E. (2003). Playing safe in coordi-
    nation games: the role of risk dominance, payoff dominance, social history, and
    reputation. *Games Econ. Behav.* (Submitted.)
Segal, M. W. (1974). Alphabet and attraction: an unobtrusive measure of the effect of
    propinquity in a field setting. *J. Personality Social Psychol.* **30**, 654–7.
Sethi, R. and Somanathan, E. (2001). Preference evolution and reciprocity. *J. Econ.
    Theory* **97**, 273–97.

Slugoski, B. R. and Turnbull, W. (1988). Cruel to be kind and kind to be cruel: sarcasm, banter and social relations. *J. Lang. Social Psychol.* **7**, 101–21.

Smith, A. (1790). *The theory of moral sentiments*. Indianapolis: Liberty Classics (reprinted 1976).

Solarz, A. (1960). Latency of instrumental responses as a function of compatibility with the meaning of eliciting verbal signs. *J. Exp. Psychol.* **59**, 239–45.

Sperber, D. and Wilson, D. (1995). *Relevance*, 2nd edn. Oxford: Blackwell.

Straub, P. G. (1995). Risk dominance and coordination failures in static games. *Q. Rev. Econ. Finance* **35**, 339–63.

Tager-Flusberg, H. (2000). Language and understanding minds: connections in autism. In *Understanding other minds: perspectives from developmental cognitive neuroscience*, 2nd edn (ed. S. Baron-Cohen, H. Tager-Flusberg and D. J. Cohen), pp. 124–49. Oxford: Oxford University Press.

Tremblay, L. and Schultz, W. (1999). Relative reward preference in primate orbitofrontal cortex. *Nature* **398**, 704–8.

Tversky, A. (1977). Features of similarity. *Psychol. Rev.* **84**, 327–52.

Van Lancker, D. (1997). Rags to riches: our increasing appreciation of cognitive and communicative abilities of the human right cerebral hemisphere. *Brain Lang.* **57**, 1–11.

Van Lange, P. A. M., Otten, W., De Bruin, E. M. N. and Joireman, J. A. (1997). Development of prosocial, individualistic, and competitive orientations: theory and preliminary evidence. *J. Personality Social Psychol.* **73**, 733–46.

Von Neumann, J. and Morgenstern, O. (1944). *Theory of games and economic behavior*. Princeton University Press.

Wichman, H. (1970). Effects of isolation and communication on cooperation in a two-person game. *J. Personality Social Psychol.* **16**, 114–20.

Wittgenstein, L. (1958). *Philosophical investigations* (tr. G. E. M. Anscombe). Oxford: Basil Blackwell.

Young, H. P. (1993). The evolution of conventions. *Econometrica* **61**, 57–84.

Zajonc, R. B. (1998). Emotions. In *The handbook of social psychology*, 4th edn (ed. D. T. Gilbert, S. T. Fiske and G. Lindzey), pp. 591–632. Boston, MA: McGraw-Hill.

14

A unifying computational framework for motor control and social interaction

Daniel M. Wolpert, Kenji Doya, and Mitsuo Kawato

Recent empirical studies have implicated the use of the motor system during action observation, imitation and social interaction. In this paper, we explore the computational parallels between the processes that occur in motor control and in action observation, imitation, social interaction and theory of mind. In particular, we examine the extent to which motor commands acting on the body can be equated with communicative signals acting on other people and suggest that computational solutions for motor control may have been extended to the domain of social interaction.

Keywords: motor control; social interaction; computational models; internal models; theory of mind

14.1 Introduction

Movement is the only way we have of interacting with the world, whether foraging for food or attracting a waiter's attention. Direct information transmission between people, through speech, arm gestures or facial expressions, is mediated through the motor system which provides a common code for communication. From this viewpoint, the purpose of the human brain is to use sensory representations to determine future actions. Moreover, in recent years the motor system has been implicated in many traditionally non-motor domains. An important idea is that the perception of the action of others, including speech, involves the motor system (Liberman and Whalen 2000). The proposal is that others' actions are decoded by activating one's own action system at a sub-threshold level and there appears to be a special neural mechanism for decoding such information. Recently, these ideas have gained empirical support in neuroscience with the finding of 'mirror neurons' that respond to both self-generated actions and the actions of others (Gallese *et al.* 1996; Rizzolatti and Arbib 1998; Chapter 7 of this volume). Human neuroimaging and magnetic stimulation studies have also shown that the areas associated with action are also active during imitation and observation (Fadiga *et al.* 1995, 2002; Iacoboni *et al.* 1999; Grezes *et al.* 2001). Moreover, pre-motor systems are activated when subjects view manipulable tools or even action verbs

(Martin *et al.* 1996; Grafton *et al.* 1997). Such studies have brought the motor system to the forefront in the investigation of action interpretation and social interaction. In this paper, we explore the parallels between the computations that occur in motor control and in action observation, imitation, social interaction and theory of mind. In particular, we examine the extent to which motor commands acting on the body can be equated with communicative signals acting on other people. We suggest that computational solutions that developed for motor control could have been extended to the domain of social interaction.

14.2 The Sensorimotor and social interaction loops

The study of motor control is fundamentally the study of sensorimotor transformations. We can view the motor system as forming a loop in which motor commands cause muscle contractions, with consequent sensory feedback, which in turn influences future motor commands (Wolpert and Ghahramani 2000) (Fig. 14.1*a*). The transformation from motor commands to their sensory consequences is governed by the physics of the musculoskeletal system, the environment and the sensory receptors. The descending motor command generates contractions in the muscles and causes the musculoskeletal system to change its configuration. However, the same motor command can have very different consequences in different situations. For example, the same motor command will generate less muscle contraction when the muscles are fatigued. Moreover, the same motor command can lead to very different changes in body configuration depending on the nature of the physical objects we interact with. To describe the variables that specify the configuration of the body, such as joint angles or hand position, we use the word *state*. In general, a state is a set of variables which vary over time and when taken together with fixed parameters of the system, such as the mass of body segments, and the equations governing the physics of the musculoskeletal system and the world are sufficient to predict the system's future behaviour. In general, the state, for example the set of activations of groups of muscles (synergies) or the position and velocity of the hand, changes rapidly and continuously within a movement. However, other key parameters change discretely, like the identity of a manipulated object, or, on a slower time-scale, like the mass of a limb. We refer to such discrete or slowly changing parameters as the *context* of the movement. Finally, dependent on sensory feedback the CNS can generate a new motor command or update the current motor command, thereby completing the sensorimotor loop.

For accurate control the CNS has to adapt the motor command to both the current context and state of the body. However, this information is not directly available to the CNS and these variables are refereed to as *hidden variables* in the engineering literature. Instead the CNS has access to sensory feedback

	motor control	social interaction
loop	(a) 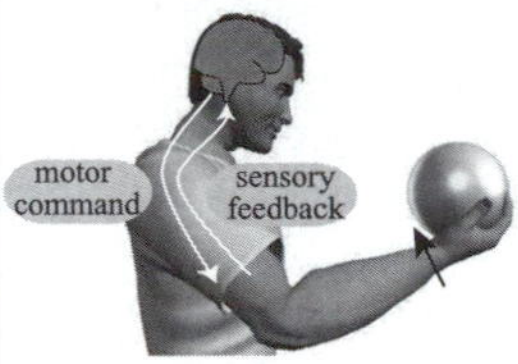	(b) 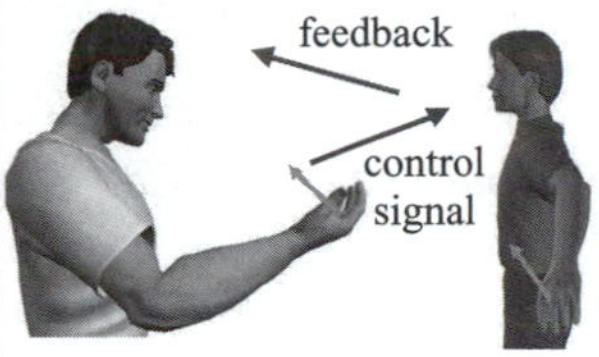
control signal	motor command	communicative actions e.g. speech, gesture
consequences	change in my body's state	change in your mental state
state	configuration of my body	mental state of your mind

Fig. 14.1 The sensorimotor and social interaction loops. The motor control loop (*a*) involves generating motor commands that cause changes in the state of my own body. Depending on this new state and the outside world I receive sensory feedback. The social interaction loop (*b*) involves me generating motor commands that cause communicative signals. These signals when perceived by another person can cause changes in their internal mental state. These changes can lead to actions which are, in turn, perceived by me.

from which it may be able to estimate the state of the body. For example, there is no sensory receptor that directly tells us the location of our hand in space, but many proprioceptive and tactile sensors from the arm can be used to make an estimate of this state variable. Similarly the weight of an object to be picked up can be estimated visually on the basis of prior experience and then updated during the handling of the object.

Motor control is, therefore, concerned with inputs and outputs from a controlled object (e.g. the arm) that is part of our own body. When interacting with another person we can think of an analogous social interaction loop in which the controlled object is the other person rather than part of our own body (Fig. 14.1*b*). Again, our motor commands cause muscle contractions and these lead to motor consequences which generate communicative signals, such as speech or gestures. When perceived by another person these can have influences on their hidden (mental) state, which constitutes the set of parameters that determine their behaviour. We can regard the other person as having a state in the same way that our own body has a state. If we know the state of someone else and have a model of their behaviour, we should be able to predict their response to a given input that we or the environment provides. Given the other person's state, the motor command we have generated, and the context provided by the environment, the other person will generate motor commands causing consequences. We can perceive these consequences and these can be used to determine our next motor command, thereby closing a social interaction loop. Therefore, in social interactions, by controlling someone else rather than our own body, we can estimate their hidden state including their mental state rather than the state of our own body.

14.3 What makes motor control and social interaction difficult?

There are several features of the neural circuitry and musculoskeletal system that significantly complicate our ability to produce accurate and fast movements. First, there are considerable *time delays* in both the transduction and transport of sensory signals to the CNS. For example, visual feedback can take around 100 ms to be processed. When this sensory delay is combined with efferent delays associated with movement, the combined delay is appreciable. As a consequence, sensory information cannot be used to guide the initial part of a movement and skilled performance requires feed-forward control. However, there is still a problem of co-registering actions with their consequences in time as these signals can be separated by several hundred milliseconds. In addition to delays, the sensory inputs and motor commands suffer from intrinsic *neural noise*, or randomness, which limits the ability of the system to perform rapid and accurate movements simultaneously (Harris and Wolpert 1998).

Not only are motor and sensory signals delayed and noisy, but the relationship between the motor commands and sensory consequences can be very complicated. The equations relating the force produced by muscles and the ensuing motion of the body are highly complex. For example, the equations that determine the effect that a single muscle acting on the elbow has on the subsequent change in elbow angle will, owing to interactions between body segments, have terms that depend in complex ways on factors such as the orientation of the body with respect to gravity, the rotation of the body in space and the rotational velocity of the shoulder joint. Moreover, the complexity of the musculoskeletal system is made worse because it has *nonlinear* properties. Linear systems are ones in which if you know how the system responds to two different sequences of force acting on it, then it is very easy to predict what will happen when the two series of forces are added and applied together. For example, a ball on a table acted on by forces is a linear system. A sequence of forces acting on the ball will cause the ball to take up a sequence of positions on the table. Another sequence of forces acting on the ball will cause the ball to take up a different sequence of positions. If we add the two sequences of forces and applied these to the ball it would follow a path determined by the sum of the positions from each sequence individually. However, the musculoskeletal system is nonlinear and this makes motor control difficult as knowing the consequence of a variety of motor commands does not allow us easily to generalize to what will happen to combinations of these motor commands.

Moreover, the relationship between motor commands and ensuing movement changes every time we interact with a novel object. This property of being ever-changing is known as *non-stationarity*. This requires that the command sent to our body be tailored to the changing interactions with the world.

Finally, the motor system has a high-dimensional state (dimension refers to number of parameters required to define the state). For example, the final control must be exerted on the 600 or so muscles in the human body. Even if we consider each, as being, for extreme simplicity, either contracted or relaxed, this leads to 2^{600} possible motor activation patterns, more than the number of atoms in the known universe. When trying to represent such high-dimensional data we run into the problem of the 'curse of dimensionality' (Bellman 1957). It is implausible that the CNS represents all possible configurations so it must instead find simplifying rules during control and learning.

When considering the social interaction loop and regarding another person as the controlled object, we encounter similar, but usually more severe, problems. First, the time delays between our action and the consequences on our own body are of the order of hundreds of milliseconds, whereas with other people the consequences can be of the order of seconds to minutes or even days. Moreover, the response of a person to our actions is not easily predicted. There is usually a complex, noisy and nonlinear relationship between our actions and the consequences. In a similar way to the nonlinearity of the arm, knowing how someone will respond to two separate actions we perform does not allow us to predict accurately the response to both actions performed simultaneously. Moreover, in the same way that motor command and sensory feedback are corrupted by noise we can regard the other person as a nonlinear system with noise. There is noise in both their perception of our actions and our perception of their response. But moreover, there may be a stochastic element in their response to the same action. Part of this is due to their internal state to which we do not have access, and part can be considered as a stochastic element in their choice of response. In addition, whereas the state of the human body has perhaps several hundred degrees of freedom, the possible degrees of freedom of another person's brain are likely to be far greater.

Finally, in the same way that the motor system has to deal with multiple contexts, such as multiple tools, social interaction requires us to interact with multiple people. Different tools have different dynamics, that is, different response to forces we apply to them. Similarly, different people will react in different ways to the same input. Therefore both control and social interaction have to take into account the context, whether it is the identity of a tool or the identity of another person.

However, although the behaviour of others given our actions are more noisy, nonlinear, delayed and of higher dimension than the response of our arm to our motor command, they may not be fundamentally different in terms of computational requirements.

14.4 Internal models of the loop transformations

On the basis of computational studies it has been proposed that the CNS internally simulates aspects of the sensorimotor loop in planning, control and learning (Kawato *et al.* 1987; Jordan 1995; Miall and Wolpert 1996; Wolpert and Flanagan 2001). The neural circuits within the CNS that perform such transformations are termed *internal models* as they are internal to the CNS and model aspects of the sensorimotor loop. Internal models that predict the sensory consequences of a motor command are known as *forward* models as they model the causal (forward) relationship between actions and their consequences. A forward model, therefore, can be used to predict how the motor system's state changes in response to a given motor command. Therefore, whereas the descending motor command acts on the actual sensorimotor system, a copy of this motor command, termed *efference copy* can pass into a forward model which acts as a neural simulator of the musculoskeletal system and environment. A forward model can, therefore, be used as a predictor or simulator of the consequences of an action. An inverse model performs the opposite transformation to a forward model, determining the motor command required to achieve some desired outcome. Here, we will use predictor and controller synonymously with forward and inverse models, respectively.

Skilled motor behaviour relies on accurate predictive models of both our own body and external objects and environments. As the dynamics of our body changes during development, and as we experience tools that have their own intrinsic dynamics, we constantly need to acquire new models and update existing models. Thus, forward models are not fixed entities but must be learned and updated through experience. Learning a predictive model is relatively straightforward. By comparing the predicted and actual outcome of a motor command a prediction error can be generated. Well-established computational learning rules can be used to translate these errors in prediction into changes in synaptic weights that will improve any future predictions of a forward model. We can consider a similar forward or predictive model for social interaction. In this case another person's response to my motor commands or communicative behaviour is modelled. Again, discrepancies between anticipated and actual behaviour can be used to refine such a model. Therefore, by monitoring one's own action and the response of others it is possible to learn a predictive model of the likely behaviour of someone in response to our actions.

Inverse models or controllers are in general more difficult to learn. Additional transformations may have to be applied to the error signal before it can be used to train a controller. For example, when we throw a dart, the error we receive is in visual coordinates. This sensory error must be converted into motor command errors suitable for updating the inverse model. The two principal methods proposed in the motor control literature for solving this problem are 'distal supervised learning' (Jordan and Rumelhart 1992) and 'feedback error learning' (Kawato 1990). Distal supervised learning uses a predictive model of the system to convert from sensory errors to the required changes to the motor command, whereas feedback error learning uses a simple feedback controller to achieve a similar conversion of errors. In motor control a controller often tries to achieve some desired state of the motor system. Similarly, an inverse social model could be used to try to achieve some hidden mental state, and hence behaviour, in another person. Again, learning such a model is difficult in social interaction, as a discrepancy between another person's internal state and/or behaviour and what you wanted does not directly allow you to determine how to change your communicative signals to get nearer to the desired outcome. As with motor control, a forward social model could be used to determine the appropriate change in our actions to achieve our desired result.

Although we can phrase the forward and inverse social models in the same computational framework as motor control this should not hide several differences which makes learning such social models immensely more difficult. First, when the brain models (either forward or inverse) the motor apparatus, regardless of noise, delay, nonlinearity, the degrees of freedom are relatively small, and although some states can be considered as hidden, the depth to which they are hidden is not severe. This is because our sensory system provides us with ample information to determine the state of our arm and we have relatively limited set of control parameters that we can apply to our 600 or so muscles. Alternatively, when trying to learn an internal model of another person, the degrees of freedom are enormous, and the hidden variables are more deeply hidden. We usually need to estimate inputs and outputs of a system to model it. The brain's inputs and outputs are sensory feedbacks and motor commands. Those of the other person's brain are not available. My communication signal transmitted to you and your perceived communication signals may be too superficial to train a good internal model of you. If these signals were sufficient for a general algorithm to learn, then we would expect there to be nothing special to human communication when compared with learning an internal model of a pet dog or a humanoid robot. So, if exactly the same computational algorithms as those used in motor control are applied for communication problems, we believe the task would be excessively difficult to solve. Another problem in terms of learning is that when learning how a system responds to a set of inputs you normally want to explore a large range of inputs to see the range of outputs. Although this is possible when trying out commands on your arm, you cannot give an arbitrary battery of inputs to another person for system identification purposes, as unlike your arm another person has the option to withdraw communication once you have provided a 'bad' input (except, perhaps, in the case of infants and their mothers).

We propose that the reason we are able to solve the problem of learning internal models of other people is because of the similarity of brains across people. We propose that the uniqueness of human communication relies on our brains being similar. This allows the brain to use this fact to train a good internal model of another person's brain. We will review how having a similar motor system (brain and musculoskeletal system) between two people enables us to use the mappings between our actions and our own mental states as *a priori* information to bootstrap any learning of another person's internal models. We will illustrate these principles for a model of motor control: the MOSAIC model that we have developed.

14.5 Multiple internal models for action production and imitation

Humans demonstrate a remarkable ability to generate accurate and appropriate motor behaviour under many different and often uncertain environmental conditions. It has been proposed that the CNS uses a modular approach in which multiple controllers coexist and are selected based on the movement context or state (Jacobs *et al.* 1991; Narendra *et al.* 1995; Narendra and Balakrishnan 1997; Ghahramani and Wolpert 1997). Therefore, when we pick up an object with unknown dynamics we need to identify the context and select the appropriate controller. One possible solution to this identification and selection problem has been proposed in the form of the MOSAIC model (Wolpert and Kawato 1998; Haruno *et al.* 2001; Doya *et al.* 2002). The idea is that the brain simultaneously runs multiple forward models that predict the behaviour of the motor system to determine the current dynamics of the body which will change when interacting with different objects. Consider a very simple example in which there are only two contexts: that a teapot to be lifted is either full or empty (Fig. 14.2). When a motor command is generated, an efference copy of the motor command is used to simulate the sensory consequences under the two possible contexts. The predictions based on an empty teapot suggest that lift-off will take place early compared with a full teapot and that the lift will be higher. These predictions are compared with actual feedback. As the teapot is, in fact, empty the sensory feedback matches the predictions of the empty teapot context. This leads to a high likelihood for the empty teapot and a low likelihood of the full teapot. Each predictor can, therefore, be regarded as a hypothesis tester for the context that it models. The smaller the error in prediction, the more likely the context. Moreover, each predictor is paired with a corresponding controller forming a predictor–controller pair. The MOSAIC model is able to learn a set of predictors to cover the experienced behaviours and also ensures that the each paired controller is the appropriate controller to use in the context for which paired predictor is tuned (Haruno *et al.* 2001). If the prediction of one of the forward models closely matches the actual sensory feedback, then its paired controller will be selected and used to determine subsequent motor commands. In computational terms, the sensory prediction error from a given forward model is

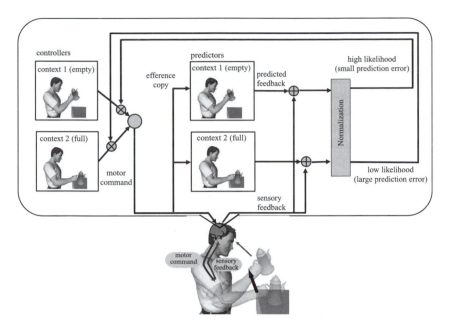

Fig. 14.2 The MOSAIC architecture. A schematic of context estimation with just two contexts: that a teapot is empty or full. In this highly simplified example, a module consists of a controller–predictor pair. In this case two controller–predictor pairs exist: one tuned for a full teapot and one for an empty teapot. The outputs of the controllers are weighted by the likelihood that each is appropriate, to determine the final motor command. When this motor command is generated, an efference copy of the motor command is used to simulate, using the two predictors, the sensory consequences under the two possible contexts. The predictions based on an empty teapot suggest that lift-off will take place early compared with a full teapot and that the lift will be higher. These predictions are compared with actual feedback and the errors are normalized to turn them into likelihood or responsibilities. As the teapot is, in fact, empty the sensory feedback matches the predictions of the empty teapot context. This leads to a high likelihood for the empty teapot and a low likelihood of the full teapot. These responsibilities are used to adjust the weightings of the controllers so as to generate motor commands appropriate for an empty teapot. In addition, the responsibilities are used to gate the learning of the predictors and controllers (not shown).

represented as a probability; if the error is small then the probability that the forward model is appropriate is high. The set of probabilities, termed *responsibilities*, from an array of forward models is used to weight the outputs of the paired controllers.

Learning by imitation is an essential part of human motor behaviour and seems very limited in other animals, even chimpanzees. Although seemingly a trivial task of 'copying' somebody's action, learning by imitation poses a series of computational challenges including:

  (i) how to map the perceptual variables (e.g. visual and auditory input) into
       corresponding motor variables;
 (ii) how to compensate for the difference in the physical properties and con-
       trol capability of the demonstrator and imitator; and
(iii) how to understand the intention of action (e.g. objective function in
       optimal control) from observation of the resulting movements (see
       Schaal *et al.* 2003).

In the MOSAIC model the consequences of a movement are compared with
multiple predictions as a form of hypothesis testing as to the dynamics of the
current state or context. Each predictor tests the hypothesis that the current
dynamic is well captured by the predictor. The set of errors are transformed
into responsibilities (probabilities) and provide rich information about the
likely state the system is in. A natural extension of the model is to compare
the predictions, not with one's own state, but with the state of a system that is
being observed. We hypothesize that, in this way, during action observation
the motor system can be used to understand the actions of others. This could
be an efficient process because our CNS has learned to predict the consequences of actions on our own body and this can be used to make accurate
prediction about others. The use of our own motor system in understanding
actions could underlie our extraordinary ability to detect and identify biological motion (Johansson 1973).

For the actor, at a given time only one or a small set of modules generates
a motor output (Fig. 14.3*a*). To use MOSAIC to imitate movements requires
three stages. First, the visual information of the actor's movement must be
converted into a format that can be used as inputs to the system such as the
motor system. This requires that the visual processing system obtains something akin to state (e.g. joint angles) over time which can then be used by the
MOSAIC (we do not deal with this visual problem here). The second stage is
that each controller in the observer generates the motor command which it
would produce given the observed trajectory and current state of the actor.
Rather than these commands acting on the observer's own musculoskeletal
system, the output of each controller forms the input to its paired predictor,
thereby generating a prediction of the next likely state (Fig. 14.3*b*).
Therefore the observer uses his own multiple modules to try to simulate the
observed percept. This next state prediction can be compared with the actor's
next state to produce prediction errors. Again, these prediction errors can be
converted into responsibilities determining which of my controllers has to be
active to generate the motion I see you perform. Therefore, the identities of the
modules which best account for the percept form a symbolic code of the hidden state of the actor. When the actor generates a continuous trajectory (by
activating modules $2 \rightarrow 1 \rightarrow 3 \rightarrow 1 \rightarrow 4 \ldots$), the observer encodes this as a symbolic stream (e.g. module $1 \rightarrow 3 \rightarrow 4 \rightarrow 2 \rightarrow 1 \ldots$) representing which module

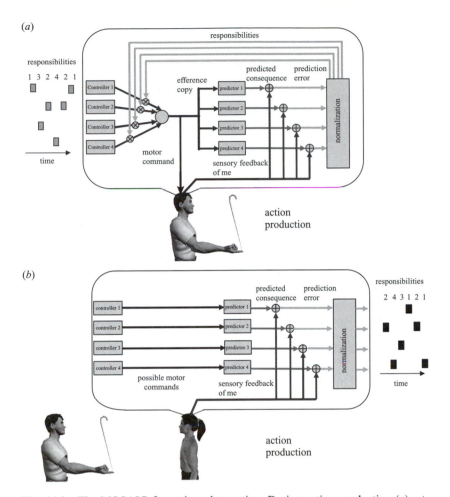

Fig. 14.3 The MOSAIC for action observation. During action production (*a*), at a given time only one or a small set of modules generates a motor output. In this example of balancing a walking stick on a finger, the modules are activated in a particular sequence such as $1 \rightarrow 3 \rightarrow 2 \rightarrow 4 \rightarrow 2 \rightarrow 1$. For action production the outputs of the controllers are combined and predictions of the consequences of the motor command are compared with sensory feedback from my own body to determine future control. For action observation (*b*) each controller in the observer generates the motor command that it would produce given the observed trajectory and current state of the observed person. Rather than these commands acting on the observer's own musculoskeletal system, the output of each controller forms the input to its paired predictor, thereby generating a prediction of the likely next state. Therefore, the observer uses her own multiple modules to try to simulate the observed percept. These predictions are compared with the observed next state of the performer, leading to the likelihood that each of the observer's controllers would have generated the behaviour. Therefore, the observer encodes this as a symbolic stream, for example $2 \rightarrow 4 \rightarrow 3 \rightarrow 1 \rightarrow 2 \rightarrow 4$, representing the sequence of modules that needs to be used to generate the observed behaviour. The observer can use this information in imitation either by replacing their usual sequence of module activation or by biasing the selection.

needs to be used to generate the observed behaviour. This symbolic representation captures a representation of the observed movement, which has fewer dimensions than would be needed to store the entire trajectory. Moreover, the movement is represented in the observer's private lexicon. If the MOSAIC of the actor and observer are identical (which is never likely to be the case) then the symbolic representations should be identical. The more different the MOSAICs the harder it may be for the observer to represent the actor's behaviour. The final stage is for the observer to use the symbolic sequence in imitation. By using the extracted symbolic sequence of module activations to activate her modules over time she is able to generate the behaviour. This information can either replace the observer's usual sequence of module activation or be used to bias it towards a better action. Preliminary simulations show that the MOSAIC can be used in this way to learn a simple acrobot task (swinging up a jointed stick to the vertical) through action observation and imitation (Doya *et al.* 2000). Therefore, the MOSAIC architecture could form the basis of a system for action production and action imitation.

This method of action observation contrasts with previous methods of imitation learning that use several heuristic methods for storing features of movement patterns, for example, points of high curvature or discontinuity (Kuniyoshi *et al.* 1994; Wada *et al.* 1995; Miyamoto *et al.* 1996). The current approach could provide a more general principle for segmenting continuous movement patterns: a local trajectory that is well predicted by a pair of controllers and predictors could be regarded as a primitive motion.

Although action observation and understanding could be achieved by purely sensory approaches we suggest that there are computational benefits to using the motor system in approaches such as with the MOSAIC model. For example, HMMs have been used extensively for automatic segmentation of motion capture data of full body motion. Multiple HMMs have the same probabilistic and modular architecture as MOSAIC, and a long history of moderately successful application to fields such as speech recognition. The essential difference between MOSAIC and HMMs is that controllers are involved. Inclusion of controllers may be beneficial for two reasons. First, the communication signals such as speech, facial expressions or body language, are generated by controllers. Thus, MOSAIC is a better model than HMM as a generative model of these communicative signals. Second, given the similarity of brains within the human species, my MOSAIC should be a much better approximation than any arbitrary recurrent or feed-forward neural network or HMM as a model of another person's brain.

14.6 Hierarchy for the control and extraction of intentions

Hierarchy plays a key role in human motor control. We can generate a variety of motor sequences in a very coherent manner despite the different conditions and contexts in which we have to act. For example, the kinematics of writing is preserved when using different effectors and when the dynamics of the pen are varied. This suggests that high-level representations of the characters may exist and that the lower levels are concerned with compensating for different dynamics. An interesting question is how such hierarchical motor control can be learned and used?

A feature lacking in the current formulation of the MOSAIC model is the hierarchical and bi-directional control of the modules' activity. To incorporate such control, we have proposed a new conceptual architecture, the HMOSAIC consisting of several layers of MOSAIC (Haruno *et al.* 2003) (Fig. 14.4).

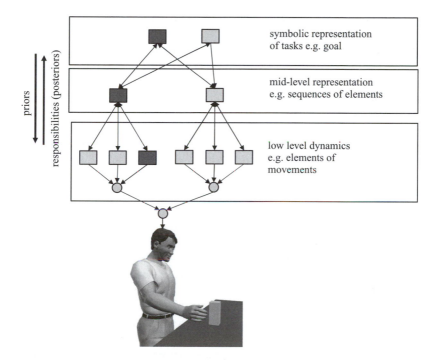

Fig. 14.4 The hierarchical MOSAIC for action generation. Three layers of a simple HMOSAIC are shown in which each block is a module, representing a predictor–controller pair, with the lowest levels represented by two flat MOSAIC structures. The input of higher-level modules is the (bottom-up) responsibility signals (posterior probability) from the subordinate modules, which represent the currently selected modules given the current behavioural situation. The output of higher-level modules is a set of (top-down) prior probabilities of the subordinate modules, which act to prioritize lower-level module selection. The HMOSAIC architecture can learn both elementary movements (lower-level chunking) and their hierarchical temporal order (mid-level sequencing) through sensorimotor learning. Progressively higher levels learn more abstract representations, with the higher-level learning goals or intentions. Therefore the activations of a higher-level goal, such as to pick up an object, would activate lower-level modules (dark) in such a way as to finally generate the appropriate commands to reach for an object.

Bi-directional information processing between layers of HMOSAIC can be phrased within a Bayesian statistical framework. The input of higher-level modules is the (bottom-up) responsibility signals (posterior probability) from the subordinate modules, which represent the currently selected modules given the current behavioural situation. The output of higher-level modules is a set of (top-down) prior probabilities of the subordinate modules, which act to prioritize lower-level module selection. More precisely, the higher control model learns to output the prior probabilities to lower modules given the current behavioural situation and possibly an abstract (symbolic) desired behaviour. By contrast, the higher predictive model learns to anticipate the posterior probability of the lower level at the next time step. The precision of the prediction is used to weight the outputs from control models as well as the learning signal for both predictive and control models. Thus, the lower- and higher-level modules interact bidirectionally during learning and control of hierarchically organized movements. The HMOSAIC architecture can learn both elementary movements (lower-level chunking) and their hierarchical temporal order (higher-level sequencing) through sensorimotor learning. Simulations have shown that the HMOSAIC can learn how to control multiple objects and learn how the object is likely to change over time, thereby learning temporal sequences (Haruno *et al.* 2003). The hierarchical architecture embodies a way of reconciling top-down plans and bottom-up constraints. This is a fundamental problem in hierarchical decision systems, often called a 'symbol grounding' problem.

Conceptually the lowest level in the hierarchy learns the elements of control for different contexts or states. The next level up learns how to put elemental sequences together: for example, learning how to control transitions between the modules, thereby learning elemental sequence patterns. Progressively higher levels learn more abstract representations, with the higher levels learning goals or intentions. Therefore the activations of a higher-level goal such as to get a drink of water, would activate lower levels in such a way as to finally generate the appropriate commands to reach for a glass of water. An important feature of the hierarchy is the tree-like structure so that higher levels could have multiple paths to activating lower levels, and the choice of path, or way of achieving a goal, can be biased by higher-level factors. By including recurrent networks within the modules at higher levels in HMOSAIC, the architecture should be able to generate arbitrary combinations of the lowest primitives, using a finite set of primitives to generate a possibly vast repertoire of actions, in a similar way to the role of recursion in language (Hauser *et al.* 2002).

In Section 14.5 we proposed that the flat MOSAIC could be used for low-level imitation of the modules which would directly reproduce the kinematics (trajectory) of a movement. However, using the HMOSAIC we could propagate up the responsibility signal during action observation to estimate which module at the various levels of the HMOSAIC would need to be active to generate the observed behaviour. Using such an architecture it may be possible to have several representations of the observed action, from the low-level kinematics of movement (which modules are active in the lowest level), to representing sequences of actions (intermediate levels) to the goal (highest level). The degree to which propagation up the hierarchy is possible depends on the extent to which a coherent account of an observed action can be made using the observer's HMOSAIC. The more similar the observer's HMOSAIC is to the actor's HMOSAIC the easier it will be to make coherent, and unique interpretations at higher levels. Therefore, a movement that has a clear goal (which is also a goal that I have represented in my HMOSAIC) could be understood at all levels and imitation of the goal, even with different effectors, would be possible. However, a meaningless movement, or one for which the observer does not have a goal, could be understood only at lower levels, with imitation slavishly replicating kinematics or sequences (see Chapter 6, this volume). The key idea is that having similar computational structures to generate movement, such as HMOSAIC, dramatically reduces the computational problems in action understanding. We have yet to simulate the hierarchical action understanding.

14.7 Communication as closing the loop

So far we have discussed the use of MOSAIC and HMOSAIC in an unidirectional manner, in that the actor pays no attention to the observer's actions. In true communication the actor (the transmitter) is responsive to misperception by the observer (the receiver). One way to close the communication loop is as follows. The transmitter uses his internal symbolic stream to generate a series of motor commands that in turn cause movements. The receiver decodes the movements he sees into his internal symbols and then also generates a series of motor commands (attempting to imitate the transmitter). The transmitter then sees these imitative movements and interprets them back into his own symbols. He can then compare the symbols he wished to transmit with the symbols he believes he has transmitted. This discrepancy error can then be used by the transmitter to determine a new sequence of motor commands in an attempt to get the receiver to internalize these symbols more accurately. So, for example, if the symbols were responsibilities he could generate an action using the original responsibilities augmented with the error. Alternatively, to learn the internal structure of the MOSAIC of others we could use the discrepancy error to update the structure of our own MOSAIC to more closely match those of others.

One of the necessary conditions for exact and rigorous communication at symbolic levels is to have an identity mapping in the closed loop of my symbols → my action → your symbols → your imitation → my perception → my interpretation of your symbols = my original symbols.

There is, therefore, no need in principle why your MOSAIC and my MOSAIC should have similar structures. However, we expect that if they have identical structures you and I will be able to communicate anything we wish. The more dissimilar the structure the more things we will get confused about during communication. In either case there is no need for the modules to be numbered or related—just the fact that you have a module somewhere that does the same job as one of mine is good enough. If discrepancies exist between the responsibilities used for generation and the responsibilities during perception, these could be used to update my MOSAIC, to make it more like yours.

Analogous to the state of our own system is the state of someone else's mind, being the set of parameters that are required to predict the behaviour of the person given inputs and their dynamics. Although in the case of our own arm we may be able to monitor fully the inputs of the system, for another person we may only know some of the inputs. Knowing the system dynamics requires us to learn how, given a particular internal state and input, the other persons will respond. A default is, as described already, to use our own HMOSAIC to estimate other people's hidden states. This allows us to use a single system to interpret the actions of all other people. However, there are situations in which it is inappropriate to assign the same set of internal state to action mappings to everyone. An alternative is to learn a new HMOSAIC for other people. One possibility is that our own HMOSAIC could be augmented by structures that aim to model the difference between our HMOSAIC and others. Such a system would allow a representation of others' internal mental state separately from our own HMOSAIC structure and may therefore form a basis for theory of mind.

14.8 Conclusion

We have explored the computational parallels between the computations that occur in motor control and in social interaction. In particular we examined how models of motor control, such as the HMOSAIC, could be used for action observation, imitation, social interaction and theory of mind. We suggest that using our motor system in action understanding is an efficient mechanism for performing the computations needed in social interaction.

This work was supported by the McDonnell Foundation, Wellcome Trust and Human Frontiers Science Programme.

References

Bellman, R. (1957). *Dynamic programming*. Princeton, NJ: Princeton University Press.
Doya, K., Katagiri, K., Wolpert, D. M. and Kawato, M. (2000). Recognition and imitation of movement patterns by a multiple predictor–controller architecture. *Technical Rep.* **IEICE TL2000–11**, 33–40.

Doya, K., Samejima, K., Katagiri, K. and Kawato, M. (2002). Multiple model-based reinforcement learning. *Neural Comput.* **14**, 1347–1369.

Fadiga, L., Fogassi, L., Pavesi, G. and Rizzolatti, G. (1995). Motor facilitation during action observation: a magnetic stimulation study. *J. Neurophysiol.* **73**, 2608–11.

Fadiga, L., Craighero, L., Buccino, G. and Rizzolatti, G. (2002). Speech listening specifically modulates the excitability of tongue muscles: a TMS study. *Eur. J. Neurosci.* **15**, 399–402.

Gallese, V., Fadiga, L., Fogassi, L. and Rizzolatti, G. (1996). Action recognition in the premotor cortex. *Brain* **119**, 593–609.

Ghahramani, Z. and Wolpert, D. M. (1997). Modular decomposition in visuomotor learning. *Nature* **386**, 392–5.

Grafton, S. T., Fadiga, L., Arbib, M. A. and Rizzolatti, G. (1997). Premotor cortex activation during observation and naming of familiar tools. *NeuroImage* **6**, 231–236.

Grezes, J., Fonlupt, P., Bertenthal, B., Delon-Martin, C., Segebarth, C. and Decety, J. (2001). Does perception of biological motion rely on specific brain regions? *NeuroImage* **13**, 775–85.

Harris, C. M. and Wolpert, D. M. (1998). Signal-dependent noise determines motor planning. *Nature* **394**, 780–4.

Haruno, M., Wolpert, D. M. and Kawato, M. (2001). Mosaic model for sensorimotor learning and control. *Neural Comput.* **13**, 2201–20.

Haruno, M., Wolpert, D. and Kawato, M. (2003). Hierarchical MOSAIC for movement generation. In *Excepta Medica International Coungress Series*, vol. 1250. (ed. T. Ono, G. Matsumoto, R. R. Llinas, A. Bethoz, R. Norgren, H. Nishijo, *et al.*). Amsterdam: Elsevier Science.

Hauser, M. D., Chomsky, N. and Fitch, W. T. (2002). The faculty of language: what is it, who has it, and how did it evolve? *Science* **298**, 1569–79.

Iacoboni, M., Woods, R. P., Brass, M., Bekkering, H., Mazziotta, J. C. and Rizzolatti, G. (1999). Cortical mechanisms of human imitation. *Science* **286**, 2526–8.

Jacobs, R. A., Jordan, M. I., Nowlan, S. J. and Hinton, G. E. (1991). Adaptive mixture of local experts. *Neural Comput.* **3**, 79–87.

Johansson, G. (1973). Visual perception of biological motion and a model for its analysis. *Perception Psychophys.* **14**, 201–11.

Jordan, M. I. (1995). Computational aspects of motor control and motor learning. In *Handbook of perception and action: motor skills* (ed. H. Heuer and S. Keele). New York: Academic Press.

Jordan, M. I. and Rumelhart, D. E. (1992). Forward models: supervised learning with a distal teacher. *Cogn. Sci.* **16**, 307–54.

Kawato, M. (1990). Feedback-error-learning neural network for supervised learning. In *Advanced neural computers* (ed. R. Eckmiller), pp. 365–72. Amsterdam: North-Holland.

Kawato, M., Furawaka, K. and Suzuki, R. (1987). A hierarchical neural network model for the control and learning of voluntary movements. *Biol. Cybern.* **56**, 1–17.

Kuniyoshi, Y., Inaba, M. and Inoue, H. (1994). Learning by watching: extracting reusable task knowledge from visual observation of human performance. *IEEE Trans. Robotics Automation* **10**, 799–822.

Liberman, A. M. and Whalen, D. H. (2000). On the relation of speech to language. *Trends Cogn. Sci.* **4**, 187–96.

Martin, A., Wiggs, C. L., Ungerleider, L. G. and Haxby, J. V. (1996). Neural correlates of category-specific knowledge. *Nature* **379**, 649–52.

Miall, R. C. and Wolpert, D. M. (1996). Forward models for physiological motor control. *Neural Networks* **9**, 1265–79.

Miyamoto, H., Schaal, S., Gandolfo, F., Koike, Y., Osu, R., Nakano, E., *et al.* (1996). A Kendama learning robot based on bi-directional theory. *Neural Networks* **9**, 1281–302.

Narendra, K. S. and Balakrishnan, J. (1997). Adaptive control using multiple models. *IEEE Trans. Automatic Control* **42**, 171–87.

Narendra, K. S., Balakrishnan, J. and Ciliz, M. K. (1995). Adaptation and learning using multiple models, switching, and tuning. *IEEE Control Systems Mag.* **15**, 37–51.

Rizzolatti, G. and Arbib, M. A. (1998). Language within our grasp. *Trends Neurosci.* **21**, 188–94.

Schaal, S., Ijspeert, A. and Billard, A. (2003). Computational approaches to motor learning by imitation. *Phil. Trans. R. Soc. Lond.* B **358**, 537–47. (DOI 10.1098/rstb.2002.1258.)

Wada, Y., Koike, Y., Vatikiotis-Bateson, E. and Kawato, M. (1995). A computational theory for movement pattern recognition based on optimal movement pattern generation. *Biol. Cybern.* **73**, 15–25.

Wolpert, D. M. and Flanagan, J. R. (2001). Motor prediction. *Curr. Biol.* **11**, R729–R732.

Wolpert, D. M. and Ghahramani, Z. (2000). Computational principles of movement neuroscience. *Nature Neurosci.* **3**(Suppl.), 1212–17.

Wolpert, D. M. and Kawato, M. (1998). Multiple paired forward and inverse models for motor control. *Neural Networks* **11**, 1317–29.

Glossary

CNS: central nervous system
HMM: hidden Markov model
HMOSAIC: hierarchical modular selection and identification for control
MOSAIC: modular selection and identification for control

Index